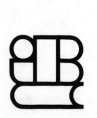

AT RISK
IN AMERICA

LU ANN ADAY

Foreword by
Odin W. Anderson

AT RISK
IN AMERICA

The Health
and Health Care Needs
of Vulnerable Populations
in the United States

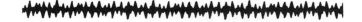

Jossey-Bass Publishers · San Francisco

Substantial discounts on bulk quantities of Jossey-Bass books are available to corporations, professional associations, and other organizations. For details and discount information, contact the special sales department at Jossey-Bass Inc., Publishers. (415) 433-1740; Fax (415) 433-0499.

For sales outside the United States, contact Maxwell Macmillan International Publishing Group, 866 Third Avenue, New York, New York 10022.

Manufactured in the United States of America

The ink in this book is either soy- or vegetable-based and during the printing process emits fewer than half the volatile organic compounds (VOCs) emitted by petroleum-based ink.

Library of Congress Cataloging-in-Publication Data

Aday, Lu Ann.
    At risk in America : the health and health care needs of vulnerable populations in the United States / Lu Ann Aday. — 1st ed.
      p.   cm. — (A joint publication in the Jossey-Bass health series, and the Jossey-Bass social and behavioral science series)
    Includes bibliographical references and index.
    ISBN 1-55542-503-8 (alk. paper)
    1. Poor—Medical care—United States.   2. Poor—Medical care—Government policy—United States.   3. Socially disadvantaged—Medical care—Untied States.   4. Socially disadvantaged—Medical care—Government policy—United States. I. Title. II. Series.
RA418.5.P6A3 1993
362.1'0425—dc20   92-32437
                                                CIP

FIRST EDITION
HB Printing   10 9 8 7 6 5 4 3 2 1   *Code 9307*

A joint publication in
**The Jossey-Bass
Health Series**
and
**The Jossey-Bass
Social and Behavioral Science Series**

CONTENTS

TABLES AND FIGURES

Tables

Figures

FOREWORD

The theory of risk was invented by actuaries and economists to calculate the costs of spreading risks over an aggregate of events from shipwrecks to the cost of medical care. In *At Risk in America: The Health and Health Care Needs of Vulnerable Populations in the United States,* Lu Ann Aday has added another risk, which she calls *vulnerability* — a social concept related to an individual's position in the social structure. In this book, vulnerability is largely related to sociomedical morbidities such as AIDS, drug and alcohol addiction, family violence, and homelessness, which make these groups more prone to ill health and disability. The vulnerable segment of the population can be made much less vulnerable by appropriate and possible social and health policies, given the political will to do so.

The author's theoretical framework is sociological, as the beginning of Chapter One illustrates: "Both the origins and remedies of vulnerability are rooted in the bonds of human communities. The parentheses that inscribe our lives (their beginnings and endings, as well as the passages within them) take form in the arms of those who care for us when we are most in need of physical help, spiritual solace, or warm companionship.

"To be vulnerable to others is to be in a position of being hurt or ignored, as well as helped, by them. . . . As members of human communities, we are all potentially vulnerable." What the author says reminds me of the Puritan aphorism, "There but for the grace of God go I."

All through human history, there has been a concept of the relationship between the individual and the group — mutual obligations and rights in some sort of balance. Today, in the United States, the author documents that there is an imbalance; too large a segment of the population is left in a state of vulnerability because of indifferent or ineffective social policy. Two different languages have characterized American social and political discourse: those of individual rights and those of the common good. The language of individualism has overridden the language of the common good.

The author has formulated a taxonomy of vulnerability and a taxonomy of programs to deal with vulnerability. They should guide the policy analysts and policy makers in putting together a social policy of wholeness so as to interrelate in one seamless web the problems of infant mortality, sickness due to lack of money and lack of insurance, housing for the inadequately housed and the homeless, and care for the mentally ill in and out of institutions. Aday demonstrates that there are common threads tying these seemingly disparate problems together for a theory of vulnerability and its mitigation.

This is an exhaustive and elaborately empirical work that is invaluable to public health, social work, economics, political science, and ethics, given the seriousness of the problems categorized in American society. The book is not a sentimental polemic; it is a social scientific effort to analyze and understand what is going on so as to approach solutions as rationally as possible in an irrational world. Implicit in the entire book is a plea for a caring, organic society.

The author is well equipped for this stupendous task. She has been trained in economics and sociology (medical) but has also steeped herself in political science and ethics. The book reveals her as a scientist and a compassionate person. I have been privileged to have had her on my research staff at the Graduate School of Business, University of Chicago.

December 1992

ODIN W. ANDERSON
professor of sociology
University of Wisconsin, Madison
and emeritus professor
Graduate School of Business
and Department of Sociology
University of Chicago

PREFACE

Policy developments earlier in the century led to the expansion of the U.S. health care system and to improved access for many of the traditionally disadvantaged segments of the U.S. population. Progress has not been without its price, however. A corresponding acceleration in the rate of expenditures for medical care has accompanied these changes. In the decade of the 1980s, public and private providers and third-party payers responded by encouraging initiatives to cut back on the resources spent on health care and to develop innovative organizational models for the cost-effective practice of medicine.

These changes have slowed or reversed many of the favorable trends of improved access for groups for whom the doors of the health care system were historically most likely to be closed—such as the poor, minorities, the uninsured, and those without a usual medical provider. Further, the increasing visibility of sociomedical morbidities, such as AIDS, drug and alcohol addiction, family violence, and homelessness, among others, has highlighted categories of individuals who are particularly vulnerable to restrictive social, economic, and health policies. The solutions to addressing the needs of these diverse groups have been fragmented and categoric—resulting in many particularly at-risk individuals slipping through the cracks of the existing health and social service systems.

The research in this area is also often categoric and fragmented, not systematically related to other bodies of information, and it frequently fails to identify issues that cut across different professional or service delivery domains. No source has pulled together, in a systematic fashion, the array of information and identified the cross-cutting policy and research issues for the seemingly growing numbers of the vulnerable.

This book provides this needed integration and synthesis. It presents (1) a framework for identifying and studying vulnerable populations; (2) data on their needs, and the trends and correlates in their growth over time; (3) issues regarding the access, cost, and quality of their care; (4) policies and programs that have been developed to address their needs; and (5) the research and policy initiatives that could be undertaken to ameliorate vulnerability.

Audience

Public health, health care, social science, social work, and policy analysis professionals, academicians, and researchers will be interested in this book. It can serve as a reference for legislative staff, policy makers, health professionals, program administrators, and students, as well as provide a framework for guiding subsequent research and program development in this area.

It can acquaint students with the literature in the field and provide a framework for them to use in identifying such groups and both their specific and common problems. The book could be used as a text for public health, health administration, medical sociology, behavioral science, and social work students, as well as for students in the health care professions in courses dealing with the operation and evaluation of the health care system.

It provides health and public health professionals the background information they need to develop or evaluate programs addressing the needs of vulnerable groups in their own states or communities. The book can serve as a reference source for policy makers and their staffs who need a quick review of the issues for selected target groups now, but who also require a vision of who the target groups are likely to be in the future. Finally, it shows what programs or policies can anticipate and address the needs of vulnerable populations and what systemic solutions should be considered to address the deepening access, cost, and quality crises in the U.S. health care system.

Overview of the Contents

Each chapter poses a question to explore with respect to the health and health care of vulnerable populations. Vulnerable populations are defined as being at risk of poor physical, psychological, and/or social health. Selected groups are highlighted throughout the book to illustrate and examine the applicability of the framework for studying vulnerability developed here. The nine vulnerable population groups, based on the primacy of the different types of needs, that will be the primary focus of the book are as follows: *physical needs* — high-risk mothers and infants, the chronically ill and disabled, persons with AIDS; *psychological needs* — the mentally ill and disabled, alcohol or substance abusers, the suicide- or homicide-prone; *social needs* — abusing families, homeless people, and immigrants and refugees. The rationale for choosing these groups is discussed in Chapter One.

The chapters are organized to facilitate an overview of the cross-cutting issues among the groups examined, as well as to provide specific details on a particular group of interest. Thus, Chapter One also describes the conceptual framework for the examination of vulnerability in subsequent chapters. The final chapter (Chapter Eleven) discusses the principles and parameters of a more community-oriented health policy to address the health and health care needs of vulnerable populations.

Each of the other chapters (Two through Ten) is divided into three main sections: (1) an introduction to the main question that will be addressed in the chapter and the approach used to assemble and organize the evidence to answer it, (2) a synopsis of the cross-cutting issues identified among all of the vulnerable populations examined, and (3) a population-specific overview of the evidence for each group. In the final section of each of these chapters, summary tables are provided and a summary paragraph precedes the presentation of detailed findings for each of the groups to highlight key findings. Readers may elect to focus on the summary or overview chapters or sections of each chapter, or to examine the evidence for a specific question or group within or across chapters.

Chapter One asks who the vulnerable are. It presents the framework for defining and studying vulnerable populations that serves as the basis for the perspective on vulnerability developed in subsequent chapters.

Chapter Two asks how many are vulnerable. It summarizes national estimates of the number and growth of vulnerable populations and highlights the extent to which there is an overlap in these groups.

Chapter Three poses the question of who is most vulnerable. Data on demographic subgroups of each of the nine major vulnerable population groups are presented, focusing particularly on breakdowns by age, sex, race, income, and education.

Chapter Four asks why these groups are vulnerable. This discussion provides an overview of the major political, cultural, social, and economic changes in the United States that have given rise to growth in the number and categories of vulnerable populations. The chapter examines the impact of resources such as social status (prestige and power), social capital (social support), and human capital (jobs, schools, income, and housing) on the vulnerability of different subgroups.

Chapter Five asks what programs there are to address the needs of vulnerable populations. It highlights major programs and services for vulnerable populations in the context of a continuum of prevention-oriented, treatment-oriented, and long-term care.

Chapter Six asks who pays for their care. The discussion focuses on the public and private third-party sources of financing that have been available to pay for the services provided.

Chapter Seven explores how good the access to care is for vulnerable populations. It reviews evidence of organizational and financial barriers to obtaining needed services.

Chapter Eight asks how much their care costs. It provides a summary of what is known about the total and out-of-pocket costs of care and the cost-benefit and cost-effectiveness of alternative program and care arrangements. This chapter illuminates the personal and societal costs of providing care to vulnerable populations and considers the efficiency of alternative programs and policies to address their needs.

Chapter Nine reviews what is known about the quality of care. It summarizes data that are available on structure, process, and outcome dimensions of the quality of care currently being provided to vulnerable populations, through the medical care, as well as other, service delivery sectors.

Chapter Ten raises the question of what still needs to be known about the health and health care of vulnerable populations. It identifies descriptive, analytical, and evaluative research priorities and presents proposals for the type of information needed to make informed decisions and how to obtain it.

Chapter Eleven asks what programs and policies are needed. This final chapter presents a community-oriented health policy paradigm, based on the perspective on vulnerability developed in previous chapters, as a basis for recommendations regarding how best to address the health and health care needs of vulnerable populations.

The book furnishes an extensive set of references. It also includes two resources — one describing the major national data sources on vulnerable populations and the other providing detailed reference information on the data tables that appear earlier in the book.

The unique contribution this book makes is to synthesize existing information on the array of vulnerable populations that have emerged in recent years and to present a framework for articulating coherent and integrated research and policy agendas to address their needs. It identifies research in progress to reflect the most up-to-date information on these issues, documents the major sources to consult on the topic, and provides recommendations regarding what still needs to be known and done to address the health and health care needs of vulnerable populations in the United States.

Acknowledgments

I gratefully acknowledge the support provided by the National Library of Medicine for the preparation of the book under grant number R01-LM05175.

Particular thanks go to those colleagues who read all or part of the draft manuscript for the book and provided invaluable comments, all of which I took seriously in making the final revisions: Ronald M. Andersen, Odin W. Anderson, Robert L. Eichhorn, Gretchen V. Fleming, Ronald N. Forthofer, D. Blair Justice, David Lairson, Stephen H. Linder, Beatrice J. Selwyn, and Carl H. Slater. An anonymous Jossey-Bass reviewer also provided an excellent and helpful critique of the original manuscript.

Special thanks go to Martha Hargraves and Chih-Wen Chung, who helped locate and scrupulously compile the extensive literature and data on the groups that are the special focus of the book. I also gratefully acknowledge the many hours that Dima Abi-Said and Adel Youssef spent in locating and copying sources, as well as the great amount of time and effort Regina Fisher devoted to formatting, typing, and revising the complex set of data tables for the book.

I am grateful for the supportive environment at the University of Texas School of Public Health (UTSPH), which allowed me the flexibility to write the book. I wish in particular to thank Stephanie Normann and the staff of the University of Texas School of Public Health Library, for ordering or facilitating my access to state-of-the-art sources in this area; Gay Robertson and Media Services, for assisting with the preparation of tables and figures for the book; and the students in my spring 1992 special topics course, "The Health and Health Care of Vulnerable Populations," who provided instructive reflections on the draft manuscript.

Finally, my thanks go to my friend Katherine V. Wilcox, who expertly mastered the bibliographical software entry and editing tasks for the extensive set of references at the end of the book and who read and critiqued each draft chapter with a keen eye for clarity.

My experience of writing the book was greatly enriched by the intellectual and social capital provided by this highly valued community of collaborators.

Houston, Texas   Lu Ann Aday
December 1992

THE AUTHOR

Lu Ann Aday is professor of behavioral sciences and management and policy sciences at the University of Texas School of Public Health. She received her B.S. degree (1968) from Texas Tech University in economics and her M.S. (1970) and Ph.D. (1973) degrees from Purdue University in sociology.

Aday's principal research interests have focused on policy-relevant research on indicators and correlates of health services utilization and access. She has conducted major national and community surveys and evaluations of national demonstrations in this area. She is the principal author of eight books: *The Utilization of Health Services: Indices and Correlates—A Research Bibliography* (1972), *Development of Indices of Access to Medical Care* (1975), *Health Care in the United States: Equitable for Whom?* (1980), *Access to Medical Care in the U.S.: Who Has It, Who Doesn't* (1984), *Hospital-Physician Sponsored Primary Care: Marketing and Impact* (1985), *Pediatric Home Care: Results of a National Evaluation of Programs for Ventilator Assisted Children* (1988), *Designing and Conducting Health Surveys: A Comprehensive Guide* (1989) and *Health Services Research: Effectiveness, Efficiency, and Equity as Indicators of System Performance* (1993). She is also the second coauthor of *Ambulatory Care and Insurance Coverage in an Era of Constraint* (1987, with R. M. Andersen, C. S. Lyttle, L. J. Cornelius, and M. Chen).

1

Who Are the Vulnerable?

Both the origins and remedies of vulnerability are rooted in the bonds of human communities. The parentheses that inscribe our lives (their beginnings and endings, as well as the passages within them) take form in the arms of those who care for us when we are most in need of physical help, spiritual solace, or warm companionship. Their presence supports and strengthens us, and the blessings of their caring seek to salve the wounds of body, mind, and spirit that accompany the odyssey of our lives.

To be vulnerable to others is to be in a position of being hurt or ignored, as well as helped, by them. The word *vulnerable* is derived from the Latin verb *vulnerare* ("to wound") and the noun *vulnus* ("wound").

As members of human communities, we are all potentially vulnerable.

Framework for Studying Vulnerable Populations

Two different mother tongues—those of "individual rights" and the "common good"—have historically characterized American social and political discourse. The semantics of the first emphasize the meanings of autonomy, independence, and individual well-being, while those of the second highlight norms of reciprocity, interdependence, and the public good. Bellah, Madsen, Sullivan, Swidler, and Tipton (1985) and Beauchamp (1988) have, however, observed that in contemporary American society, the first language of individualism has come to override the second mother tongue of community. Excessive individualism may, they argue, be "destroying those social integuments [ties] that de Tocqueville saw as moderating its more destructive potentialities" (Bellah et al., 1985, p. viii).

In his book *Foundations of Social Theory* (1990), James Coleman points out that to formulate meaningful theories or explanations of social phenomena,

This publication was supported in part by grant number R01-LM05175 from the National Library of Medicine. Its contents are solely the responsibility of the author and do not necessarily represent the official views of the National Library of Medicine.

both the macro (collective) and the micro (individual) levels of observation and analysis and their interrelationships must be examined. Focusing on individuals' characteristics, attitudes, or behaviors (violence-proneness) may fail to reveal the impact that larger social influences or trends (media violence) have on the individuals themselves. Correspondingly, theories regarding relationships between largely collective phenomena (the prevalence of media violence and rates of violent crime) that fail to illuminate the dynamics of these social forces for individuals fall short of developing fully meaningful explanations of the phenomena. The measurement of collective phenomena at the individual level of analysis (methodological individualism) also tends to bias the explanations of these phenomena toward individual motivations and actions.

The approach to studying the health and health care of vulnerable populations undertaken here examines the ethical, conceptual, and political contributions of the community (macro) and individual (micro) perspectives and their interrelationships in illuminating the concept of vulnerability. (See Figure 1.1.) In the discussion that follows, a framework for studying vulnerability will be presented and described with respect to how it contributes to understanding the origins and consequences of vulnerability to poor physical, psychological, and/or social health.

Ethical Norms and Values

An individual perspective on the origins of poor physical, psychological, or social health views personal autonomy and the associated individual rights as the principal ethical norms and values for guiding decision making regarding the amelioration of risk. Good health is viewed primarily as a function of personal life-style choices, and poor health outcomes result because individuals fail to assume adequate personal responsibility for their health and well-being (Knowles, 1977).

A community perspective on the origins of health needs focuses on the differential risks that exist for different groups as a function of the availability of opportunities and resources for maximizing their health. Norms of reciprocity, trust, and social obligation acknowledge the webs of interdependence and mutual support and caring that are essential for minimizing the risks of poor physical, psychological, or social health. Poor health results because communities fail to invest in and assume responsibility for the collective well-being of their members (Tesh, 1988).

Concept: Health Status

Health can be measured along a continuum. *Good health* is at the positive end of the continuum, defined by the World Health Organization (WHO) concept of health as a "state of complete physical, mental, and social well-being" (World Health Organization, 1948, p. 1). *Death* is at the negative end, as the total absence of health, defined by population-specific mortality (death)

Figure 1.1. Framework for Studying Vulnerable Populations.

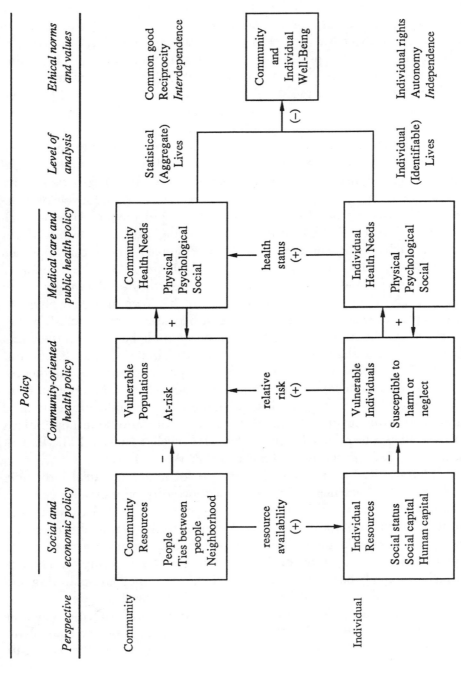

Note: (+) indicates direct relationship (likelihood of outcome *increases* as predictor increases); (–) indicates inverse relationship (likelihood of outcome *decreases* as predictor increases).

rates. *Needs* are those departures from full physical, mental, and social health that people experience in the course of their lives.

Though a variety of indicators of the different WHO dimensions of health (physical, mental, and social) have been developed, physical health has been generally characterized as the physiological and physical status of the body, and mental or psychological health as the state of mind, including basic intellectual functions such as memory and feelings. Physical and mental indicators tend to "end at the skin," while indicators of social health extend beyond the individual to include both the quantity and quality of social contacts with other people (Ware, 1986, pp. 205–206).

The magnitude and seriousness of individual or community needs along each of these dimensions may differ depending on how they are defined and measured. Health needs can, for example, be based on (1) clinicians' judgments, (2) patients' perceptions, or (3) observed or reported levels of functioning. The first approach — clinical or diagnostic judgments of disease (such as hypertension or diabetes) — utilizes relevant diagnostic tests or procedures administered by medical or mental health professionals. The second approach involves individuals' perceptions of illness, which are based on self-reported symptoms, on individuals' assessments of whether they think of their health as excellent, good, or poor, or on other aspects of their own subjective physical, mental, or social well-being. The third approach focuses on individuals' abilities to perform certain functions or activities, based on behavioral, rather than perceptual or clinical, criteria. Need characterized in this way underlies conceptions of the "sick role" — a sociological concept that points out that people change their usual behavior in certain ways (go to bed, take time off from work, and so on) when they are sick. All of these conceptualizations are used in measuring the health and health care needs of vulnerable populations (Bergner, 1989; Freeman & Levine, 1989; McDowell & Newell, 1987; Patrick & Bergner, 1990; Twaddle & Hessler, 1977; Ware, 1987).

Community health needs assessments focus on statistical indicators of the rates of prevalence or incidence of morbidity or mortality (such as infant mortality rates, HIV seroprevalence, percent of the elderly with limitations in activities of daily living, and so on). Individual health needs assessments measure the health status of identifiable community residents or patients (based on symptoms or diagnoses of illness, for example). The former has principally been the focus of public health policy and planning and the latter of personal medical care service delivery and practice.

Often anecdotes regarding identifiable individual tragedies (such as a schoolchild dying of AIDS or an infant in need of a kidney transplant) are more likely to compel policy makers' attention than are the aggregate statistical indicators of suffering.

Concept: Relative Risk

Vulnerable populations are at risk of poor physical, psychological, and/or social health. Underlying this definition of vulnerability is the epidemiological concept of *risk*, in the sense that there is a probability that an individual will become ill within a stated period of time. Community and corresponding individual characteristics are *risk factors* associated with the occurrence of poor physical, psychological, and/or social health. Risk factors refer to those attributes or exposures (smoking, drug use, and lead paint poisoning, for example) that are associated with or lead to increases in the probability of occurrence of health-related outcomes.

Relative risk refers to the ratio of the risk of poor health among groups that are exposed to the risk factors versus those who are not (Last, 1983). Relative risk reflects the differential vulnerability of different groups to poor health. The *differential vulnerability hypothesis* argues that negative or stressful life events (such as unemployment or related loss of income or personal resources) hurt some people more than others. Findings based on this hypothesis show that the mental health and well-being of low socioeconomic status (SES) groups tend to be more adversely affected by stressful or negative events than is the case for those with higher SES. They also indicate that historical and current social status differences help to explain these discrepancies (Hamilton, Broman, Hoffman, & Renner, 1990; McLeod & Kessler, 1990; Ulbrich, Warheit, & Zimmerman, 1989).

The concept of risk asssumes that there is always a chance that an adverse health-related outcome will occur. Correspondingly, we are all potentially at risk of poor physical, psychological, and/or social health. People may, however, be more or less at risk of poor health at different times in their lives, while some individuals and groups are apt to be more at risk than others at any given point in time.

Being in poor physical health (such as having a debilitating chronic illness) may also make one more vulnerable (at risk) of poor psychological (depression) or social health (few supportive social contacts). The risk of harm or neglect would be increased for those who are in poor health and have few material (economic) and nonmaterial (psychological or social) resources to assist them in coping with illness.

Concept: Resource Availability

The beginning point for understanding the factors that increase the risk of poor health originates in a macro-level look at the availability and distribution of community resources (Figure 1.1). Individuals' risks vary as a function of the opportunities and material and nonmaterial resources associated with (1) the personal characteristics (age, sex, and race/ethnicity) of the individuals themselves; (2) the nature of the ties between them (family members, friends, and neighbors, for example); and (3) the schools, jobs, incomes, and housing that characterize the neighborhoods in which they live. The corresponding rewards and resources available to individuals as a function of these social arrangements include (1) social status (prestige and power); (2) social capital (social support); and (3) human capital (productive potential).

Social status is associated with positions individuals occupy in society as a function of age, sex, or race/ethnicity, and the socially defined opportunities and rewards, such as prestige and power, they have as a result. Minorities often have poorer health and fewer material and nonmaterial resources to meet their needs than do majority race individuals. The prevalence of certain types of illnesses and the need to depend on others for assistance due to poor health differs at different stages of life (infancy, adolescence, adulthood, and old age). Women report higher rates of many types of illnesses than men, which has been variously attributed to their differing health needs, the stress associated with the complex of deferential and demanding roles women play, and the greater social acceptability for women to admit their vulnerability. However, men may also be placed at greater risk of poor health outcomes as a function of working in hazardous jobs, or being influenced by societal sex-role expectations regarding heavy drinking or the use of violence to settle disputes. Those individuals with a combination of statuses (poor, minority elderly women or young males) that put them at a high risk of having both poor health and few material and nonmaterial resources are in a highly vulnerable position (Kaplan, 1989).

Social capital resides in the quantity and quality of interpersonal ties between people. Families provide social capital to members in the form of social networks and support and associated feelings of belonging, psychological well-being, and self-esteem. The value of social capital to individuals (single mothers) is that it provides resources (such as having someone to count on for child care) they can use to achieve other interests (going to school or working). Social support has been found to be an important resource for individuals in coping with and minimizing the impact of negative life events or adversity on their physical and mental health. Physical, psychological, and social well-being are directly enhanced for people who have supportive social networks. Communities constitute the reservoir in which social capital resources are both generated and drawn on by individual community members. Those who are likely to have the least social capital (or the fewest social ties to count on) are people living alone or those in female-headed families, those who are not married or in an otherwise committed intimate relationship, people who do not belong to any voluntary organizations (such as churches or volunteer interest groups), or those who have weak or nonexistent social networks of family or friends (Coleman, 1990; Gore, 1989).

Human capital refers to investments in people's skills and capabilities (such as vocational or public education) that enable them to act in new ways (master a trade) or enhance their contributions to society (enter the labor force). Social capital can also enhance the generation of human capital through, for example, family and community support for encouraging students to stay in school. Neighborhoods that have poor schools, high rates of unemployment, and substandard housing reflect low levels of investments in the human capital (or productive potential) of the people who live there.

Similarly, individuals who are poorly educated, unemployed, and poorly housed are likely to have the fewest resources for coping with illness or other personal or economic adversities (Coleman, 1990; Warner & Luce, 1982).

The relative importance and relationship of predictors of risk of poor physical, psychological, or social health are summarized in Figure 1.2.

Figure 1.2. Predictors of Populations at Risk.

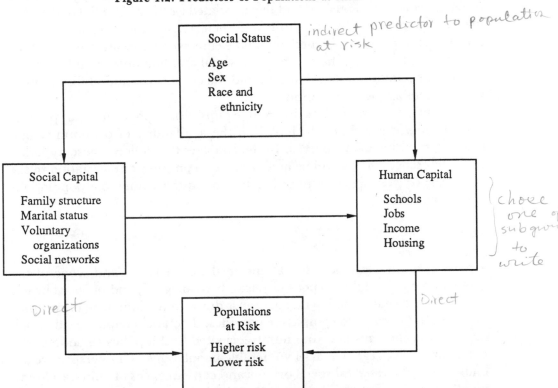

indirect predictor to population at risk

Direct

choose one of subgroups to write

Direct

Social status differences for different age, sex, or racial and ethnic subgroups are made manifest in the differential availability of personal and political power and associated human and social capital resources to different subgroups. These disparities are reinforced either informally through socially defined norms and behavioral expectations or formally through legally sanctioned differences in access to human resources (such as schools, jobs, income, or housing)—for children versus adults, men versus women, or whites versus minorities, for example. The purposive blocking of access to resources for certain groups relative to others on the basis of these ascribed characteristics constitutes the discrimination associated with age, gender, and/or race in U.S. society.

The webs of mutual dependencies that define the social life of families, friendship networks, churches, volunteer service organizations, self-help groups, neighborhood or civic organizations, and related community groups generate social capital or support. This can be both invested in and drawn on to achieve individuals' personal *and* purposive aims — enhancing feelings of self-esteem or a sense of belonging, creating child-care alternatives, or calling on others for assistance when ill, for example.

The social status and social capital resources of individuals and groups in a community influence the level of investments that are likely to be made in the schools, jobs, housing, and the associated earning potential of the families and individuals living within it. When neighborhood residents come together and seek or are invited to become empowered to work toward shared interests and/or goals, the prospect for social and human capital formation within the community is enhanced, and the corollary vulnerability of individual members within it diminished.

Table 1.1 summarizes different groups' risk of poor physical, psychological, and/or social health, based on the availability of community and associated individual resources. In the chapters that follow, these hypothesized differences in risk will be analyzed based on subgroup variation in the incidence or prevalence of poor health among the vulnerable populations being examined.

Policy

To begin to both envision and attend to the dimensions and scope of the problem of vulnerability to poor physical, psychological, and/or social health in the United States, policy makers must draw on the language of community and the normative compass it provides. The final chapter of the book outlines the elements of a community-oriented health policy to address the health and health care needs of vulnerable populations. This perspective acknowledges the essential social origins and consequences of vulnerability to poor physical, psychological, and/or social functioning. It encourages, invests in, and empowers U.S. families and communities to be full participants in shaping their collective health and well-being. A community-oriented point of view seeks to produce networks of cooperation and support, rather than wedges of bureaucratic division and indifference between individuals and institutions, to form communities of caring for the vulnerable. And finally, community-oriented health policy builds explanatory bridges in exploring the roles that both social and economic, as well as medical care and public health, policies play in ameliorating the health risks and consequences of vulnerability.

Health Needs of Vulnerable Populations

The vulnerable populations that are the primary focus of this book are those for whom the risk of poor physical, psychological, or social health has or

Table 1.1. Comparisons of Relative Risk.

Community and Individual Resources	Relative Risk	
	Higher risk	Lower risk
The people: social status		
Age	Infants Children Adolescents Elderly	Working-age adults
Sex	Females	Males
Race and ethnicity	African Americans Hispanics Native Americans Asian Americans	Whites
The ties between people: social capital		
Family structure	Living alone Female-headed families	Extended families Two-parent families
Marital status	Single Separated Divorced Widowed	Married/mingles
Voluntary organizations	Nonmember	Member
Social networks	Weak	Strong
The neighborhood: human capital		
Schools	Less than high school	High school +
Jobs	Unemployed Blue collar	White collar
Income	Poor Near Poor	Nonpoor
Housing	Substandard	Adequate +

Note: The terms to designate the race and ethnicity categories in this table will be used in talking about these groups in general. When presenting specific data in the text on these groups, the designation (such as black or Asian) in the original source from which the data were derived will generally be used. *Mingles* are individuals who are not married but are living with a sexual partner. Voluntary organizations include churches, volunteer interest groups, and civic or neighborhood organizations.

is quite likely to become a reality: high-risk mothers and infants, chronically ill and disabled, persons with AIDS, mentally ill and disabled, alcohol or substance abusers, suicide- or homicide-prone, abusing families, the homeless, and immigrants and refugees. These groups are arrayed in Table 1.2, based on their principal health needs. The impact of the availability of material and nonmaterial resources in contributing to their vulnerability to (risk of) poor health, as well as the role of their poor health in leading to vulnerability to subsequent harm or neglect, will be explored.

Table 1.2. Principal Health Needs of Vulnerable Populations.

Physical	*Psychological*	*Social*
High-risk mothers and infants	Mentally ill and disabled	Abusing families
Chronically ill and disabled	Alcohol or substance abusers	Homeless
Persons with AIDS	Suicide- or homicide-prone	Immigrants and refugees

The major reasons for choosing to focus on these groups in examining the health and health care needs of vulnerable populations are as follows: (1) their needs are serious and in many cases debilitating or life-threatening ones; (2) they require an extensive set of medical and nonmedical services; (3) the growth in their number and the seriousness of their needs are placing greater demands on the medical care, public health, and related service delivery sectors; (4) their complex and multifaceted needs are, however, not adequately met through existing financing or service delivery arrangements; and (5) federal, state, and local policy makers are increasingly concerned about how to deal with the demands they place on existing systems of care, as well as about how to aid the growing number of Americans at risk of serious physical, psychological, and/or social health problems.

Poor health along one dimension (physical) is quite likely to be compounded with poor health along others (psychological and/or social, for example). Health needs are greatest for those who have problems along more than one of these dimensions. A categorization of groups, based on their cross-cutting needs, appears in Table 1.3. This categorization is intended to illuminate the overlapping, multifaceted nature of needs experienced by many of the most vulnerable.

Topics in Studying Vulnerability

The framework introduced in Figure 1.1 provides a conceptual, empirical, and normative point of reference for understanding the origins and consequences of poor health. The framework can guide the development of coherent and relevant research and policy agendas in addressing the health and health care needs of what appear to be a growing number of vulnerable populations. The major topics regarding these groups that will be covered in the chapters that follow and the relationships among them are summarized in Figure 1.3.

Figure 1.3. Topics in Studying Vulnerable Populations.

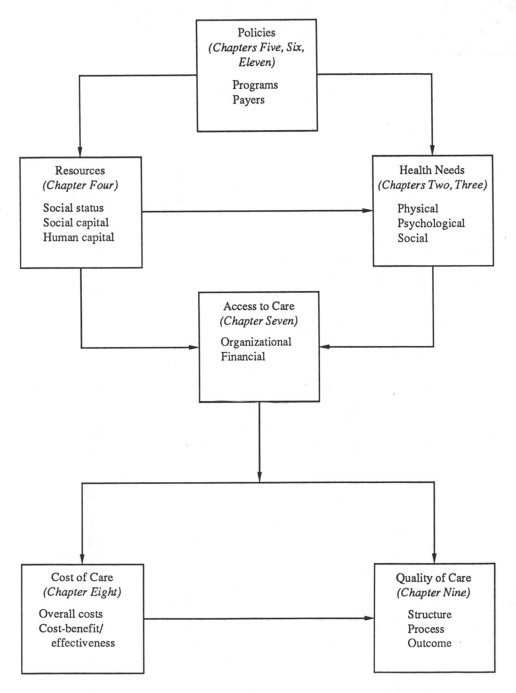

Note: Chapter Ten reviews the research needed on these and related topics.

Table 1.3. Cross-Cutting Health Needs of Vulnerable Populations.

Vulnerable Populations	Vulnerable Populations								
	High-risk mothers and infants	Chronically ill and disabled	Persons with AIDS	Mentally ill and disabled	Alcohol or substance abusers	Suicide- or homicide-prone	Abusing families	Homeless	Immigrants and refugees
High-risk mothers and infants	X	Chronically ill/technology-dependent children	Pediatric AIDS cases	Developmentally disabled infants	Fetal alcohol syndrome/crack babies	Child homicides	Battered pregnant women and infants	Pregnant homeless women	Pregnant refugee women
Chronically ill and disabled	Chronically ill/technology-dependent children	X	HIV-positive individuals	Chronically mentally ill	Chronic alcoholics/drug addicts	Suicidal long-term care patients	Abused handicapped or elderly	Homeless with chronic disease	Refugees with chronic disease
Persons with AIDS	Pediatric AIDS cases	HIV-positive individuals	X	Central nervous system-impaired PWAs	IV drug user PWAs	Suicidal PWAs/prisoners with AIDS	Homophobic families/AIDS boarder babies	Homeless adults, runaways with AIDS	Refugees with AIDS
Mentally ill and disabled	Developmentally disabled infants	Chronically mentally ill	Central nervous system-impaired PWAs	X	Mentally ill substance abusers	Suicidal/criminally insane	Dysfunctional families	Homeless mentally ill	Refugees with post-traumatic distress

	Fetal alcohol syndrome/ crack babies	Chronic alcoholics/ drug addicts	IV drug user PWAs	Mentally ill substance abusers	Alcohol/ drug-related suicides or homicides	Addictive families	Alcoholic/ drug abusing homeless	Alcoholic/ drug abusing refugees
Alcohol or substance abusers	X							
Suicide- or homicide-prone	Child homicides	Suicidal long-term care patients	Suicidal PWAs/ prisoners with AIDS	Suicidal/ criminally insane	X	Violent families	Suicidal/ violence-prone homeless	Suicidal/ violence-prone refugees
Abusing families	Battered pregnant women and infants	Abused handicapped or elderly	Homophobic families, AIDS boarder babies	Dysfunctional families	Violent families	X	Runaways	Maltreated refugee children
Homeless	Pregnant homeless women	Homeless with chronic disease	Homeless adults, runaways with AIDS	Homeless mentally ill	Alcoholic/ drug abusing homeless	Runaways	X	Political detainees
Immigrants and refugees	Pregnant refugee women	Refugees with chronic disease	Refugees with AIDS	Refugees with post-traumatic distress	Suicidal/ violence-prone refugees	Maltreated refugee children	Political detainees	X

The assumption underlying the framework (Figure 1.1) and approach to these topics (Figure 1.3) is that social and economic, as well as medical care and public health, programs and policies are intended to address the health and health care needs of vulnerable populations and the availability of community and individual resources to meet them. The characteristics of existing programs and services and how they are financed will be described and their current success evaluated along a number of dimensions. These include organizational and financial barriers to access; the overall costs and cost-benefit or cost-effectiveness; and the structure, process, and outcome measures of quality of these programs and services. This analysis will provide a knowledge base for recommendations regarding how to better design programs and policies to address the needs of vulnerable populations, and how to improve on the access, cost, and quality of their care.

In each of the chapters that follows, to highlight the cross-cutting findings in response to the question posed in the chapter, a summary of common themes across groups will precede a detailed review of the evidence presented separately for each group (listed in Table 1.2). This approach is intended to apply and verify the utility of the framework for organizing and interpreting the array of disparate evidence on the health and health care needs of vulnerable populations—both those examined here in detail and others that may subsequently trouble our national conscience.

2

How Many Are Vulnerable?

Vulnerable populations are an increasingly immediate and visible reality of the experiences that touch our lives. The homeless reach out to us at the intersections near our homes and in front of the neighborhood stores from which we emerge with our abundance. Persons with AIDS are the young-sters who sit next to our children in school, the co-workers with whom we have shared coffee and committee assignments, as well as the friend's son who has come home to die. Alcohol, substance, and other abuses emerge as a part of our own, not just others', experiences when we seek to illumi-nate and speak the secrets our families have sought to keep. Chronic or mental illness takes on a painful, personal reality with the news that an elderly par-ent or a beloved partner has Alzheimer's disease or cancer. The experience of vulnerability is or can be a part of all of our lives.

In this chapter, aggregate statistical data on the number and growth of the vulnerable populations that are a focus of this book are presented. These data provide a look at the national level regarding how manyAmericans are at risk of poor physical, psychological, and/or social health, and whether their numbers have increased over time. An inventory of the major national data sources available on these populations is provided in Resource A.

Many of the groups described here (high-risk mothers and infants, chronically ill and disabled, and persons with AIDS, among others) are the focus of the Year 2000 Public Health Service Objectives for improving the nation's health (PHS, 1990). When available, the health objectives for those groups, and the extent they have been or are likely to be achieved, will be discussed. See Resource B for detailed table source notes.

Cross-Cutting Issues

In this chapter, data are presented on the prevalence and trends in the number of individuals in the following groups: high-risk mothers and infants, the chronically ill and disabled, persons with AIDS, the mentally ill and disabled, alcohol or substance abusers, suicide or homicide victims, abusing families, the homeless, and immigrant and refugee populations. These and other vulnerable populations are at risk of poor physical, psychological, and/or social health, which may be measured in a variety of ways.

Prevalence

Two main problems in estimating the number (or prevalence) of people who are vulnerable are that (1) the quality and completeness of the data for identifying them are limited, and (2) the categories of vulnerable populations for which data are reported are not mutually exclusive, but overlapping, in that many experience problems in more than one area of functioning.

The data sources used for identifying the groups examined here included clinical diagnoses of disease, patient self-reports of illness, vital statistics inventories on births and deaths, and health and social service agency records on clients. These different sources tend to yield varying estimates of those in need *within* a particular group, which also makes direct comparisons of the magnitude of need *across* groups problematic. Different universes (or groups) of individuals are used as the basis for different estimates. Further, estimates based on survey data (such as the prevalence of alcohol or substance abuse or family violence) may also have systematic biases resulting from only selected groups or individuals being included in or responding to the survey, as well as variable (standard) errors associated with the size and complexity of the sample design. Between-group and over-time differences for which explicit standard errors or tests of statistical significance are not reported should be interpreted with caution. Trend data that document increases in certain types of problems (such as child abuse and neglect) are also confounded with the increased visibility and likelihood of reporting these types of events. Methodological problems underlying estimates of the number and growth of vulnerable populations are discussed in Chapter Ten and noted in the tables presented in this and the next chapter.

A mix of indicators of need, based on clinical diagnoses, subjective perceptions of illness, and/or behavioral limitations are available. The most direct indicators of the need for assistance with functioning are those measuring limitations in activities of daily living or cognitive impairment among the chronically physically and/or mentally ill. The most immediate evidence of direct neglect or injury includes case reports and rates of family abuse or violence. For other major categories of the vulnerable examined here, vulnerability is implicit in the potential or actual harm to vital interests mirrored in other indicators of poor physical, psychological, and/or social health or functioning (low birthweight; deaths due to AIDS, drug-related causes, suicide, or homicide; and homelessness, for example).

As displayed in Table 1.3, many people have more than one type of health problem. Low-birthweight babies may have congenital defects or other adverse outcomes associated with prematurity that result in long-term physical or mental impairment. Particularly high-risk categories of mothers and infants include those in which the mother or her sex partner(s) used drugs or were HIV positive. Pregnant women with abusive partners or those who are homeless or fleeing political persecution are particularly at risk of poor outcomes for themselves and their unborn children. Accurate national estimates on the number of these and other groups with a multiplicity of cross-cutting needs are not readily available. An examination of data for discrete subcategories should not obscure this mosaic of physical, psychological, and social needs that characterizes the lives of many of the vulnerable.

Trends

The variety of indicators of vulnerable populations examined here indicates that during the 1980s, the incidence of serious physical, psychological, and/or social needs was exacerbated (at worst) and unameliorated (at best) for millions of Americans.

AIDS emerged as a new and deadly threat from a handful of cases classified as gay-related immune disorder in the early 1980s to what now may be over a million Americans who are HIV positive. The number of homeless has increased an average of 20 percent a year, so that estimates now range from up to one million men, women, or children homeless on any given night to twice that number who may be homeless sometime during the year. Over five million people have immigrated to the United States since the beginning of the decade—an increasing proportion of whom are refugees carrying with them the physical, psychological, and social wounds of war. The number of children abused by family members or other intimates has burgeoned to an estimated 1.6 to 1.7 million per year, and with the greater use of firearms, intentional acts of violence toward oneself or others are becoming increasingly deadly in their consequences.

Though fewer Americans smoke, drink, and use illicit drugs in general than was the case in the 1980s, the use of cocaine (and particularly crack) among hard-core addicts has resulted in increases in the numbers of drug-related deaths. Previously favorable trends in reducing the numbers or rates of high-risk mothers and newborns slowed or reversed during the past decade. The dependency needs of the chronically physically and mentally ill are becoming more—not less—visible as families and communities increasingly face the challenge of health and mental health policy–motivated discharge and deinstitutionalization decisions.

Population-Specific Overview

The discussion that follows presents data on each of the populations being examined.

High-Risk Mothers and Infants

High-risk mothers and infants include very young women who become pregnant, expectant mothers who fail to have adequate care during their pregnancy, infants who are premature or underweight at birth, and the mothers and babies who die at a time when the beginning rather than the end of life is promised.

The trends during the past decade reflect a troublesome slowdown or in some cases reversal of previously favorable progress in reducing the numbers of vulnerable mothers and newborns. The current reality falls far short of the Year 2000 Objectives for these groups, and the trends portend, at best, slow progress toward and, at worst, a retreat from moving toward those goals. (See Table 2.1.)

Low Birthweight. Between 1970 and 1980, the proportion of low-birthweight (LBW) infants (less than 2,500 grams or 5.5 pounds) and very-low-birthweight (VLBW) infants (less than 1,500 grams or 3.3 pounds) declined from 7.94 to 6.84 percent, and from 1.17 to 1.15 percent, respectively. This represented a 14 percent and 2 percent *decrease* during the 1970s. In 1989, the rates were 7.05 percent and 1.28 percent, however, reflecting a 3 percent and 11 percent *increase* over the 1980s. An important factor contributing to the high level of low birthweight is the incidence of preterm births (those born before thirty-seven completed weeks of gestation). The proportion of babies born preterm rose to 10.6 percent in 1989, compared to 10.2 percent in 1988 and 9.4 percent in 1981 (NCHS, 1991a).

The Year 2000 Objectives for the nation provide for an incidence of no more than 5 percent of all live births being a LBW infant and no more than 1 percent VLBW. The 1989 rates of 7.05 percent and 1.28 percent are then higher than the national objectives, and they appear to be increasing, rather than declining (NCHS, 1989e).

Infant Mortality. Low birthweight is one of the leading correlates of infant death (McCormick, 1985). The total number of infant deaths per 1,000 live births in 1989 (9.8) was half that in 1970 (20.0). Similarly, the neonatal mortality rate (deaths of infants under twenty-eight days) was 6.2 in 1989 compared to 15.1 in 1970, and the postneonatal mortality rate (deaths of infants ages twenty-eight days up to one year) was 3.6 in 1989 relative to 4.9 in 1970. The largest decline in these rates occurred between 1970 and 1980. The rate of total infant mortality declined 37 percent to 12.6 per 1,000 live births in 1980. There was a 44 percent decrease in neonatal mortality to 8.5, and a 16 percent decrease in postneonatal mortality to 4.1. The corresponding rates of decline between 1980 and 1989 were lower — 22 percent, 27 percent, and 12 percent, respectively. Provisional data indicate that the total infant mortality rate is continuing to decrease — to 9.1 in 1990 (NCHS, 1991b). The Year 2000 Objectives are for no more than 7.0 total infant

Table 2.1. Indicators of High-Risk Mothers and Infants.

Indicators	Year													
	1970	1975	1980	1981	1982	1983	1984	1985	1986	1987	1988	1989
Low Birthweight[1]												
Percent of live births less than 2,500 grams	7.94	7.39	6.84	6.81	6.75	6.82	6.72	6.75	6.81	6.90	6.93	7.05
Percent of live births less than 1,500 grams	1.17	1.16	1.15	1.16	1.18	1.19	1.19	1.21	1.21	1.24	1.24	1.28
Infant Mortality[2]												
Deaths per 1,000 live births												
Total	20.0	16.1	12.6	11.9	11.5	11.2	10.8	10.6	10.4	10.1	10.0	9.8
Neonatal	15.1	11.6	8.5	8.0	7.7	7.3	7.0	7.0	6.7	6.5	6.3	6.2
Postneonatal	4.9	4.5	4.1	3.9	3.8	3.9	3.8	3.7	3.6	3.6	3.6	3.6
Prenatal Care[3]												
Percent of mothers who received prenatal care in third trimester or no prenatal care	7.9	6.0	5.1	5.2	5.5	5.6	5.6	5.7	6.0	6.1	6.1	6.4
Teen Births[4]												
Live births per 1,000 females												
10–14 years	1.2	1.3	1.1	1.1	1.1	1.1	1.2	1.2	1.3	1.3	1.3	1.4
15–17 years	38.8	36.1	32.5	32.1	32.4	32.0	31.1	31.1	30.6	31.8	33.8	36.5
18–19 years	114.7	85.0	82.1	81.7	80.7	78.1	78.3	80.8	81.0	80.2	81.7	86.4
Maternal Mortality[5]												
Deaths per 100,000 live births all ages, crude	21.5	12.8	9.2	8.5	7.9	8.0	7.8	7.8	7.2	6.6	8.4	7.9

Source: NCHS reports; see Resource B for specific references to table items marked with superscript numerals.

deaths, 4.5 neonatal deaths, and 2.5 postneonatal deaths per 1,000 live births. Though infant death rates have declined substantially over the last twenty years, they continue to exceed these target goals.

Prenatal Care. Obtaining no or inadequate prenatal care puts mothers and infants at a considerably higher risk of adverse pregnancy outcomes (Institute of Medicine, 1988d). The percentage of women who had no prenatal care or who did not seek care until the last trimester of their pregnancy declined from 7.9 percent in 1970 to 5.1 percent in 1980. Since 1980, however, the percentage increased to 5.6 percent in 1983 and 1984, and further to 6.4 percent in 1989. The Year 2000 Objectives provide for a goal of 90 percent of women seeking care in the first trimester of their pregnancy. However, the actual rate has remained stable at around 76 percent since 1979 (NCHS, 1990b).

Births to Teen Mothers. The rates of births to teenage mothers declined from 1970 to 1980 but have not changed substantially since then. As a matter of fact, between 1986 and 1989, the number of live births per 1,000 young women fifteen to seventeen years of age increased almost 20 percent — from a low of 30.6 in 1986 to 36.5 in 1989.

Maternal Mortality. The number of women who died of pregnancy- or birth-related complications per 100,000 live births declined from 21.5 in 1970 to 6.6 in 1987. In 1988, the rate rose sharply to 8.4, 27 percent higher than the rate in the previous year. Data for 1989 show that the rate had declined to 7.9. This figure nonetheless remains more than twice that of the Year 2000 Objective of a maximum of 3.3 maternal deaths per 100,000 live births.

Chronically Ill and Disabled

The prevalence of long-term chronic disease (such as heart disease, cancer, or stroke, among others) is reflected in reports of how many people are living with these problems, how seriously they are limited in their abilities to go about their normal daily activities as a result, and ultimately how many die from these illnesses and associated complications.

Deaths due to major chronic illness have declined over the past twenty years for some conditions (such as heart disease and stroke), but not for others (chronic obstructive pulmonary disease and cancer). Estimates of the number of Americans who have to limit their usual daily activities in some way due to chronic illness range as high as 32 million. (See Table 2.2.)

Death Rates for Chronic Diseases. Heart disease has been the leading cause of death over the past twenty years, followed by cancer and stroke. The number of deaths due to heart disease declined 39 percent from 253.6 per 100,000 in 1970 to 155.9 in 1989. Though still short of the Year 2000 Objective of 20.0, the rate for strokes has declined by more than half to 28.0 in 1989, compared to 66.3 in 1970. The death rates for cirrhosis and diabetes have also declined over this same period—from 14.7 to 8.9 and from 14.1 to 11.5, respectively. On the other hand, the cancer death rate remains high and has, in fact, increased over this same period—from 129.8 to 133.0. This figure is higher than the Year 2000 Objective of 130 deaths per 100,000. Deaths from chronic obstructive pulmonary disease have also increased—from 13.2 to 19.4.

Prevalence of Chronic Conditions. Hypertension and arthritis are the most frequently reported chronic conditions among the noninstitutionalized population. The prevalence of these conditions has not changed substantially since 1982. (The questions asked in prior years to elicit this information were not comparable [NCHS, 1986e].) The rates for arthritis were 127.3 per 1,000 persons in 1989, compared to 133.0 in 1982. For hypertension, the corresponding rates were 113.6 and 116.9. The rank ordering of the prevalence of other major chronic conditions has not changed substantially over this period. The numbers of conditions per 1,000 persons in 1989 were as follows: hearing impairment (83.1), heart disease (75.9), asthma (47.7), visual impairment (32.4), diabetes (26.6), stroke (10.8), and emphysema (8.2).

Limitation in Major Activity Due to Chronic Conditions. The percent of the U.S. noninstitutionalized population having to limit their activities due to chronic illness has remained around 13 to 14 percent since the 1970s (or thirty-two million Americans in 1989). Based on the National Center for Health Statistics National Health Interview Survey, the usual activities for the respective age groups are as follows: children under five—play; six to seventeen—school; adults eighteen to sixty-four—work; sixty-five and over—self-care. The relative distribution of types of activity limitation have been similar over this time period. In 1989, the distribution of types of limitation was as follows: limited but not in major activity (4.1 percent), limited in amount or kind of major activity (5.2 percent), or unable to carry on major activity (3.9 percent). Approximately twenty-two million people were limited in or unable to carry out their major activity.

Limitation in Activities of Daily Living (ADLs) and Instrumental Activities of Daily Living (IADLs). Surveys of the functional impact of illness, particularly for the elderly, have focused on estimates of the numbers of individuals who are unable to carry on basic personal care activities (such as bathing, transferring to a bed or chair, dressing, toileting, feeding, walking—also referred to as activities of daily living or ADLs). They have also covered home management activities (such as using a telephone, handling money, shopping, and preparing meals—instrumental activities of daily living or IADLs). The questions asked to obtain this information and the types of activities inventoried vary across studies, so comprehensive trend data on ADLs and IADLs are not available.

Table 2.2. Indicators of Chronically Ill and Disabled.

Indicators	Year											
	1970	1975	1980	1981	1982	1983	1984	1985	1986	1987	1988	1989
Age-Adjusted Death Rates for Selected Chronic Diseases per 100,000 Persons[1]												
Heart disease	253.6	217.8	202.0	195.0	190.5	188.8	183.6	180.5	175.0	169.6	166.3	155.9
Stroke	66.3	53.7	40.8	38.1	35.8	34.4	33.4	32.3	31.0	30.3	29.7	28.0
Cancer	129.8	129.4	132.8	131.6	132.5	132.6	133.5	133.6	133.2	132.9	132.7	133.0
Chronic obstructive pulmonary disease*	13.2		15.9	16.3	16.2	17.4	17.7	18.7	18.8	18.7	19.4	19.4
Cirrhosis	14.7	13.7	12.2	11.4	10.5	10.2	10.0	9.6	9.2	9.1	9.0	8.9
Diabetes	14.1	11.4	10.1	9.8	9.6	9.9	9.5	9.6	9.6	9.8	10.1	11.5
Number of Selected Chronic Conditions per 1,000 Persons (Self-Reported)[2]												
Heart disease					74.5	82.8	84.2	82.6	78.1	82.4	84.1	75.9
Hypertension					116.9	121.3	124.0	125.1	122.6	118.6	121.5	113.6
Stroke					9.7	9.2	12.0	11.6	11.9	11.4	10.4	10.8
Visual impairment					38.3	35.2	34.3	36.4	35.3	33.3	34.7	32.4
Hearing impairment					87.1	90.3	91.5	90.7	87.7	88.0	90.8	83.1
Arthritis					133.0	131.3	132.9	128.6	130.8	131.8	129.9	127.3
Emphysema					10.2	8.9	9.4	8.9	8.5	8.5	7.9	8.2
Asthma					34.8	38.3	36.2	36.8	41.0	40.1	41.2	47.7
Diabetes					25.4	24.5	26.1	26.2	27.9	27.8	25.8	26.6
Age-Adjusted Degree of Activity Limitation Due to Chronic Conditions (percent)[3]												
Limited but not in major activity		3.5	3.4	3.3		4.1	3.9	4.2	4.2	4.0	4.0	4.1
Limited in amount or kind of major activity		7.2	6.9	6.8		6.0	5.7	5.5	5.4	5.2	5.3	5.2
Unable to carry on major activity		3.3	3.5	3.6		3.6	3.7	3.7	3.7	3.7	3.8	3.9
Total with activity limitation		13.9	13.7	13.7		13.8	13.3	13.4	13.3	12.9	13.1	13.4

Limitation in Activities of Daily Living (ADLs) or Instrumental Activities of Daily Living (IADLs), 65+, Living in the Community, 1987[a][b]

Percent with at least one ADL (personal care activities)	11.4
Number of ADLs	
1	5.2
2–3	3.8
4+	2.4
Percent with at least one IADL (home management activities)	17.5
Number of IADLs	
1	5.0
2–3	5.7
4+	6.8
Percent with at least one ADL or IADL	19.5

Limitation in Activities of Daily Living (ADLs) or Instrumental Activities of Daily Living (IADLs), Living in Nursing Homes, 1985[c][d]

Percent with at least one ADL	90.2
Number of ADLs	
1	11.2
2–3	17.9
4+	61.1
Percent with at least one IADL	84.8

[a]Chronic obstructive pulmonary disease was not coded in the same way in 1975.

[b]ADLs: bathing, transferring to a bed or chair, dressing, toileting, feeding, walking. IADLs: use of telephone, handling money, shopping, getting about the community, preparing meals, doing light housework.

[c]ADLs: bathing, transferring to a bed or chair, dressing, toileting, continence, eating. IADLs: use of telephone, handling money, securing personal items, care of personal possessions.

Source: NCHS reports; Leon & Lair, 1990. See Resource B for specific references.

According to the 1987 National Medical Expenditure Survey, about one in ten (11.4 percent) of the noninstitutionalized elderly (those living in private residences) had limitations in personal care activities (ADLs), and 17.5 percent had IADL limitations. About two out of ten community-dwelling elderly (19.5 percent) reported having at least one type of activity limitation (ADL or IADL). The prevalence of activity limitation is much higher among the institutionalized nursing home population. Based on the 1985 National Nursing Home Survey, around 90 percent had at least one ADL and 85 percent had one or more IADLs. The majority (61.1 percent) had four or more ADL limitations. Combined estimates of the institutionalized and noninstitutionalized elderly population in 1984 and 1985 showed that 29 percent, or eight million elderly, were functionally dependent in terms of needing help with at least one personal care or home management activity (Hing & Bloom, 1991).

Estimates of the number of children under eighteen, working-age adults eighteen to sixty-four, and elderly living in the community with substantial limitations in function have also been derived from the 1984 Survey of Income Program Participation (SIPP). Around 3.7 percent (2.3 million children) had serious physical or mental limitations. Serious limitations for adults referred to needing assistance with two or more functions, including selected ADLs, IADLs, or sensory or physical functions, such as seeing, hearing, speaking, walking, lifting, or climbing stairs without resting. Using this more inclusive (or less restrictive) definition, 8.1 percent (11.6 million) of working-age adults and a much higher percent of elderly (44.0 percent, or 11.6 million community-dwelling elderly) experienced serious limitations (Office of Assistant Secretary for Planning and Evaluation, 1989).

Persons with AIDS

Acquired immunodeficiency syndrome (AIDS) emerged on the public health landscape early in the 1980s, mysterious in its origins, debilitating and universally fatal in its consequences, and seemingly contained within the confines of the gay ghettos in which its inflictions were first felt (as gay-related immune disorder or GRID).

During the past decade over 200,000 Americans have contracted AIDS; around two-thirds have died from it and the rest are expected to. Further, around one million Americans are estimated to have the precursor to AIDS — human immunodeficiency virus (HIV) infection — and its ravages have increasingly extended to heterosexuals in general, particularly those who use drugs, and to their children. (See Table 2.3.)

AIDS Cases. Prior to 1983, there were fewer than 800 reported cases of AIDS. In 1983 alone, however, over 2,000 new cases were reported. This number more than doubled from 1983 to 1984 and then again between 1984 and 1985. Through March 1992, 218,301 cases of AIDS had been reported in

Table 2.3. Indicators of Persons with AIDS.

Indicators	1984	1985	1986	1987	1988	1989	1990	1991	Cumulative total
AIDS Cases¹*									
Total number	4,441	8,219	13,150	21,120	30,769	33,649	43,352	45,506	206,392
Under 13 (children)	50	130	183	321	571	596	788	683	3,471
13+	4,391	8,089	12,967	20,799	30,198	33,053	42,564	44,823	202,921
Number by transmission category, 13+ (Percent distribution)									
Male homosexual/bisexual	2,855 (65.0)	5,449 (67.4)	8,551 (65.9)	13,556 (65.2)	17,872 (59.2)	19,673 (59.5)	24,053 (56.5)	23,960 (53.4)	118,362 (58.3)
Intravenous drug use	777 (17.7)	1,398 (17.3)	2,244 (17.3)	3,542 (17.0)	6,903 (22.8)	7,216 (21.8)	10,161 (23.9)	11,155 (24.9)	45,753 (22.5)
Male homosexual/bisexual and intravenous drug use	411 (9.4)	584 (7.2)	982 (7.6)	1,553 (7.5)	2,027 (6.7)	2,146 (6.5)	2,445 (5.7)	2,366 (5.3)	13,135 (6.5)
Hemophilia/coagulation disorder	38 (0.9)	73 (0.9)	123 (0.9)	206 (1.0)	297 (1.0)	284 (0.9)	338 (0.8)	324 (0.7)	1,713 (0.8)
Born in Caribbean/African countries	112 (2.6)	140 (1.7)	216 (1.7)	261 (1.2)	365 (1.2)	369 (1.1)	413* (1.0)	510* (1.1)	2,523* (1.2)
Heterosexual	56 (1.3)	143 (1.8)	338 (2.7)	647 (3.1)	1,173 (3.9)	1,501 (4.5)	2,799 (6.6)	3,387 (7.6)	11,936 (5.9)
Sexual contact with intravenous drug user	42 (1.0)	107 (1.3)	236 (1.8)	443 (2.1)	852 (2.8)	1,061 (3.2)	1,600 (3.8)	1,798 (4.0)	6,366 (3.1)
Transfusion	49 (1.1)	169 (2.1)	298 (2.3)	625 (3.0)	815 (2.7)	739 (2.2)	846 (2.0)	706 (1.6)	4,347 (2.1)
Undetermined	93 (2.1)	133 (1.6)	215 (1.6)	409 (2.0)	746 (2.5)	1,125 (3.4)	1,922 (4.5)	2,925 (6.5)	7,675 (3.8)

Table 2.3. Indicators of Persons with AIDS, cont'd.

Indicators	1984	1985	1986	1987	1988	1989	1990	Cumulative total
Deaths Among AIDS Cases[2]†								
Total number	3,322	6,584	11,329	15,125	19,120	24,847	25,747	122,203
Under 13 (children)	50	106	149	269	281	326	323	1,701
13+	3,272	6,478	11,180	14,856	18,839	24,521	25,424	120,502
Number by transmission category, 13+ (Percent distribution)								
Male homosexual/bisexual	2,028 (62.0)	4,171 (64.4)	7,184 (64.2)	8,921 (60.0)	11,207 (59.5)	14,614 (59.6)	15,312 (60.2)	73,387 (60.9)
Intravenous drug use	637 (19.5)	1,193 (18.4)	2,020 (18.1)	3,089 (20.8)	4,172 (22.1)	5,489 (22.4)	5,314 (20.9)	24,847 (20.6)
Male homosexual/bisexual and intravenous drug use	314 (9.6)	485 (7.5)	837 (7.5)	1,113 (7.5)	1,235 (6.6)	1,494 (6.1)	1,531 (6.0)	8,012 (6.6)
Hemophilia/coagulation disorder	26 (0.8)	75 (1.2)	107 (1.0)	158 (1.1)	191 (1.0)	209 (0.8)	231 (0.9)	1,129 (0.9)
Born in Caribbean/African countries	80 (2.4)	109 (1.7)	146 (1.3)	190 (1.3)	183 (1.0)	233 (1.0)	181 (0.7)	1,356 (1.1)
Heterosexual	44 (1.3)	126 (1.9)	269 (2.4)	457 (3.1)	705 (3.7)	1,007 (4.1)	1,272 (5.0)	4,624 (3.8)
Sexual contact with intravenous drug user	38 (1.2)	89 (1.4)	184 (1.6)	320 (2.2)	501 (2.6)	720 (2.9)	833 (3.3)	3,146 (2.6)
Transfusion	64 (2.0)	193 (3.0)	359 (3.2)	533 (3.6)	597 (3.2)	590 (2.4)	528 (2.1)	3,156 (2.6)
Undetermined	79 (2.4)	126 (1.9)	258 (2.3)	395 (2.6)	549 (2.9)	885 (3.6)	1,055 (4.1)	3,991 (3.3)

Indicators	Year						
	1984	1985	1986	1987	1988	1989	1990
Median (Range) Percent Positive HIV Prevalence[3]‡							
Sexually transmitted disease clinics						2.2 (0.0–38.5)	2.1 (0.0–39.0)
Drug treatment centers						4.1 (0.0–48.2)	3.9 (0.0–49.3)
Women's health clinics						0.2 (0.0–2.6)	0.2 (0.0–2.5)
Tuberculosis clinics						3.4 (0.0–46.3)	5.9 (0.0–58.3)
Childbearing women						0.15 (0.0–0.58)	0.15 (0.0–0.66)
Civilian applicants for military service						0.12	0.12
Blood donors						0.0084	0.0051
Job Corps entrants						0.36	0.34
Sentinel hospital patients						0.9 (0.1–7.7)	0.9 (0.1–7.6)
National Clinical Laboratory Survey						0.89	
Ambulatory Sentinel Practice Network							0.2

*Estimates for 1984–1989 exclude residents of U.S. territories. The AIDS case definition was changed in September 1987 to allow for the presumptive diagnosis of AIDS-associated diseases and conditions and to expand the spectrum of human immunodeficiency virus-associated disease reportable as AIDS. Estimates for 1990, 1991, and cumulative total include residents of U.S. territories, which represent approximately 3 percent of the cumulative total of AIDS cases. The cumulative total includes cases prior to 1984. Estimates for the transmission category "Born in Caribbean/African countries" are classified as a subset of the "Heterosexual" category in CDC (1992a).

†Estimates exclude residents of U.S. territories. The cumulative total includes deaths from 1981 through 1991. Estimates for 1991 are not complete due to reporting delays.

‡The estimates reported for each year are actually cumulative, generally beginning in 1988 for each site.

Source: NCHS and CDC reports; see Resource B for specific references.

the United States, including 211,337 in the fifty states and 6,964 in the U.S. territories (CDC, 1992b). The number of children under thirteen with AIDS reported annually has steadily increased — from thirty-four in 1983 to around 700 in 1990 and 1991. In the early years of the AIDS epidemic, the principal mode of transmission for adults was through male homosexual/bisexual contact. Since 1988, however, transmission through intravenous (IV) drug use in general and in connection with heterosexual sexual contacts with IV drug users has increased. The principal mode of transmission for children is perinatally through mothers who have or are at risk for HIV infection, due mainly to their own or their sex partners' use of drugs.

AIDS Deaths. Over 130,000 people have died of AIDS since the beginning of the epidemic. By 1988, HIV/AIDS had become the third leading cause of death among men twenty-five to forty-four years of age; by 1989, it was estimated to be second. In 1988, it ranked eighth among causes of death among women in this age group, and in 1991 it was ranked among the top five causes (CDC, 1991). Most deaths have occurred among homosexual/bisexual men and among women and heterosexual men who are intravenous drug users. There is some evidence that the short-term survival rates for AIDS have increased in recent years — possibly due to the introduction of the drug azidothymidine (AZT) (Lemp, Payne, Neal, Temelso, & Rutherford, 1990).

HIV Prevalence. Approximately one million people in the United States are believed to have the HIV virus (CDC, 1990d). Plans for a CDC national survey of households to measure the prevalence of HIV infection were abandoned because of concerns that those with high-risk behaviors would be unlikely to participate in such a survey (APHA, 1991a). CDC has, however, conducted seroprevalence studies in a number of different institutional sites. Average prevalence rates among individuals seen at these sites varied, from highest to lowest: tuberculosis clinics (5.9 percent), drug treatment centers (3.9 percent), sexually transmitted disease clinics (2.1 percent), sentinel hospital patients (0.9 percent), Job Corps entrants (0.34 percent), Ambulatory Sentinel Practice Network (0.20 percent), women's health clinics (0.20 percent), childbearing women (0.15 percent), civilian applicants for military service (0.12 percent) and blood donors (0.0051 percent). Based on current prevalence estimates and annual incidence of AIDS cases, it is estimated that there will be around 61,000 to 98,000 new cases in 1993 (CDC, 1990d), which begins to approximate the Year 2,000 Objectives ceiling of no more than 98,000 new cases each year.

Mentally Ill and Disabled

Sources of data to estimate the magnitude of mental illness in the United States include community surveys that ask people whether they have had certain mental health problems, as well as patient census or visit data obtained from institutions that care for the mentally ill.

Data on the prevalence of mental illness in U.S. communities indicate that three out of ten Americans may have experienced a mental health problem sometime in their life, and about half that number currently report having a problem. (See Table 2.4.) From 1.7 to 2.4 million Americans (around 900,000 of whom are institutionalized in mental health services organizations or nursing homes) have been estimated to be chronically mentally ill. That is, they have emotional disorders that seriously interfere with their ability to function in the primary activities of daily life (such as self-care, interpersonal relationships, working or going to school) and require prolonged mental health care as a result (Goldman & Manderscheid, 1987).

Community Prevalence Rates. The best source of data on the prevalence of mental illness among those who may or may not actually be under treatment is the Epidemiological Catchment Area (ECA) surveys conducted during the early 1980s in five U.S. cities (New Haven, Conn.; Baltimore; St. Louis; Durham, N.C.; and Los Angeles). Based on combined data for all five ECA communities using the Diagnostic Interview Schedule (DIS) to screen for mental illness, specifically designed for that study, around 15.4 percent of the population were estimated to have experienced at least one mental disorder during the past month. This estimate varied across sites, however — from a low of 12.9 percent in St. Louis to 19.3 percent in Durham and 19.8 percent in Baltimore. These between-site differences were principally due to variations in the rates of phobia reported, which varied from approximately 11 percent in Durham and Baltimore to around 4 to 5 percent in the other sites.

The overall rates increased from 15.4 percent having experienced a mental disorder within the past month, to 19.1 percent having had a problem within the past six months (six-month prevalence), and to 32.2 percent ever having experienced a mental health problem (lifetime prevalence). The most common current, specific disorders, in order of one-month prevalence rates, included phobia (6.2 percent), dysthymia or long-term seriously depressed mood (3.3 percent), alcohol/abuse dependence (2.8 percent), and major depressive episode (2.2 percent). All other disorders were found in less than 2 percent of the population. Substance abuse disorders were relatively more common long-term disorders, based on six-month and lifetime prevalence rates: six-month prevalence — phobia (7.7 percent), alcohol/abuse dependence (4.7 percent), dysthymia (3.3 percent), major depressive episode (3.0 percent); lifetime prevalence — alcohol/abuse dependence (13.3 percent), phobia (12.5 percent), drug abuse/dependence (5.9 percent), major depressive episode (5.8 percent).

Treated Rates — Inpatient Psychiatric Services. As Table 2.5 illustrates, the number of people under care in psychiatric facilities provides a profile of

Table 2.4. Indicators of Mentally Ill and Disabled: Community Prevalence Rates.

DIS/DSM-III Disorders per 100 Persons, 18+ Years[1]*	One-Month[†]					All sites combined[‡]		
	New Haven, Conn., 1980–1981 (N = 5,034)	Baltimore, 1981–1982 (N = 3,481)	St. Louis, 1981–1982 (N = 3,004)	Durham, N.C. 1982–1983 (N = 3,921)	Los Angeles, 1983–1984 (N = 3,131)	One-Month	Six-Month	Lifetime
Any DIS disorder covered	14.5 (0.7)§	19.8 (0.9)	12.9 (0.9)	19.3 (0.9)	15.4 (0.6)	15.4 (0.4)	19.1 (0.4)	32.2 (0.5)
Any DIS disorder except phobia	11.5 (0.6)	11.7 (0.7)	10.7 (0.9)	11.1 (0.7)	11.9 (0.6)	11.2 (0.3)	14.0 (0.4)	25.2 (0.5)
Substance use disorders	3.8 (0.4)	5.3 (0.5)	3.2 (0.4)	2.8 (0.4)	4.5 (0.4)	3.8 (0.2)	6.0 (0.3)	16.4 (0.4)
Alcohol abuse/dependence	3.0 (0.4)	4.3 (0.5)	2.0 (0.3)	2.4 (0.4)	3.2 (0.4)	2.8 (0.2)	4.7 (0.2)	13.3 (0.4)
Drug abuse/dependence	1.0 (0.2)	1.4 (0.3)	1.5 (0.2)	0.6 (0.2)	1.7 (0.2)	1.3 (0.1)	2.0 (0.1)	5.9 (0.2)
Schizophrenic/schizophreniform disorders	0.7 (0.2)	1.0 (0.2)	0.6 (0.2)	1.3 (0.3)	0.4 (0.1)	0.7 (0.1)	0.9 (0.1)	1.5 (0.1)
Schizophrenia	0.7 (0.2)	0.8 (0.2)	0.5 (0.2)	1.2 (0.3)	0.3 (0.1)	0.6 (0.1)	0.8 (0.1)	1.3 (0.1)
Schizophreniform disorder	0.0 (0.0)	0.2 (0.1)	0.1 (0.0)	0.1 (0.1)	0.1 (0.0)	0.1 (0.0)	0.1 (0.0)	0.1 (0.0)
Affective disorders	5.6 (0.4)	4.3 (0.4)	5.8 (0.6)	3.5 (0.3)	5.7 (0.5)	5.1 (0.2)	5.8 (0.3)	8.3 (0.3)
Manic episode	0.5 (0.1)	0.4 (0.1)	0.6 (0.2)	0.2 (0.1)	0.1 (0.1)	0.4 (0.1)	0.5 (0.1)	0.8 (0.1)
Major depressive episode	2.5 (0.3)	1.8 (0.3)	2.6 (0.4)	1.5 (0.2)	2.4 (0.2)	2.2 (0.2)	3.0 (0.2)	5.8 (0.3)
Dysthymia‖	3.2 (0.3)	2.1 (0.3)	3.8 (0.4)	2.2 (0.2)	4.2 (0.4)	3.3 (0.2)	3.3 (0.2)	3.3 (0.2)
Anxiety disorders	6.1 (0.5)	12.5 (0.7)	5.1 (0.5)	12.2 (0.8)	5.9 (0.4)	7.3 (0.3)	8.9 (0.3)	14.6 (0.4)
Phobia	5.1 (0.5)	11.1 (0.6)	4.0 (0.4)	11.0 (0.8)	5.2 (0.3)	6.2 (0.2)	7.7 (0.3)	12.5 (0.3)
Panic	0.4 (0.1)	0.7 (0.1)	0.6 (0.2)	0.5 (0.2)	0.6 (0.2)	0.5 (0.1)	0.8 (0.1)	1.6 (0.1)
Obsessive-compulsive	1.2 (0.2)	1.7 (0.3)	1.1 (0.2)	2.1 (0.4)	0.7 (0.2)	1.3 (0.1)	1.5 (0.1)	2.5 (0.2)
Somatization disorder	0.1 (0.0)	0.1 (0.1)	0.1 (0.1)	0.4 (0.1)	0.0 (0.0)	0.1 (0.0)	0.1 (0.0)	0.1 (0.0)
Personality disorder, antisocial personality	0.3 (0.1)	0.5 (0.1)	0.8 (0.2)	0.4 (0.2)	0.4 (0.1)	0.5 (0.1)	0.8 (0.1)	2.5 (0.2)
Cognitive impairment (severe)	1.2 (0.1)	1.4 (0.2)	1.0 (0.2)	3.3 (0.3)	1.2 (0.2)	1.3 (0.1)	1.3 (0.1)	1.3 (0.1)

*DIS/DSM-III refers to the Diagnostic Interview Schedule, based on American Psychiatric Association, Committee on Nomenclature and Statistics, *Diagnostic and Statistical Manual of Mental Disorders* (1980).

†Rates for each site are standardized to the age, sex, and race characteristics of the population eighteen and older in its catchment area.

‡Rates are standardized to the age, sex, and race distribution of the 1980 noninstitutionalized population of the U.S. eighteen and older.

§Numbers in parentheses refer to the standard errors of the estimates.

‖Was asked about only as a lifetime disorder. The one-month, six-month, and lifetime rates are therefore considered to be the same.

Source: Table 3 (p.980) and Table 4 (p.981) in Regier et al., (1988). *Archives of General Psychiatry, 45,* 977–986. Copyright 1988, American Medical Association.

See Resource B for further detail.

Table 2.5. Indicators of Mentally Ill and Disabled: Treated Rates—Inpatient Psychiatric Services.

Principal Diagnoses, 1986[1]*	Total, All Inpatient Services	State and County Mental Hospitals	Private Psychiatric Hospitals	VA Medical Centers	Nonfederal General Hospitals	Multiservice Mental Health Organizations
Number (Percent Distribution) of Total Persons Under Care						
Alcohol-related disorders	10,008 (6.2)	2,740 (2.9)	500 (3.0)	2,484 (18.8)	4,036 (12.5)	248 (5.3)
Drug-related disorders	4,829 (3.0)	1,460 (1.5)	591 (3.6)	527 (4.0)	1,981 (6.1)	† †
Affective disorders	34,722 (21.6)	11,719 (12.4)	8,158 (49.7)	2,130 (16.1)	11,845 (36.8)	870 (18.6)
Schizophrenia	69,994 (43.5)	54,277 (57.5)	2,184 (13.3)	5,359 (40.6)	6,115 (19.0)	2,059 (44.0)
Personality disorders	3,893 (2.4)	2,400 (2.5)	601 (3.7)	255 (1.9)	550 (1.7)	† †
Adjustment disorders	6,301 (3.9)	2,458 (2.6)	650 (4.0)	113 (0.9)	2,835 (8.8)	245 (5.2)
Organic disorders	9,001 (5.6)	6,603 (7.0)	470 (2.9)	793 (6.0)	954 (3.0)	181 (3.9)
Number (Percent Distribution) of Total Admissions						
Alcohol-related disorders	236,917 (14.8)	53,788 (16.5)	15,715 (7.6)	57,506 (32.1)	99,044 (12.5)	10,864 (12.1)
Drug-related disorders	105,096 (6.6)	20,768 (6.4)	14,525 (7.0)	16,785 (9.4)	48,437 (6.1)	4,581 (5.1)
Affective disorders	490,991 (30.8)	54,571 (16.7)	100,254 (48.3)	27,301 (15.2)	291,680 (36.7)	17,185 (19.2)
Schizophrenia	369,402 (23.1)	118,852 (36.5)	23,588 (11.4)	47,298 (26.4)	151,407 (19.1)	28,257 (31.5)
Personality disorders	29,910 (1.9)	6,360 (2.0)	2,230 (1.1)	4,135 (2.3)	13,588 (1.7)	3,597 (4.0)
Adjustment disorders	121,330 (7.6)	20,408 (6.3)	13,413 (6.5)	7,019 (3.9)	69,914 (8.8)	10,576 (11.8)
Organic disorders	47,796 (3.0)	10,412 (3.2)	4,795 (2.3)	6,018 (3.4)	23,420 (2.9)	3,151 (3.5)

*Percentages do not sum to 100 percent because only selected diagnoses are reported.

†Estimate based on five or fewer sample cases or estimate has a relative standard error of 50 percent or higher. Therefore, estimate not shown.

Source: Rosenstein, Milazzo-Sayre, & Manderscheid, 1990; see Resource B for further detail.

who is being treated for mental illness at a particular point in time (in this case, on April 1, 1986), while admission rates refer to the number of people admitted or readmitted over an extended period (usually annually). The former provides a cross-sectional profile of the long-term continuing patient population, and the latter a more dynamic picture of the types of patients served in the mental health system on an acute basis.

Based on a 1986 NIMH survey of specialty mental health outpatient and inpatient institutions, 160,862 people were receiving inpatient care. Overall, schizophrenia (43.5 percent) was the most frequently reported diagnosis, followed by affective disorders (forms of major depression) (21.6 percent). Schizophrenia was most frequently reported for patients in state and county hospitals (57.5 percent), VA medical centers (40.6 percent), and multiservice mental health organizations (44.0 percent). Affective disorders were the most frequently reported diagnoses in private psychiatric hospitals (49.7 percent) and nonfederal general hospitals (36.8 percent). The percent under care for alcohol-related disorders was highest in the VA (18.8 percent) and nonfederal general hospitals (12.5 percent) and lowest in state and county (2.9 percent) and private psychiatric (3.0 percent) hospitals.

There were 1.6 million inpatient psychiatric admissions in 1986. Affective disorders were the most frequent reasons for admission (30.8 percent), followed by schizophrenia (23.1 percent) and alcohol-related disorders (14.8 percent). Comparisons of the admissions and under-care populations showed that persons with schizophrenia comprised a much higher percentage of those under care (43.5 percent) than admissions (23.1 percent) for all institutions, except for private psychiatric hospitals and nonfederal general hospitals, for which there was little or no difference. The admission rate for alcohol-related disorders was particularly high in the VA (32.1 percent) compared to the other institutions (from 7.6 to 16.5 percent).

Treated Rates — Outpatient Psychiatric Services. In 1986, 1.4 million people were under psychiatric care in outpatient mental health facilities (including state and county mental hospitals, private psychiatric hospitals, VA medical centers, nonfederal general hospitals, multiservice mental health organizations, freestanding outpatient clinics, and residential treatment centers for emotionally disturbed children). Affective disorders (22.3 percent), schizophrenia (21.6 percent), and adjustment disorders (reflecting problems in coping at home or work, for example) (16.6 percent) accounted for about 60 percent of all clients under care. Schizophrenic patients were most likely to be cared for in state and county mental hospitals (36.5 percent). Affective disorders was the most common diagnosis among patients seen at private psychiatric hospitals (26.5 percent). Nonfederal general hospitals saw the highest percent of clients with adjustment disorders (22.4 percent). (See Table 2.6.)

There were 2.1 million admissions to outpatient psychiatric facilities in 1986. Adjustment disorders were somewhat more frequent among those

Table 2.6. Indicators of Mentally Ill and Disabled: Treated Rates—Outpatient Psychiatric Services.

Principal diagnoses, 1986¹†	Total, All Outpatient Services*	State and County Mental Hospitals	Private Psychiatric Hospitals	VA Medical Centers	Nonfederal General Hospitals	Multiservice Mental Health Organizations	Freestanding Outpatient Clinics
Number (Percent Distribution) of Total Persons Under Care							
Alcohol-related disorders	68,181 (4.9)	1,082 (1.9)	2,753 (5.9)	4,584 (6.3)	6,056 (3.2)	47,099 (6.2)	6,330 (2.6)
Drug-related disorders	26,195 (1.9)	‡ ‡	‡ ‡	4,170 (5.7)	4,542 (2.4)	9,524 (1.2)	4,824 (2.0)
Affective disorders	308,110 (22.3)	10,912 (19.7)	12,434 (26.5)	17,962 (24.6)	48,158 (25.3)	169,795 (22.2)	46,364 (19.1)
Schizophrenia	298,808 (21.6)	20,236 (36.5)	5,136 (11.0)	19,929 (27.2)	33,943 (17.8)	177,733 (23.2)	41,011 (16.9)
Personality disorders	81,731 (5.9)	‡ ‡	2,196 (4.7)	1,342 (1.8)	10,761 (5.7)	48,515 (6.3)	14,884 (6.1)
Adjustment disorders	229,801 (16.6)	4,072 (7.3)	7,212 (15.4)	2,987 (4.1)	42,692 (22.4)	120,166 (15.7)	50,811 (20.9)
Social conditions	77,069 (5.6)	1,241 (2.2)	3,024 (6.5)	1,693 (2.3)	5,518 (2.9)	49,764 (6.5)	15,708 (6.5)
Number (Percent Distribution) of Total Admissions							
Alcohol-related disorders	202,444 (9.5)	‡ ‡	9,047 (10.5)	11,117 (18.6)	17,864 (5.7)	131,928 (11.3)	28,961 (7.0)
Drug-related disorders	65,452 (3.1)	833 (1.4)	2,535 (2.9)	6,389 (10.7)	7,434 (2.4)	40,639 (3.5)	7,559 (1.8)
Affective disorders	306,874 (14.4)	7,042 (12.1)	18,147 (21.0)	11,295 (18.9)	68,105 (21.6)	146,007 (12.5)	49,207 (11.8)
Schizophrenia	166,737 (7.8)	12,174 (21.0)	3,045 (3.5)	10,267 (17.2)	29,569 (9.4)	88,595 (7.6)	21,688 (5.2)
Personality disorders	136,903 (6.4)	2,667 (4.6)	‡ ‡	1,188 (2.0)	19,483 (6.2)	79,228 (6.8)	31,950 (7.7)
Adjustment disorders	491,169 (23.1)	9,569 (16.5)	18,051 (20.9)	6,966 (11.7)	83,592 (26.5)	270,623 (23.1)	99,081 (23.8)
Social conditions	197,553 (9.3)	1,752 (3.0)	5,808 (6.7)	750 (1.3)	15,146 (4.8)	117,738 (10.1)	55,808 (13.4)

*Includes estimates for residential treatment centers for emotionally disturbed children.

†Percentages do not sum to 100 percent because only selected diagnoses are reported.

‡Estimate based on five or fewer sample cases or estimate has a relative standard error of 50 percent or higher. Therefore, estimate not shown.

Source: Rosenstein, Milazzo-Sayre, & Manderscheid, 1990; see Resource B for further detail.

admitted (23.1 percent) than among those under care (16.6 percent). The
VA had the highest admission rate for alcohol-related disorders (18.6 percent).

Treated Rates — Nursing Homes. Findings from the 1985 National Nursing
Home Survey revealed that nearly two-thirds (65.3 percent) of nursing home
residents had at least one mental disorder. The most prevalent disorder was
organic brain syndrome (OBS), including Alzheimer's disease. Almost half
(46.7 percent) of the total nursing home population was diagnosed as having this disorder. Among those residents with one or more disorders, more
than 70 percent (71.5 percent) had OBS, 20 percent had schizophrenia and
other psychoses, 17.1 percent had depressive disorders, and 16.8 percent had
anxiety disorders. Mental retardation (8.5 percent), alcohol and drug abuse
(6.0 percent), and other mental illnesses (1.8 percent) accounted for the re-
mainder of the diagnoses among mentally ill nursing home residents. (See
Table 2.7.)

Table 2.7. Indicators of Mentally Ill and Disabled: Treated Rates — Nursing Homes.

Mental Disorders, 1985[1]	Residents with Mental Disorders		Percent of All Residents with Mental Disorders
	Number	Percent	
Total*	974,300	100.0	65.3
Mental retardation	83,200	8.5	5.6
Alcohol and drug abuse	58,700	6.0	3.9
Organic brain syndromes (including Alzheimer's disease)	696,800	71.5	46.7
Depressive disorders	167,000	17.1	11.2
Schizophrenia and other psychoses	195,400	20.0	13.1
Anxiety disorders	163,700	16.8	11.0
Other mental illnesses	17,700	1.8	1.2

*Figures may not add to totals because of rounding.
Source: Strahan, 1990; see Resource B for further detail.

Alcohol or Substance Abusers

Alcohol and substance users differ from abusers in that the latter have developed a long-term physical and/or psychological dependency on (or addiction to) drugs, alcohol, and/or tobacco. National surveys of households
and high school seniors provide data on those who have used or are currently using (and may be abusing) these substances. Vital statistics and emergency room and medical examiner data on alcohol or drug-related medical
emergencies or deaths more directly reflect the life-threatening consequences
for those who routinely and/or seriously abuse these substances.

The percent of the U.S. population in general that smokes, drinks,
or uses illicit drugs has declined over the past decade. The number using
cocaine daily as well as those dying from the effects of it has increased,

however—confirming a growth in a subgroup of users who are seriously addicted to this particular drug. (See Table 2.8.)

Household Population, 12+ Years. Based on the National Household Survey on Drug Abuse, which covers the population age twelve and older living in households in the contiguous United States, the prevalence rates for use of any illicit drug (the percent who used it at least once within the thirty days prior to the survey) decreased steadily from 1985 to 1991—from 23 million (12.1 percent) in 1985 to 14.5 million (7.3 percent) in 1988 to around 13 million (6.2 percent) in 1991.

Marijuana remains the most commonly used illicit drug. Approximately 67.7 million Americans (33.4 percent) have tried marijuana at least once in their lifetime. Rates of use of marijuana in the past month have continued to decline since the period of its peak use during the late 1970s. The prevalence of cocaine use increased steadily from the early 1970s to mid 1980s. During the three-year period from 1988 to 1991, however, the number of current cocaine users decreased substantially from 2.9 million (1.5 percent) to 1.8 million (0.9 percent), which represents a 69 percent decrease from the 1985 prevalence rate of 2.9 percent (or 5.8 million users). However, among those who used cocaine in the past year, 855,000 used it once a week or more in 1991 compared to 662,000 in 1990 (NIDA, 1991c, 1991d, 1991e, 1991g).

The rates of cigarette and alcohol use declined from 1985 to 1991. Current cigarette use dropped from 32 percent in 1985 to 29 percent in 1988 and 27 percent in 1991. The current alcohol use rates also declined from 59 percent in 1985 to 53 percent in 1988 to 51 percent in 1991 (NIDA, 1991c, 1991d, 1991e, 1991g).

High School Seniors. In 1991, 16.4 percent of all high school seniors said they had used an illegal drug at least once during the past month—down from a high of 38.9 percent in 1978 and 1979. Marijuana was and continues to be the most frequently used drug. Around 14 percent reported having smoked marijuana in the past month—down from a high of 37.1 percent in 1978. Over a period from 1980 to 1991, the current prevalence of inhalant use ranged from 2.5 to 3.5 percent. Hallucinogen use ranged from a high of 5.3 percent in 1979 to 2.3 percent in 1990. The percent having used cocaine in the past month increased sharply from 1.9 percent in 1975 to 5.2 percent in 1980, and peaked at 6.7 percent in 1985. The rates of reported use of cocaine have declined since 1985, however, to a low of 1.4 percent in 1991. Crack cocaine use also declined sharply from 1988 (1.6 percent) to 1991 (0.7 percent) (University of Michigan, 1991, 1992).

The prevalence of cigarette smoking among high school seniors is similar to that for the U.S. household population twelve years of age and older. In 1991, 27 percent of people 12+ years of age, compared to 28 percent of U.S. high school seniors, reported having smoked cigarettes in the past

Table 2.8. Indicators of Alcohol or Substance Abusers.

Indicators	Year								
	1974	1976	1977	1979	1982	1985	1988	1990	1991
Household Population, 12–17 Years (%)[1] Drug Use									
Marijuana and hashish									
Past year	18.5	18.4	22.3	24.1	20.6	19.7	12.6	11.3	10.1
Past month	2.0	12.3	16.6	16.7	11.5	12.0	6.4	5.2	4.3
Hallucinogens									
Past year	4.3	2.8	3.1	4.7	3.6	2.7	2.8	2.4	2.1
Past month	1.3	0.9	1.6	2.2	1.4	1.2	0.8	0.9	0.8
Cocaine									
Past year	2.7	2.3	2.6	4.2	4.1	4.0	2.9	2.2	1.5
Past month	1.0	1.0	0.8	1.4	1.6	1.5	1.1	0.6	0.4
Any illicit drug use*									
Past year				26.0	22.0	23.7	16.8	15.9	14.8
Past month				17.6	12.7	14.9	9.2	8.1	6.8
Alcohol use									
Past year	51.0	49.3	47.5	53.6	52.4	51.7	44.6	41.0	40.3
Past month	34.0	32.4	31.2	37.2	30.2	31.0	25.2	24.5	20.3
Cigarette use									
Past year				13.3†	24.8	25.8	22.8	22.2	20.1
Past month	25.0	23.4	22.3	12.1†	14.7	15.3	11.8	11.6	10.8
Household Population, 18–25 Years (%)[1] Drug Use									
Marijuana and hashish									
Past year	34.2	35.0	38.7	46.9	40.4	36.9	27.9	24.6	24.6
Past month	25.2	25.0	27.4	35.4	27.4	21.8	15.5	12.7	13.0
Hallucinogens									
Past year	6.1	6.0	6.4	9.9	6.9	4.0	5.6	3.9	4.8
Past month	2.5	1.1	2.0	4.4	1.7	1.9	1.9	0.8	1.2

Cocaine									
Past year	8.1	7.0	10.2	19.6	18.8	16.3	12.1	7.5	7.7
Past month	3.1	2.0	3.7	9.3	6.8	7.6	4.5	2.2	2.0
Any illicit drug use*									
Past year				49.4	43.4	42.6	32.0	28.7	29.2
Past month				37.1	30.4	25.7	17.8	14.9	15.4
Alcohol use									
Past year	77.1	77.9	79.8	86.6	87.1	87.2	81.7	80.2	82.8
Past month	69.3	69.0	70.0	75.9	70.9	71.4	65.3	63.3	63.6
Cigarette use									
Past year	48.8	49.4	47.3	46.7†	47.2	44.3	44.7	39.7	41.2
Past month				42.6†	39.5	36.8	35.2	31.5	32.2

Household Population, 26+ Years (%)[1] Drug Use

Marijuana and hashish									
Past year	3.8	5.4	6.4	9.0	10.6	9.5	6.9	7.3	6.8
Past month	2.0	3.5	3.3	6.0	6.6	6.1	3.9	3.6	3.3
Hallucinogens									
Past year	‡	‡	‡	0.5	0.8	1.0	0.6	0.4	0.6
Past month	‡	‡	‡	‡	‡	‡	‡	0.1	0.1
Cocaine									
Past year	‡	0.6	0.9	2.0	3.8	4.2	2.7	2.4	2.5
Past month	‡	‡	‡	0.9	1.2	2.0	0.9	0.6	0.8
Any illicit drug use*									
Past year				10.0	11.8	13.3	10.2	10.0	9.6
Past month				6.5	7.5	8.5	4.9	4.6	4.5
Alcohol use									
Past year	62.7	64.2	65.8	72.4	72.0	73.6	68.6	66.6	69.1
Past month	54.5	56.0	54.9	61.3	59.8	60.6	54.8	52.3	52.5
Cigarette use									
Past year	39.1	38.4	38.7	39.7†	38.2	36.0	33.7	31.9	32.0
Past month				36.9†	34.6	32.8	29.8	27.7	28.2

Table 2.8. Indicators of Alcohol or Substance Abusers, Cont'd.

Indicators	Year											
	1980	1981	1982	1983	1984	1985	1986	1987	1988	1989	1990	1991
High School Seniors (%)[2] Drug Use												
Marijuana and hashish												
Past year	48.8	46.1	44.3	42.3	40.0	40.6	38.8	36.3	33.1	29.6	27.0	23.9
Past month	33.7	31.6	28.5	27.0	25.2	25.7	23.4	21.0	18.0	16.7	14.0	13.8
Inhalants§												
Past year	7.9	6.1	6.6	6.2	7.2	7.5	8.9	8.1	7.1	6.9	7.5	6.9
Past month	2.7	2.5	2.5	2.5	2.6	3.0	3.2	3.5	3.0	2.7	2.9	2.6
Hallucinogens‖												
Past year	10.4	10.1	9.0	8.3	7.3	7.6	7.6	6.7	5.8	6.2	6.0	6.1
Past month	4.4	4.5	4.1	3.5	3.2	3.8	3.5	2.8	2.3	2.9	2.3	2.4
Cocaine (Crack)⁺												
Past year	12.3	12.4	11.5	11.4	11.6	13.1	12.7	10.3	7.9	6.5	5.3	3.5
							(4.1)	(3.9)	(3.1)	(3.1)	(1.9)	(1.5)
Past month	5.2	5.8	5.0	4.9	5.8	6.7	6.2	4.3	3.4	2.8	1.9	1.4
								(1.3)	(1.6)	(1.4)	(0.7)	(0.7)
Any illicit drug use#												
Past year	53.1	52.1	49.4	47.4	45.8	46.3	44.3	41.7	38.5	35.4	32.5	29.4
Past month	37.2	36.9	32.5	30.5	29.2	29.7	27.1	24.7	21.3	19.7	17.2	16.4
Alcohol use												
Past year	87.9	87.0	86.8	87.3	86.0	85.6	84.5	85.7	85.3	82.7	80.6	77.7
Past month	72.0	70.7	69.7	69.4	67.2	65.9	65.3	66.4	63.9	60.0	57.1	54.0
Cigarette use												
Past month	30.5	29.4	30.0	30.3	29.3	30.1	29.6	29.4	28.7	28.6	29.4	28.3
Daily use	21.3	20.3	21.1	21.2	18.7	19.5	18.7	18.7	18.1	18.9	19.1	18.5
Alcohol-Related Mortality Rates[3]												
Age-adjusted rate per 100,000	7.5	7.0	6.4	6.1	6.2	6.2	6.4	6.0	6.3			

Indicators	1988		1989		1990		1991	
	Jan.-June	July-Dec.	Jan.-June	July-Dec.	Jan.-June	July-Dec.	Jan.-June	July-Sept.
Emergency Room Drug Abuse Reports (Number)[*]								
Total episodes	203,356	213,606	223,252	202,651	189,555	181,653	196,787	104,479
Cocaine mentions	49,597	55,135	57,428	52,585	41,306	39,049	47,652	28,700

Year

*Refers to using one or more of the following: marijuana, cocaine, inhalants, hallucinogens, PCP, heroin, or nonmedical psychotherapeutics.

†Includes only persons who ever smoked at least five packs.

‡Low precision—no estimate shown.

§Adjusted for underreporting of amyl and butyl nitrites.

‖Adjusted for underreporting of PCP.

⁺Numbers in parentheses refer to crack cocaine use.

#Refers to using one or more of the following: marijuana, cocaine, hallucinogens, heroin, or any use of other opiates, stimulants, barbiturates, methaqualone (excluded since 1990), or tranquilizers not under a doctor's orders. Estimates for the period 1982–1991 are based on revisions to the questionnaire that attempted to exclude the inappropriate reporting of nonprescription stimulants.

Source: NIDA, University of Michigan, and IHS publications; see Resource B for specific references.

month. The percent of current smokers among high school students declined sharply from 36.7 percent in 1975 to 30.5 percent in 1980, but then did not change substantially over the period from 1980 to 1991. The percent of high school seniors reporting having drunk an alcoholic beverage in the past month was lowest in 1991 (54.0 percent)—down from a high of 72.1 percent in 1978 (University of Michigan, 1991, 1992).

Alcohol-Related Mortality Rates. The rates of death attributable to alcohol-related causes declined from 7.5 in 1980 to 6.3 in 1988. The average annual per capita consumption of pure alcohol also declined over this same period from a high of 2.76 gallons in 1980–1981 to a low of 2.54 gallons in 1987—principally due to the decline in the consumption of spirits (hard liquor) (ADAMHA, 1990).

Emergency Room Drug Abuse Reports. Reports of drug-related visits to an emergency room (ER) in participating cities through the Drug Abuse Warning Network (DAWN) showed that the number of drug-related ER visits increased steadily from the first half of 1988 (203,356) to the first half of 1989 (223,252), and then began to decline through 1990. A similar pattern was observed for cocaine-related visits. The 1991 DAWN data indicated that the number of drug-related, as well as cocaine-related, visits to hospital emergency rooms had once again begun to increase, which has been attributed to the serious health consequences that are beginning to be experienced by hard-core drug users (NIDA, 1992). The number of drug-related deaths in general and cocaine-related deaths in particular also did not diminish over this period. The wider availability of crack cocaine (which is smoked rather than inhaled), as well as increases in the number of cocaine users using it daily, contributed to these higher numbers of deaths during a period in which cocaine use in the general population appeared to be declining (GAO, 1991a; NIDA, 1990a, 1990c).

Suicide- or Homicide-Prone

The ultimate harm resulting from violent and intentional acts to injure oneself or others is reflected in suicide and homicide rates. These estimates are derived from what medical examiners report as the cause of death on the victims' death certificates.

Though suicide death rates did not change substantially from 1950 to 1980, the homicide rate doubled during this period and has fallen only slightly since. Firearms have become an increasingly important and deadly contributor to both suicide and homicide statistics. (See Table 2.9.)

Suicide. Suicide is the eighth leading cause of death in the United States. The Year 2000 Objectives for the nation are to reduce suicides to no more than 10.5 per 100,000 people. In 1989, the age-adjusted rate was 11.3. Suicide

Table 2.9. Indicators of Suicide- or Homicide-Prone.

Indicators	Year														
	1950	1960	1970	1980	1981	1982	1983	1984	1985	1986	1987	1988	1989
Age-Adjusted Death Rates per 100,000 Resident Population[1]													
Suicide	11.0*	10.6*	11.8	11.4	11.5	11.6	11.4	11.6	11.5	11.9	11.7	11.4	11.3
Homicide and Legal Intervention	5.4*	5.2*	9.1	10.8	10.4	9.7	8.6	8.4	8.3	9.0	8.6	9.0	9.4

*Includes deaths of nonresidents of the United States.
Source: NCHS reports; see Resource B for specific references.

rates have changed little since 1950. Suicide attempts are estimated to occur eight times more often than suicide deaths, with ratios of attempts to completed suicides being much higher for females (25 to 1) compared to males (3 to 1). Injuries resulting from gunshots cause the majority of suicidal deaths. Unsuccessful suicide attempts principally entail poisoning by pill ingestion or the infliction of minor lacerations (NCHS, 1991c; PHS, 1990; Rosenberg, Gelles, et al., 1987; Rosenberg, Smith, Davidson, & Conn, 1987).

Homicide and Legal Intervention. Homicide is the tenth leading cause of death in the United States. The Year 2000 Objectives are to reduce homicides to no more than 7.2 per 100,000. In terms of this objective, homicide is defined as death due to injuries purposely inflicted by another person — not including deaths caused by law enforcement officers or legal execution (which constitute around 0.2 per 100,000 deaths). The age-adjusted rate in 1989, including those due to legal intervention, was 9.4 (or 23,000 deaths). Since 1950, these rates have ranged from a low of 5.2 (1960) to a high of 10.8 (1980). Firearms are an increasingly important contributor to homicide-related deaths. Firearms are involved in approximately 60 percent and knives in 20 percent of homicides.

A Year 2000 Objective related to both suicide and homicide is to reduce weapon-related violent deaths to no more than 12.6 per 100,000. Age-adjusted rates in 1987 were 12.9 for firearms and 1.9 for knives (NCHS, 1991c; PHS, 1990).

Suicide and homicide rates differ a great deal for different age, sex, and race groups, which will be discussed in Chapter Three.

Abusing Families

Perhaps the most vulnerable individuals are those who are intentionally harmed by close family members or friends. Estimates of the number of children, elderly adults, and spouses who are abused by their family or other intimates are based on cases reported to relevant protective service agencies and on the informed opinions of people who head these agencies. They are also based on what family members say when asked about the occurrence of such incidents in their homes — which may or may not actually be reported to any official agency or authority.

Reports of family abuse and neglect have increased dramatically over the last twenty years. Around 1.6 to 1.7 million children and a corresponding number of elderly adults were estimated to be affected annually in the late 1980s. Rates of child abuse reported to protective service agencies tend to be lower than those reported in national surveys of violent behavior within families. The incidence of hidden violence, not reflected in any of these estimates, may be even higher. (See Table 2.10.)

Child Abuse and Neglect Reports. Since 1976, the National Study on Child Neglect and Abuse Reporting has collected annual data on official reports of child maltreatment from state level Child Protective Services (CPS) programs. With the exception of seven states among fifty-four jurisdictions reporting (the fifty states, the District of Columbia, Guam, Puerto Rico, and the Virgin Islands), the estimates include duplicate reports — that is, the same child and/or family may have more than one report filed in a given year. For those states that were able to provide both duplicated and unduplicated counts in 1987, 73 percent of the children were reported only once during the calendar year. Further, approximately 37 to 40 percent of the reported cases were substantiated — that is, a degree of certainty was established that the child was in fact at risk and that some level of intervention was warranted. (It cannot necessarily be assumed, however, that the absence of substantiation means that no maltreatment occurred.)

In 1987, an estimated 2,178,000 reports were filed for child abuse and neglect in 1,404,000 families. The rate of reporting was estimated at 34.0 per 1,000 U.S. children. This is substantially higher than the number (669,000) and rate (10.1) reported in 1976. Though the number of reports continued to climb between 1982 and 1987, the percentage annual increase in the rate per 1,000 children decreased from 17 percent from 1982 to 1983 to 4 percent from 1986 to 1987 (American Humane Association, 1989).

Based on 1986 data available from sixteen states, the major types of maltreatment were as follows: deprivation of necessities (54.9 percent), sexual maltreatment (15.7 percent), minor physical injury (13.9 percent), unspecified physical injury (11.1 percent), emotional maltreatment (8.3 percent), major physical injury (2.6 percent), and other maltreatment (7.9 percent). The percent of sexual abuse cases increased between 1983 and 1986, from approximately 9 to 16 percent.

The rates of reported child abuse tend to be lower than those obtained from national surveys of the incidence of violent behaviors within families (discussed later in this chapter).

Child Abuse and Neglect Incidence Rates. Another source of child abuse and neglect rates, the Study of the National Incidence and Prevalence of Child Abuse and Neglect, differs from the National Study on Child Neglect and Abuse Reporting in the following ways: it is based on a national probability sample of community professionals in twenty-nine U.S. counties regarding cases their agencies had handled, rather than a routine reporting system; it includes Child Protective Service as well as non-CPS agencies; estimates are based on unduplicated counts of individual children; and data were collected at only two points in time (1980 and 1986).

Based on the 1980 Study of the National Incidence and Prevalence of Child Abuse and Neglect, 625,000 (or 9.8 per 1,000) children were identified as having been abused or neglected. Using the same definition, based on whether a child had actually experienced demonstrable harm (the "harm standard"), in 1986, there was a 49 percent increase in the number of children to 931,000 (14.8 per 1,000). The largest increase between 1980 and

Table 2.10. Indicators of Abusing Families.

Indicators	1975	1976	1977	1978	1979	1980	1981	1982	1983	1984	1985	1986	1987	1988
Child Abuse and Neglect Reports[1]*														
Number of reports in 1,000s		669	838	836	988	1,154	1,225	1,262	1,477	1,727	1,928	2,086	2,178	
Rate per 1,000 U.S. children		10.1	12.8	12.9	15.4	18.1	19.4	20.1	23.6	27.3	30.6	32.8	34.0	
Child Abuse and Neglect Incidence Rates[2]†														
Number of children in 1,000s (revised definition, 1986)						625						931 (1,424)		
Rate per 1,000 U.S. children (revised definition, 1986)						9.8						14.8 (22.6)		
Domestic Elder Abuse[3]														
Number of reports in 1,000s‡												117	128	140
Number of "reportable" incidents in 1,000s (estimated)												1,600	1,800	2,000
Family Violence (Rates of Severe Violence)*§														
Parent-to-child (Number per 1,000 children)	36										19			
Husband-to-wife (Number per 1,000 wives)	38										30			
Wife-to-husband (Number per 1,000 husbands)	46										44			

*Estimates include substantiated and unsubstantiated reports of child maltreatment provided by state Child Protective Service personnel. Except for a small number of states (five to ten), the counts may be duplicated: a child may be reported more than once in the year.

†Numbers in parentheses for 1986 are estimates based on a broader definition, including children who are at risk of harm but who may not necessarily have actually been harmed.

‡The number of reports may be duplicated: an elderly individual may be reported more than once in the year, and some reports may involve more than one victim.

§Children ages three to seventeen are included in the rates for children. "Very severe" parent-to-child violence includes the following "conflict tactics": kicked, bit, or hit with fist; beat up; used gun or knife. "Severe" husband-to-wife and wife-to-husband violence include the following: kicked, bit, or hit with fist; hit or tried to hit with something; beat up; threatened with gun or knife; or used gun or knife.

Source: American Humane Association, 1989; Sedlak, 1991; Tatara, 1990; Gelles & Straus, 1988. See Resource B for more detailed references.

1986 by type of abuse was in the category of sexual abuse, for which rates almost tripled (from 0.7 to 1.9).

The 1986 study also included a broader definition, which reflected the incidence of children who were at risk of maltreatment but had not yet actually been harmed. Incorporating this "endangerment standard" as well, 1,424,400 (22.6 per 1,000) children had been or were at risk of abuse or neglect. The total number (2,086,000) of duplicated reports of child abuse and neglect in 1986, adjusted for the estimated percentage of unduplicated reports (80 percent), approximated the count of abused and neglected children (1,424,400) identified that year (American Humane Association, 1988; National Center on Child Abuse and Neglect, 1988; Sedlak, 1991).

The Year 2000 Objectives provide that the rates of maltreatment overall and for each specific type of maltreatment fall below the rates in the 1986 Study of the National Incidence and Prevalence of Child Abuse and Neglect. The incidence rates of abuse and neglect in that study, using the more inclusive definition, are 9.4 and 14.6 per 1,000 children, respectively. The incidence of specific types of abuse (more than one of which may have been reported for a given child) were as follows: physical abuse (4.9), sexual abuse (2.1), and emotional abuse (3.0) (National Center on Child Abuse and Neglect, 1988; PHS, 1990; Sedlak, 1991).

Domestic Elder Abuse. A Survey of States on the Incidence of Elder Abuse was conducted in 1988, based on a structured survey form sent to state Adult Protective Services (APS) and State Units on Aging (SUA) in fifty-four jurisdictions. The estimated unduplicated number of reports of elder abuse, neglect, or exploitation in domestic (home or noninstitutionalized) settings identified for the 1986–1988 fiscal years (FY) were as follows: 117,000 (FY 1986), 128,000 (FY 1987), and 140,000 (FY 1988). Somewhat over half of these reports were substantiated. The distribution of specific types of maltreatment that occurred in twenty-four states during FY 1988 was as follows: neglect (37.2 percent), physical abuse (26.3 percent), financial/material exploitation (20.0 percent), emotional abuse/neglect (11.0 percent), sexual abuse (1.6 percent), other types or unknown (3.9 percent).

Based on an estimate by the National Aging Resource Center on Elder Abuse that only one in fourteen incidents of elder abuse is actually reported, the number of "reportable" cases were estimated to be much greater than the actual number of reports—1.6 million (FY 1986), 1.8 million (FY 1987), and 2.0 million (FY 1988). This approximates the number of children (1.6 to 1.7 million) that were estimated to be abused or neglected in those same years (Tatara, 1990).

Family Violence. The National Surveys of Family Violence, conducted in 1976 and 1986, attempted to identify incidents of intrafamily violence that may not have been reported to CPS, APS, or other agencies. The 1976 study used a personal interview survey and the 1986 study a telephone interview about violent incidents that had occurred within the family during the previous year (1975 and 1985, respectively).

A range of methodological and societal changes make interpretations of comparisons between the 1976 and 1986 studies problematic, though both suggest that the incidents of family violence actually reported to authorities are far less than the number that actually occur. The rates of very severe parent-to-child violence (parent kicked, bit, or hit child with fist; beat up the child; or used a gun or knife), based on that study, were 36 per 1,000 children aged three to seventeen in 1975 and nineteen per 1,000 children in 1985. The corresponding rates of severe violence between spouses were as follows: husband-to-wife—38 per 1,000 wives (1975) and 30 per 1,000 (1985); wife-to-husband—46 per 1,000 husbands (1975) and 44 per 1,000 (1985). The rate of very severe family violence estimated for children in 1985 (19.0 per 1,000 children), based on this survey, is twice the rate of abuse (9.4 per 1,000 children) actually reported to agencies in 1986, according to the Study of the National Incidence and Prevalence of Child Abuse and Neglect (Gelles & Straus, 1988; National Center on Child Abuse and Neglect, 1988; Straus, Gelles, & Steinmetz, 1981).

Homeless

Varying estimates of the number of homeless exist, depending on how homelessness is defined (whether doubling up with relatives in hard times counts), when the data are gathered (during the day versus at night, or in the summer versus winter months), as well as where one looks for them (in shelters versus on the streets).

Based on data from a variety of sources, it appears that around one million men, women, and children do not have a place to call "home" on any given night, and up to twice as many are in this situation at some point during the year. (Estimates from different sources are reported in Table 2.11, and the methodological problems underlying these estimates are more fully discussed in Chapter Ten.)

The earliest projections of the number of homeless, published in 1982 and 1983 by a homeless advocacy group, the Community for Creative Non-Violence, estimated that there were two to three million homeless on any given night (Hombs & Snyder, 1982, 1983). The following year (1984), using several different extrapolation techniques, the U.S. Department of Housing and Urban Development estimated many fewer homeless. Estimates ranged from 192,000 to 586,000 nationwide, with the most likely number estimated to be between 250,000 to 350,000 (USDHUD, 1984).

Later studies tended to confirm estimates in the hundreds of thousands rather than the millions. In 1986, Freeman and Hall (1986), applying a street-to-shelter ratio, estimated there were some 287,000 homeless. Based on estimates from fifty U.S. cities, and varying the rates for large, medium, and small cities, in 1987 Tucker (1987) projected 700,000 indi-

Table 2.11. Indicators of Homeless.

| | Year | | |
Indicators	1984	1987	1988
Homeless (Estimated Numbers)			
U.S. Department of Housing and Urban Development	250,000–300,000		
Urban Institute		496,000–600,000* (1+ million)‡	
National Alliance to End Homelessness			736,000† (1.3–2.0 million)‡

*Numbers refer to the count of homeless at a given time (March 1987).

†Numbers refer to a reestimated count of the homeless at a given time, using USDHUD (1984) data, adjusted for an estimated 20 percent average annual rate of growth in the homeless.

‡Numbers in parentheses refer to the estimated number of people homeless at some time during the year.

Source: U.S. Department of Housing and Urban Development, 1984; Burt & Cohen, 1989; National Alliance to End Homelessness, 1988.

viduals to be homeless. In the same year, using a nationally representative random sample of homeless adults who used soup kitchens and shelters in cities of 100,000 or more, the Urban Institute projected the number of homeless in March 1987 to be 496,000 to 600,000 (Burt & Cohen, 1989).

In 1988, the National Alliance to End Homelessness recomputed the 1984 HUD figures, applying different rates of homelessness to the city and suburbs — resulting in a revised estimate of 355,000 (rather than 250,000 to 300,000) homeless individuals in 1984. Based on reports from local officials regarding increases in the demand for shelter services, the Alliance estimated an annual growth rate of 20 percent in the number of homeless — yielding an estimated upper bound on the number of any given night to be 736,000 in 1988 (National Alliance to End Homelessness, 1988).

The number who experienced homelessness some time during the year is estimated to be around twice the number homeless on any given night. Based on the Urban Institute data, there were then a maximum of 1.2 million people homeless some time during 1987 (Burt & Cohen, 1989). According to the National Alliance to End Homeless projections, around 1.3 to 2 million people experienced homelessness during 1988 (National Alliance to End Homelessness, 1988). A 1989 report from the Partnership for the Homeless pointed out that "most attempts at estimating the homeless by cities and localities have concluded that homeless comprise from 0.7 to 1.1 percent of their respective populations" — confirming that "there may be as many as two million homeless across the nation" (Partnership for the Homeless, 1989, p. 3).

The numbers reported for different years do not necessarily accurately reflect trends in the growth of the number of homeless because of differ-

ences in the definitions, data gathering methods, and bases for projections
used — though several studies have documented steady increases (of around
20 percent per year on average) in the demands for emergency and associated
homeless shelters and services in U.S. cities since 1985 (National Alliance
to End Homelessness, 1988; Partnership for the Homeless, 1987, 1989; U.S.
Conference of Mayors, 1991).

Immigrants and Refugees

National data on the number and characteristics of people currently living
in the United States who voluntarily left their home countries, as well as
those who were pushed out by political, military, or economic hardship, are
available from the U.S. Immigration and Naturalization Service (INS, 1990;
U.S. Bureau of the Census, 1991c). Studies of the specific health and health
care needs of these immigrant and refugee populations are generally local
in nature or limited to subgroups of emigres.

Over five million people have legally immigrated to the United States
in the past decade, and many in addition have entered the United States
illegally. An increasing portion of both groups are fleeing political or military conflicts in their countries of origin, and many have experienced the
death of or separation from family members, as well as serious physical or
psychological problems, as a result. (See Table 2.12.)

Table 2.12. Indicators of Immigrants and Refugees.

Indicators	Year		
	1961–1970	*1971–1980*	*1981–1989*
Total Number[1]			
Immigrants	3,321,700	4,493,300	5,801,600
Refugees	212,843	539,447	916,256

Source: U.S. Bureau of the Census, 1991c; see Resource B for further detail.

Immigrants. Immigrants are aliens admitted for legal permanent residence
in the United States. The procedures for admission depend on whether the
alien is residing inside or outside the United States at the time of application for permanent residence. Eligible aliens residing outside the United States
are issued immigrant visas by the U.S. Department of State. Eligible aliens
residing in the United States are allowed to change their status from temporary to permanent residents, by applying to the Immigration and Naturalization Service. Nonresident aliens admitted to the United States for a temporary period are considered nonimmigrants, rather than immigrants.

The number of immigrants to the United States has increased steadily over the last three decades: 1961–1970 (3,321,700); 1971–1980
(4,493,300); 1981–1989 (5,801,600).

Immigrants have an official legal (documented) status—that of aliens who are admitted for the purpose of obtaining permanent residence. There are, in addition, an imprecise number of illegal (undocumented) aliens. Some estimates have put the number of undocumented aliens at two to four times the number of legal immigrants (Bean, Edmonston, & Passel, 1990; Rumbaut, Chavez, Moser, Pickwell, & Wishik, 1988).

Refugees. Refugees are considered nonimmigrants when initially admitted into the United States. A series of acts have specified the provisions (the length of time in residence, for example) required to permit certain groups of refugees to seek permanent residence (immigrant) status—such as the Cuban Refugee Act (1966), Indochinese Refugee Act (1977), and Refugee-Parolee Act (1978). The Refugee Act of 1980, effective April 1, 1980, provided for a uniform admission procedure for all countries, based on the United Nations' definition of *refugees* and *asylees* as having "a well-founded fear of persecution." Under this act, refugees are eligible for immigrant status after one year of residence in the United States. Authorized admission ceilings are set annually by the president in consultation with the Congress.

Asylees differ from refugees, in that refugees petition for entrance from outside U.S. borders, while asylees enter the U.S. first, often without documentation, and then petition to remain. They may stay in the United States indefinitely in a temporary status and are entitled to work, but they are not entitled to certain social services benefits as are refugees. Up to 5,000 asylees may adjust to immigrant status each year (Bean, Vernez, & Keely, 1989; U.S. Bureau of the Census, 1991c).

The number of refugees, as well as the proportion they represent of the total immigrant population, has increased steadily over the last three decades: 1961–1970 (212,843); 1971–1980 (539,447); 1981–1989 (916,256). The proportions they represented of the total immigrant population for the respective time periods were 6 percent, 12 percent, and 16 percent.

Additional information on the origins and health needs of these and other vulnerable populations will be provided in Chapters Three and Four.

3

Who Is *Most* Vulnerable?

In general, the level of vulnerability that people experience varies according to the stages of their lives. At times, serious health problems force people to turn to others for help. Infants and very young children are all potentially vulnerable because of being totally dependent on parents or other caretakers to meet their most fundamental physical and psychological needs. As people grow older, they may have to ask family members or friends to help them with tasks such as shopping or keeping track of finances, as well as even more basic self-care needs, such as eating, dressing, or getting out of bed. Minorities, the poor, and those with less education tend to experience more health problems in general over the course of their lives, based on an array of indicators of need, than do their more socioeconomically advantaged counterparts.

This chapter presents current national data on the varying health needs of people of differing age, sex, race, income, and education groups, as well as discusses changes that have taken place over time for these groups, based on the indicators highlighted in the previous chapter. A variety of factors influence whether some groups are more vulnerable than others. (See Figure 1.2.) This chapter sheds light on who is most vulnerable, and the next chapter explores why — for these and a variety of other subcategories of vulnerable populations.

Cross-Cutting Issues

Comparisons between groups focus on those characteristics for which data are available at the national level: age, sex, race and ethnicity, income, and/or education. These comparisons strongly confirm the predictions presented earlier (Table 1.1) regarding which groups were most and least vulnerable. Further, the longitudinal (trend) data demonstrate that the problems of many of the most vulnerable worsened rather than diminished during the past decade.

50

Age

The 1980s were particularly harsh for vulnerable newborns, especially those who had the compound disadvantage of being born in socioeconomically adverse circumstances. Very young, minority, poor, and less educated mothers were much less likely to have adequate prenatal care. They were also more likely to bear low-birthweight babies who had high risks of congenital physical or mental impairments as well as perinatal drug addiction or AIDS — as a consequence of the mother's or her sex partner's use of intravenous drugs.

Older children, adolescents, and young adults fared no better during this same period. The number of children with developmental, emotional, and behavioral problems has been and is likely to continue to increase as the number of high-risk, impaired newborns who survive also grows. Compared to white youth, young minority women are much more likely to give birth to babies who die, and young minority males are many times more likely themselves to die a violent death. Young males, particularly Native American youth, are most likely to drink, smoke, and use drugs, and also to die as a result of these addictions. The number of children who are reported to be abused or neglected by their families has multiplied dramatically over the past decade, and the face of the homeless is an increasingly youthful one, as the number of families with children and the number of runaway youth living on the streets increase.

The elderly, particularly the oldest old, are more often plagued with chronic illness and associated impairments, which limit their ability to function independently. A higher proportion of the elderly also suffer from serious cognitive impairments, and many elderly nursing home residents have Alzheimer's or related organic brain disorders. White elderly men are significantly more likely to take their own lives, and dependent elderly women are more likely to be abused by their caretakers than are elderly men.

Sex

In general, men are more likely to die from chronic disease than are women. Among those living with chronic illness, however, elderly women are much more likely to experience serious problems in being able to continue to care for themselves. The prevalence of mental illness is in general higher for women than men. However, men's mental health problems are more often manifested in substance abuse and antisocial behavior, whereas women are more apt to be depressed, anxious, or experience physical (somatic) symptoms.

Women's health and health care needs are also compounded with their childbearing and childrearing roles. Mothers who have inadequate prenatal care or experience drug addiction, AIDS, spousal abuse, homelessness, or the fears associated with being in the country illegally are also very likely to be in a position of bearing or caring for children who are also extremely needy and vulnerable.

Race and Ethnicity

Data on the health and health care needs of Hispanics, Native Americans, and Asians are somewhat more limited than for whites and African Americans (reported as blacks in most statistical reports). However, based on the major indicators of need for which data are available, African-American, Hispanic, and Native American men, women, and children are much more likely to be in poor health than are majority whites.

African-American women are more apt to have high-risk pregnancies and to die in childbirth or from chronic disease or AIDS than their white female counterparts. African-American men are also more likely to be chronically ill and to be at risk of AIDS, death from intentional acts of violence, and homelessness than are white males.

Hispanic women are less likely to have adequate prenatal care, but more likely to bear normal-birthweight babies and experience fewer infant deaths, in contrast to African-American women. On the other hand, as with African Americans, Hispanic men, women, and children are much more likely to contract AIDS through intravenous drug use, and young Hispanic males are much more apt to die from firearm-related homicides than are whites.

A higher proportion of Native American women have inadequate prenatal care and experience infant (particularly postneonatal) deaths than do white women. Native American youths are also much more apt to be substance users and abusers, and to die violently from both suicides and homicides.

By a number of criteria for which data are available (infant mortality rates, AIDS prevalence, and substance use and abuse), Asian Americans are at much lower risk than are other minorities. These risks do, however, differ for different socioeconomic groups. Socioeconomically disadvantaged Asian-American populations, particularly some categories of Southeast Asian refugees, are likely to be very socially isolated and in poor physical and mental health.

Income/Education

More years of formal schooling and higher incomes are directly associated with better health. Women with a high school education are much more likely to have adequate prenatal care and to bear normal-birthweight babies who survive past infancy than those who have not finished high school. People of lower socioeconomic status (less education, lower incomes, or employed in low-status jobs) are more likely to have serious chronic physical or mental health problems. Economic factors play a major role in family abuse and neglect, and the vast majority of the homeless are extremely poor. The problems of vulnerability in general appear to be exacerbated for the urban underclass—poor and poorly educated minorities who live in economically depressed urban areas.

Population-Specific Overview

Variation in the prevalence of poor physical, psychological, and social health will be examined for different population subgroups.

High-Risk Mothers and Infants

Very young, minority, and poorly educated mothers are much less likely to have adequate prenatal care and more likely to bear low-birthweight or very-low-birthweight infants. The rates of teenage pregnancy, preterm and low-birthweight babies, inadequate prenatal care, and infant and maternal mortality are two to three times higher among African-American women compared to white women. This racial disparity shows no signs of diminishing and may, in fact, be widening (Table 3.1).

Low Birthweight. Teenage mothers, especially those less than fifteen years of age, are most likely to give birth to low-birthweight or very-low-birthweight infants. The percentages of LBW and VLBW infants born to these mothers in 1989—13.4 percent and 3.1 percent—was around twice the national average of 7.05 percent and 1.28 percent, respectively.

Black mothers are more than twice as likely to give birth to low birthweight infants than are white mothers. The relative risk for black mothers increased rather than declined from 1980 to 1989. The percentage of LBW infants to whites in 1980 was 5.7 percent compared to 12.7 percent for black women. The corresponding rates in 1989 were 5.7 percent and 13.5 percent. The relative risk of black mothers having VLBW infants was even greater in 1989 compared to 1980. The proportion of VLBW infants born to white mothers increased 5 percent, from 0.90 in 1980 to 0.95 in 1989. For blacks, the proportion increased around 16 percent, from 2.5 to 2.9. The percent of other racial/ethnic groups with low-birthweight/very-low-birthweight infants was more similar to that of whites: Hispanics (6.2/1.05); Native Americans (6.3/1.0).

Mothers with a high school or college education are less likely to have low- or very-low-birthweight infants, compared to those who have less than a high school education (NCHS, 1988d, 1990d, 1990h).

Infant Mortality. The total infant, neonatal, and postneonatal mortality rates for blacks have been around twice that of whites, and this disparity appears to be widening rather than diminishing. In 1980, the total black infant mortality rate per one thousand live births (22.2) was 2.0 times that of the white

Table 3.1. Indicators of High-Risk Mothers and Infants by Demographic Subgroups.

Indicators	Mother's Age							Mother's Race			
	<15	15–19	20–24	25–29	30–34	35–39	40+	White	Black	Hispanic	Native American
Low Birthweight[1]											
Percent of live births less than 2,500 grams											
1980	14.6	9.4	6.9	5.8	5.9	7.0	8.3	5.7	12.7	6.1	6.4
1989	13.4	9.3	7.2	6.2	6.5	7.2	8.5	5.7	13.5	6.2	6.3
Percent of live births less than 1,500 grams											
1980	3.4	1.7	1.1	1.0	1.0	1.1	1.4	.90	2.5	0.98	0.92
1989	3.1	1.8	1.3	1.1	1.2	1.4	1.5	.95	2.9	1.05	1.00
Infant Mortality[2]											
Deaths per 1,000 live births											
Total											
1980								10.9	22.2		13.8*
1989								8.1	18.6	8.5	9.7†
Neonatal											
1980								7.4	14.6		6.6*
1989								5.1	11.9	5.4	4.6†
Postneonatal											
1980								3.5	7.6		7.2*
1989								2.9	6.7	3.1	5.1†

Prenatal Care[3]
Percent of mothers who received prenatal
care in third trimester or no prenatal care

1980	20.1	10.3	5.5	3.1	3.0	4.9	8.6	4.3	8.9	12.0	15.2
1989	21.0	12.5	8.4	4.7	3.6	4.1	6.1	5.2	11.9	13.0	13.4

Teen Births[4]
Live births per 1,000 females[‡]

10–14 years											
1980								0.6	4.3		
1989								0.7	5.0		
15–17 years											
1980								25.2	73.6		
1989								27.5	82.4		
18–19 years											
1980								72.1	138.8		
1989								72.6	160.8		

Maternal Mortality[5]
Deaths per 100,000 live births all ages, crude

1980								6.7	21.5		9.0*
1989								5.6	18.4		7.1†

*Rates for 1980 are actually three-year rates (1979–1981) centered in 1980.
†Rates for 1989 are actually three-year rates (1986–1988) centered in 1987.
‡These estimates refer to the race of the child.
Source: NCHS and IHS reports; see Resource B for specific references.

rate (10.9). In 1989, the black rate (18.6) was 2.3 times the rate for whites (8.1). The black neonatal mortality rate in 1980 (14.6) was 2.0 times the white rate (7.4). In 1989, the black rate (11.9) was 2.3 times that of whites (5.1). Postneonatal rates for blacks were also correspondingly higher compared to whites in both 1980 (7.6 versus 3.5) and 1989 (6.7 versus 2.9). The infant mortality rate for Native Americans (9.7) was also higher than that for whites, while the rates for Hispanics (8.5) were similar. The postneonatal mortality rate for Native Americans (5.1), in particular, was considerably higher than that of whites (2.9).

Though mother's education is not available on the death certificates, analyses of linked birth and death records for selected states in 1983 and 1984 showed that infant mortality rates (total, neonatal, and postneonatal) were higher for mothers with less than twelve years of schooling and lower for those with sixteen years or more (Kleinman, Fingerhut, & Prager, 1990).

Prenatal Care. In 1989, very young teenage mothers were three times more likely not to seek prenatal care or to wait until the last trimester to do so (21.0 percent), compared to the national average (6.4 percent). The proportion of very young teens with late or no prenatal care has remained relatively unchanged since 1980 (20.1 percent).

The percentage of black (11.9 percent), Hispanic (13.0 percent), and Native American (13.4 percent) women not having adequate prenatal care was more than twice that of whites (5.2 percent). The percentage of both white and black women who had inadequate care was higher in 1989 compared to 1980, though the rate of increase was higher for black women (34 percent increase, from 8.9 to 11.9 percent) than white (21 percent increase, from 4.3 to 5.2 percent) women.

In 1988, the percentage of women with inadequate prenatal care was highest for those with no high school education (15.2 percent) and lowest for those with sixteen years or more of schooling (1.2 percent) (NCHS, 1990h).

Teen Births. The proportion of births to white teens remained relatively stable from 1980 to 1989. However, the birth rates per 1,000 women for all age categories of black teenagers increased over this same period, particularly for those eighteen to nineteen, for whom there was a 16 percent increase (from 138.8 in 1980 to 160.8 in 1989). In both 1980 and 1989, the birth rates for blacks were two to three times those of whites among teens age fifteen or older, but the racial disparities for very young teens (ten to fourteen years of age) were even greater.

Maternal Mortality. The ratio of maternal deaths for "other race" women has always been greater than for white women, though vital statistics data have only recently distinguished black and other racial subgroups. In 1989, black mothers were more than three times as likely to die in childbirth as were white mothers. The number of maternal deaths per 100,000 live births was 18.4 for blacks compared to 5.6 for whites. Maternal death rates for Native Americans (7.1) were also higher compared to whites (NCHS, 1990a).

Chronically Ill and Disabled

The prevalence and the magnitude of limitation in daily activities, as well as deaths, due to chronic disease increase steadily with age. Generally, men are more likely than women to die from major chronic illnesses such as heart disease, stroke, and cancer, though among those living with such illnesses, elderly women have more problems in being able to carry out their normal daily routines. African Americans—particularly African-American men—are more likely to experience serious disabilities as well as to die from chronic illness than are either white men or women (Table 3.2).

Death Rates for Chronic Diseases. In 1989, heart disease was the major cause of death due to chronic illness among both infants and the elderly. Cancer was the principal cause of death for people of other ages. The age-adjusted death rates per 100,000 persons for heart disease, stroke, and cancer were, however, highest among black men and lowest for white women.

The age-adjusted death rate for cirrhosis among black men (20.5) was much higher than for white men (11.9), black women (8.5), or white women (5.0). The death rates among Native Americans for cirrhosis (30.4) and diabetes (25.8) were more than twice the rates for whites. White men had the highest death rate due to chronic obstructive pulmonary disease (26.8), and black women the highest death rate from diabetes (24.2).

Prevalence of Chronic Conditions. In 1989, the most prevalent chronic condition among people under forty-five years of age was asthma (48.8 per 1,000). The rates were highest for those under eighteen (61.0), blacks (57.4), and males (51.2). The prevalence of hypertension was also much higher among blacks in this age group (55.5) compared to whites (32.8).

For adults forty-five to sixty-four, the most common chronic conditions were arthritis (253.8) and hypertension (229.1). Arthritis was most prevalent among blacks (320.7) and women (300.9). The rates of hypertension in this age group were also much higher for blacks (383.5) compared to whites (213.0).

Among the elderly, the most common conditions were arthritis (483.0), hypertension (380.6), hearing impairments (286.5), and heart disease (278.9). The rates of hypertension and arthritis were generally higher among elderly women and blacks. Heart disease and hearing impairments were more common among elderly men and whites.

Limitation in Major Activity Due to Chronic Conditions. The proportion of people who must limit their major activities in some way due to a chronic

Table 3.2. Indicators of Chronically Ill and Disabled by Demographic Subgroups.

Indicators	Age											Race by Sex				
												White		Black		Native
	<1	1–4	5–14	15–24	25–34	35–44	45–54	55–64	65–74	75–84	85+	Male	Female	Male	Female	American
Age-Adjusted Death Rates for Selected Chronic Diseases per 100,000 Persons[1]																
Heart disease																
1980	22.8	2.6	0.9	2.9	8.3	44.6	180.2	494.1	1218.6	2993.1	7777.1	277.5	134.6	327.3	201.1	138.1
1989	19.7	1.9	0.8	2.6	7.9	32.3	124.2	376.7	911.8	2400.6	6701.6	205.9	106.6	272.6	172.9	
Stroke																
1980	4.4	0.5	0.3	1.0	2.6	8.5	25.2	65.2	219.5	788.6	2288.9	41.9	35.2	77.5	61.7	26.4
1989	3.2	0.3	0.2	0.6	2.1	6.4	18.4	48.8	144.7	519.8	1631.0	28.0	24.1	54.1	44.9	
Cancer																
1980	3.2	4.5	4.3	6.3	13.7	48.6	180.0	436.1	817.9	1232.3	1594.6	160.5	107.7	229.9	129.7	91.3
1989	2.7	3.4	3.3	5.1	12.1	43.1	157.2	445.1	852.6	1338.1	1662.3	157.2	110.7	230.6	130.9	
Chronic obstructive pulmonary disease																
1980	1.6	0.4	0.2	0.3	0.5	1.6	9.8	42.7	129.1	224.4	274.0	26.7	9.2	20.9	6.3	13.8
1989	1.2	0.4	0.3	0.5	0.7	1.7	9.2	49.8	148.9	313.8	403.5	26.8	15.2	24.9	10.9	
Cirrhosis																
1980	0.9	0.1	0.0	0.3	3.5	13.5	30.9	41.6	43.1	30.6	19.9	15.7	7.0	30.6	14.4	30.4
1989	0.0	0.0	0.0	0.2	2.2	9.9	19.0	31.3	35.7	34.2	23.1	11.9	5.0	20.5	8.5	
Diabetes																
1980	0.1	0.1	0.1	0.3	1.5	3.5	9.6	26.7	64.9	131.1	221.9	9.5	8.7	17.7	22.1	25.8
1989	0.0	0.0	0.1	0.4	1.6	3.9	11.2	32.1	72.4	145.1	245.6	11.0	9.6	22.6	24.2	

Number of Selected Chronic Conditions per 1,000 Persons (Self-reported)[2]

Indicators	Age by Sex, Race																
	Under 45							45-64					65+				
	<18	18-44	Male	Female	White	Black	Total	Male	Female	White	Black	Total	Male	Female	White	Black	Total
Heart disease																	
1982	17.2	34.7	23.0	32.3	28.8	22.2	27.7	165.7	110.7	140.8	123.9	136.8	268.8	248.6	268.9	162.2	256.8
1989	17.1	36.1	24.0	33.8	29.8	30.2	28.9	139.8	99.7	119.8	128.2	118.9	298.3	265.2	286.5	220.5	278.9
Hypertension																	
1982	2.9*	58.9	37.2	36.1	34.2	53.1	36.6	227.5	262.1	234.7	366.8	245.7	330.0	432.2	379.2	510.2	390.4
1989	2.2	56.0	35.0	36.0	32.8	55.5	35.5	220.3	237.2	213.0	383.5	229.1	309.6	431.1	367.4	517.7	380.6
Stroke																	
1982	0.2*	0.5*	0.3*	0.5*	0.3*	1.1*	0.4*	16.9	13.9	15.1	18.1*	15.3	56.0	58.2	55.7	65.7*	57.3
1989	0.8*	1.9	1.1*	1.9	1.7	0.8*	1.5	14.6	15.9	13.6	27.8*	15.3	61.4	53.9	56.3	70.9	57.0
Visual impairment																	
1982	13.1	31.2	32.4	15.6	24.7	20.7	24.0	71.2	37.3	52.6	68.4	53.4	120.5	87.6	98.3	122.0	101.1
1989	9.0	27.2	27.1	13.5	21.8	14.8	20.3	63.2	28.5	45.5	54.5	45.1	92.2	74.5	81.1	77.0	81.9
Hearing impairment																	
1982	19.7	48.8	46.2	28.4	40.2	21.6	37.2	195.7	94.9	149.3	81.7	142.7	352.4	263.3	304.6	277.5	299.7
1989	15.6	47.8	44.8	26.4	38.0	23.8	35.6	168.7	90.2	136.7	64.5	127.7	341.1	247.7	297.7	174.5	286.5
Arthritis																	
1982	2.7*	55.3	26.8	41.9	34.4	37.0	34.4	204.8	340.6	277.0	296.1	276.2	407.1	557.1	493.4	522.9	495.8
1989	1.4*	48.9	24.7	36.9	32.1	26.2	30.8	202.5	300.9	247.7	320.7	253.8	392.4	547.4	483.2	522.6	483.0
Emphysema																	
1982	*	1.9*	1.9*	0.4*	1.3*	*	1.1*	39.6	12.6	27.2	12.4*	25.4	69.0	20.4	42.8	18.9*	40.3
1989	0.2*	1.2*	0.7*	0.9*	0.9*	0.2*	0.8*	22.6	12.4	18.6	11.0*	17.2	56.7	21.8	38.8	16.7*	36.3
Asthma																	
1982	40.1	29.0	36.8	30.1	33.3	38.6	33.4	34.2	38.1	36.5	37.2*	36.3	38.5	42.3	39.0	48.7*	40.8
1989	61.0	41.3	51.2	46.3	47.6	57.4	48.8	34.9	47.6	43.6	23.8*	41.5	43.6	57.0	49.9	69.3	51.5
Diabetes																	
1982	1.4*	9.2	5.5	6.7	6.4	5.2*	6.1	55.9	59.0	49.5	122.9	57.6	77.8	96.6	82.1	164.5	88.9
1989	1.8*	10.7	5.5	9.0	7.0	8.3	7.3	64.9	52.1	52.6	100.2	58.2	73.9	98.3	80.2	165.9	88.2

Table 3.2. Indicators of Chronically Ill and Disabled by Demographic Subgroups, Cont'd.

Indicators	Age						Sex		Race			Income†				
	<5	5–14	15–44	45–64	65–74	75+	M	F	White	Black	Hispanic	<$14,000	$14–24,999	$25–34,999	$35–49,999	$50,000+
Age-Adjusted Degree of Activity Limitation Due to Chronic Conditions (percent)3§																
Limited but not in major activity																
1983	0.5	1.8	2.7	5.9	13.5	16.8	3.8	4.5	4.2	3.8		5.4	4.5	4.3	3.7	3.7
1989	0.6	1.6	2.7	5.6	13.5	18.5	3.9	4.4	4.2	4.0		5.5	4.5	3.8	3.5	3.4
Limited in amount or kind of major activity																
1983	1.1	4.1	3.9	10.2	13.3	17.7	5.6	6.4	5.9	7.5		9.6	6.8	6.6	5.1	4.1
1989	1.1	4.2	3.7	7.7	11.0	15.3	5.0	5.4	5.3	5.7		8.4	5.9	4.9	4.1	3.3
Unable to carry on major activity																
1983	0.5	0.3	1.9	8.2	10.7	9.9	4.6	2.7	3.3	6.2	8.3‡	8.0	5.2	3.5	2.1	1.6
1989	0.6	0.5	2.4	8.8	10.4	9.6	4.6	3.3	3.6	6.7		9.3	4.5	2.9	2.3	1.7
Total with activity limitation																
1983	2.1	6.2	8.5	24.3	37.6	44.4	13.9	13.6	13.4	17.5	11.1‡	23.0	16.6	14.4	11.0	9.4
1989	2.3	6.4	8.9	22.2	35.0	43.4	13.5	13.1	13.1	16.3		23.2	14.8	11.7	9.9	8.4

Table header: **Age by Sex** and **Race**

	65–69 Male	65–69 Female	65–69 Total	70–74 Male	70–74 Female	70–74 Total	75–79 Male	75–79 Female	75–79 Total	80–84 Male	80–84 Female	80–84 Total	85+ Male	85+ Female	85+ Total	Total	White	Black	Hispanic
Limitation in Activities of Daily Living (ADLs) or Instrumental Activities of Daily Living (IADLs), 65+, Living in the Community, 1987‖																			
Percent with at least one ADL (personal care activities)	5.0	6.5	5.9	6.3	9.2	7.9	8.7	13.3	11.5	17.4	19.3	18.6	26.3	38.4	34.5		11.1	15.5	7.8
Number of ADLs																			
1	1.7	2.9	2.4	2.3	4.3	3.4	4.2	7.6	6.2	7.4	8.3	8.0	13.0	16.9	15.6		5.1	6.0	3.7*
2–3	1.8	2.4	2.1	2.3	3.5	3.0	2.7*	3.7	3.3	6.6	7.9	7.5	9.2	9.9	9.7		3.6	6.4	4.1*
4+	1.4	1.3	1.3	1.7	1.5	1.5	1.8	2.0	2.0	3.4*	3.1	3.2	4.1*	11.7	9.2		2.4	3.2	0.0*
Percent with at least one IADL (home management activities)	6.9	9.5	8.4	7.8	14.7	11.6	12.1	20.8	17.3	25.8	34.4	31.4	50.1	56.4	54.4		17.2	23.5	12.5
Number of IADLs																			
1	2.3	3.0	2.7	1.7	5.0	3.5	4.5	6.6	5.7	9.4	10.3	10.0	11.9	9.7	10.4		5.0	4.8	3.9*
2–3	1.8*	2.8	2.4	1.7	5.8	3.9	3.1	7.6	5.8	5.3*	13.7	10.8	17.9	17.0	17.3		5.6	7.2	5.1
4+	2.8	3.7	3.4	4.5	3.9	4.2	4.6	5.9	5.9	11.1	10.4	10.6	20.3	29.8	26.7		6.5	11.5	3.5*
Percent with at least one ADL or IADL	8.0	11.3	9.9	9.2	16.5	13.2	15.5	22.9	19.9	29.5	36.6	34.1	51.5	59.3	56.8		19.1	26.3	14.1

Table 3.2. Indicators of Chronically Ill and Disabled by Demographic Subgroups, Cont'd.

Indicators	Age					Sex		Race	
		65+							
	<65	65-74	75-84	85+	Total	Male	Female	White	Black
Limitation in Activities of Daily Living (ADLs) or Instrumental Activities of Daily Living (IADLs), Living in Nursing Homes, 1985#									
Percent with at least one ADL	73.5	86.8	91.4	95.2	92.4	84.0	92.7	90.1	92.4
Number of ADLs									
1	11.7	14.0	11.6	9.6	11.1	12.3	10.7	11.5	7.3
2-3	19.7	18.5	18.3	16.8	17.7	18.8	17.6	17.8	19.9
4+	42.1	54.3	61.4	68.8	63.7	53.0	64.3	60.9	65.2
Percent with at least one IADL	75.1	81.4	84.4	89.0	86.0	79.6	86.8	84.6	87.6

*Estimates for which the numerator has a relative standard error of 30 percent.

†Family income categories for 1983 are less than $10,000; $10,000–$14,999; $15,000–$19,999; $20,000–$34,999; $35,000+.

‡Estimates for race (Hispanic) are for 1979–1980 and are not age-adjusted.

§These comparisons begin with 1983 because of changes initiated in the 1982 NCHS questionnaire.

‖ADLs = bathing, transferring to a bed or chair, dressing, toileting, feeding, walking. IADLs = use of telephone, handling money, shopping, getting about the community, preparing meals, doing light housework. Estimates for which the estimate has a relative standard error of 30 percent are indicated with an asterisk.

#ADLs = bathing, transferring to a bed or chair, dressing, toileting, continence, eating. IADLs = use of telephone, handling money, securing personal items, care of personal possessions.

Source: NCHS and IHS reports; Leon & Lair, 1990. See Resource B for specific references.

health problem increases with age. In 1989, the percentage of different age groups who were limited to some extent were as follows: less than five years of age (2.3), five to fourteen (6.4), fifteen to forty-four (8.9), forty-five to sixty-four (22.2), sixty-five to seventy-four (35.0), over seventy-five (43.4). Men were somewhat more likely to be limited in their major activity (9.6 percent) than were women (8.7 percent).

Rates of activity limitation were higher for blacks (16.3 percent) than whites (13.1 percent). Blacks (6.7 percent) were almost twice as likely as whites (3.6 percent) to be unable to carry on their major activities. People in families with incomes under $14,000 were most likely (23.2 percent) and those in families with incomes of $50,000 or greater least likely (8.4 percent) to have to limit what they did because of a chronic illness.

Limitation in Activities of Daily Living (ADLs) and Instrumental Activities of Daily Living (IADLs). In 1987, among elderly people living in the community, the prevalence of ADL or IADL limitations was much greater among the oldest old, eighty-five years of age or older (56.8 percent), than among the youngest old, sixty-five to sixty-nine years of age (9.9 percent). Elderly women were also more likely to report having either ADL or IADL limitations than were men.

The proportion of black elderly with at least one ADL or IADL limitation (26.3 percent) was also higher than for either white (19.1 percent) or Hispanic elderly (14.1 percent).

Similar patterns were observed, based on 1985 data, for the elderly living in nursing homes. The oldest old, women and blacks were most likely to experience ADL or IADL limitations, though the disparities were less dramatic than among the community-dwelling elderly.

Persons with AIDS

Early in the AIDS epidemic, homosexual or bisexual males were most likely to be affected. But more and more mothers and children are now at risk due to women or their sex partners using intravenous drugs. Higher proportions of African Americans and Hispanics, compared to whites, are likely to be HIV positive, to develop and die of AIDS, and to have contracted the disease through drug use or sexual contact with drug users (Table 3.3).

AIDS Cases. The percent distribution of blacks and Hispanics with AIDS (29 percent and 16 percent of all cases, respectively) is around twice the percent they represent in the U.S. population as a whole (12 percent and 9 percent, respectively).

The disproportionate concentration of AIDS in minority populations is particularly significant for children: around eight out of ten are nonwhite. A higher proportion of pediatric AIDS cases are boys (54.0 percent). The vast majority of black (92.4 percent), Hispanic (86.9 percent), and Native

Table 3.3. Indicators of Persons with AIDS by Demographic Subgroups.

| | Age <13 years | | | | | | | Age 13+ years | | | | | | |
| | Sex | | Race | | | | | Sex | | Race | | | | |
Indicators	Male	Female	White	Black	Hispanic	Native American	Other	Male	Female	White	Black	Hispanic	Native American	Other
Aids Cases, 1991*														
Total number	1,873	1,598	739	1,844	854	8	17	181,696	21,225	109,646	58,193	33,024	314	1,258
(Percentage)	(54.0)	(46.0)	(21.3)	(53.1)	(24.6)	(0.2)	(0.5)	(90.0)	(10.0)	(54.0)	(28.7)	(16.3)	(0.2)	(0.6)
Number by transmission category (Percent distribution)														
Male homosexual/bisexual								118,362		83,205	20,540	13,240	172	936
								(65.1)		(75.9)	(35.3)	(40.1)	(54.8)	(74.4)
IV drug use								35,048	10,705	9,285	22,983	13,274	58	56
								(19.3)	(50.4)	(8.5)	(39.5)	(40.2)	(18.5)	(4.4)
Male homosexual/bisexual and IV drug use								13,135		7,547	3,578	1,925	41	28
								(7.2)		(6.9)	(6.1)	(5.8)	(13.1)	(2.2)
Hemophilia/coagulation disorder			112	22	26		3	1,671	42	1,402	137	140	8	18
			(15.1)	(1.2)	(3.0)		(17.6)	(1.0)	(0.2)	(1.3)	(0.2)	(0.4)	(2.5)	(1.4)
Mother with/at risk for HIV infection			465	1,704	742	8	8							
			(63.0)	(92.4)	(86.9)	(100.0)	(47.0)							
IV drug use			224	833	365	2	2							
			(30.3)	(45.2)	(42.7)	(25.0)	(11.8)							
Sexual contact with IV drug user			91	269	238	1	2							
			(12.3)	(14.6)	(27.9)	(12.5)	(11.8)							
Heterosexual								4,687	7,249	2,513	7,091	2,242	13	46
								(2.6)	(34.2)	(2.3)	(12.2)	(6.8)	(4.1)	(3.6)
Sexual contact with IV drug user								1,882	4,484	1,342	3,321	1,656	10	19
								(1.0)	(21.1)	(1.2)	(5.7)	(5.0)	(3.2)	(1.5)
Transfusion			152	65	66		6	2,679	1,668	2,993	767	479	6	90
			(20.6)	(3.5)	(7.7)		(35.3)	(1.5)	(7.8)	(2.7)	(1.3)	(1.4)	(1.9)	(7.2)
Undetermined			10	53	20			6,114	1,561	2,701	3,097	1,724	16	84
			(1.4)	(2.9)	(2.3)			(3.4)	(7.4)	(2.5)	(5.3)	(5.2)	(5.1)	(6.7)

Indicators	Age						Sex		Race				
	<15	15–24	25–34	35–44	45–54	55+	Male	Female	White	Black	Hispanic	Native American	Other
Cumulative Total of Deaths Among AIDS Cases, 1991*	1,866	3,968	47,179	50,914	19,292	9,811	119,370	13,863	72,480	38,264	21,253	203	819
Percent	1.4	3.0	35.4	38.2	14.5	7.4	89.6	10.4	54.5	28.8	16.0	0.2	0.6

Indicators	Age					Sex		Race				
	<15	15–24	25–34	35–44	45+	Male	Female	White	Black	Hispanic	Native American	Other
Median (Range) Percent Positive HIV Prevalence, 1988–1990†												
Sexually transmitted disease clinics						(1.1–32.4)	(0.7–2.6)					
Drug treatment centers						4.80	3.50					
Women's health clinics							0.20 (0.0–2.5)	0.10 (0.0–6.9)	0.40 (0.0–3.4)	0.10 (0.0–2.5)		
Tuberculosis clinics						7.40	1.20					
Childbearing women							0.15 (0.0–0.66)					
Civilian applicants for military service						0.13	0.06	0.05	0.33	0.18	0.08	0.04
Blood donors						0.0232	0.0073					
Job Corps entrants	0.2	0.5	1.9	2.0	0.4	0.36	0.31					
Sentinel hospital patients						1.40	0.30	0.80	1.20	0.70		
Ambulatory Sentinel Practice Network						.70	0.06					

*Estimates include residents of U.S. territories.

†These estimates are cumulative, generally for 1988–1990 for each site.

Source: CDC reports; see Resource B for specific references.

American (100 percent, $N = 8$) children contracted the disease perinatally from mothers who were HIV-infected. Drug use or sexual contact with a drug user were the main reasons the vast majority (69 percent) of mothers were at risk (CDC, 1992a). Having hemophilia or a blood transfusion was a more common means of getting the disease among white and Asian, compared to black and Hispanic, children.

About nine out of ten adult cases of AIDS are men. The number of women with AIDS has increased steadily, however. This has corresponded to the progression of the disease to the heterosexual and bisexual populations—particularly among drug users and their sexual partners (CDC, 1990a). Almost three-fourths of the cases of AIDS among women are due to intravenous drug use (50.4 percent) or having sexual contact with a drug user (21.1 percent). Two-thirds (65.1 percent) of the cases among males were through male homosexual or bisexual transmission, 19.3 percent were through intravenous drug use, and 7.2 percent through a combination of these methods of transmission.

The mode of transmission varies considerably among racial/ethnic groups. Minority women particularly are much more likely than white women to have contracted AIDS through drug-related activity. Among blacks (39.5 percent) and Hispanics (40.2 percent) in general, intravenous drug use was five times more likely to be the way they got the disease, compared to whites (8.5 percent). Native Americans (18.5 percent) were twice as likely to contract the illness in this way. The prevalence of AIDS cases related to IV drug use among Hispanics is greatest among Puerto Ricans. The overall prevalence of AIDS among Asian Americans remains low (around 1 percent); however, the number of new cases reported for this group has increased in recent years (OMH, 1990).

AIDS Deaths. HIV/AIDS deaths have been greatest among persons twenty-five to forty-four years of age. Nine out of ten of those who had died of AIDS were men, though this pattern is likely to change as more women contract HIV infection. By 1991, it had become one of the top five causes of death among women twenty-five to forty-four (CDC, 1991).

Though the short-term survival rates for AIDS have increased overall, blacks continue to have lower survival rates than whites, which could relate to the stage at which care is sought, as well as the accessibility of AZT or related medical care (Cargill & Smith, 1990; Friedman et al., 1987).

HIV Prevalence. A survey of HIV seroprevalence among hospital patients confirmed that the risk of AIDS is concentrated among adults twenty-five to forty-four years of age. Prevalence is also higher among men than women. Prevalence rates were twice as high, for example, among male (0.13 percent) compared to female (0.06 percent) military recruits.

Seroprevalence surveys, for which data by race are available, consistently show that the prevalence of HIV antibodies is greatest among blacks.

The average prevalence rate among patients at women's health clinics was 0.40 percent for black women, compared to less than 0.10 percent for both white and Hispanic women. Among civilian applicants for military service, compared to whites (0.05 percent), the seroprevalence among black recruits was six times greater (0.33 percent), more than three times greater among Hispanics (0.18 percent), and almost twice as great among Native Americans (0.08 percent) (CDC, 1992c).

Based on a national HIV seroprevalence survey of women giving birth to infants in the United States in 1989, an estimated 1.5 per 1,000 women were infected with HIV. The rates were even higher in some areas—New York (5.8), Washington, D.C. (5.5), New Jersey (4.9), and Florida (4.5). Assuming that HIV was transmitted perinatally for 30 percent of the births to HIV-infected mothers during the one-year study period, approximately 1,800 newborns would have been HIV positive (Gwinn et al., 1991).

Mentally Ill and Disabled

The prevalence of different types of mental disorders, as well as where people get treatment for them, vary for age, sex, and race groups. Children are more likely to have developmental or behavioral problems. Substance abuse, schizophrenia, affective disorders, and anxiety disorders are more prevalent among adults under sixty-five years of age than among children or the elderly. Relative to younger adults, the noninstitutionalized elderly are much more apt to experience severe cognitive impairment, and elderly nursing home residents with mental disorders are more likely to have organic brain syndrome (including Alzheimer's). Though the prevalence of mental illness in general is greater for women, substance abuse and antisocial personality disorders are much more prevalent among men. Nonwhites are more likely to receive inpatient and outpatient psychiatric care in state and county mental hospitals than are whites, while private psychiatric hospitals are more likely to see whites than blacks, especially on an outpatient basis.

Community Prevalence Rates. Though data for children under eighteen are not available from the Epidemiological Catchment Area (ECA) surveys, in 1980 the Office of Technology Assessment (OTA) estimated that approximately 12 percent, or 7.5 million of 63 million children, had emotional or other problems that warranted mental health treatment, including developmental, behavior, emotional, psychophysiological, or adjustment disorders (OTA, 1986).

Based on ECA survey data, the proportion of noninstitutionalized adults with a mental disorder of any kind in a one-month period was higher for people eighteen to twenty-four (16.9 percent) and twenty-five to forty-four (17.3 percent) than those forty-five to sixty-four (13.3 percent) or sixty-five years of age or older (12.3 percent) (Table 3.4).

Table 3.4. Indicators of Mentally Ill and Disabled by Demographic Subgroups: Community Prevalence Rates.

	One-Month[1][‡][§]						Lifetime[2][§]							
	Age				Sex		Race							
							New Haven, Conn. (%)		Baltimore (%)		St. Louis (%)		Los Angeles (%)	
DIS/DSM-III Disorders per 100 Persons, 18+ years*	18–24	25–44	45–64	65+	Male	Female	Black N=334	Nonblack N=2,708	Black N=1,182	Nonblack N=2,299	Black N=1,158	Nonblack N=1,846	Mexican Americans N=1,243	Non-Hispanic whites N=1,309
Any DIS disorder†	16.9 (1.0)	17.3 (0.6)	13.3 (0.7)	12.3 (0.6)	14.0 (0.4)	16.6 (0.5)	30.5 (3.1)	28.6 (1.0)	45.1 (1.8)	34.7 (1.1)++	34.9 (1.9)	30.1 (1.4)+	34.6 (1.4)+	35.2 (1.7)
Any DIS disorder except cognitive impairment, substance use, and antisocial personality	11.0 (0.8)	13.0 (0.5)	10.7 (0.6)	7.4 (0.5)	7.6 (0.5)	14.5 (0.5)								
Substance use disorders	6.8 (0.7)	4.8 (0.3)	2.1 (0.3)	0.9 (0.2)	6.3 (0.4)	1.6 (0.2)							18.4 (1.2)	22.0 (1.2)
Alcohol abuse/dependence	4.1 (0.6)	3.6 (0.3)	2.1 (0.3)	0.9 (0.2)	5.0 (0.4)	0.9 (0.1)	14.3 (2.4)	11.1 (0.6)	14.6 (1.1)	13.2 (0.8)	14.7 (1.6)	16.0 (1.1)	17.3 (1.2)	14.8 (1.1)
Drug abuse/dependence	3.5 (0.5)	1.5 (0.2)	0.1 (0.0)	0.0 (0.0)	1.8 (0.2)	0.7 (0.1)	6.4 (1.3)	5.7 (0.5)	7.3 (0.9)	4.9 (0.5)+	6.4 (1.0)+	5.3 (0.7)	3.7 (0.4)	13.2 (0.9)
Schizophrenic/ schizophreniform disorders	0.8 (0.2)	1.1 (0.2)	0.5 (0.1)	0.1 (0.0)	0.7 (0.1)	0.7 (0.1)							0.5 (0.2)	0.9 (0.3)
Schizophrenia	0.7 (0.2)	0.9 (0.1)	0.4 (0.1)	0.1 (0.0)	0.6 (0.1)	0.6 (0.1)	2.1 (0.7)	1.9 (0.3)	2.4 (0.5)	1.2 (0.2)+	1.0 (0.3)	1.0 (0.3)	0.4 (0.2)	0.8 (0.3)
Schizophreniform disorders	0.1 (0.1)	0.1 (0.1)	0.0 (0.0)	0.0 (0.0)	0.1 (0.0)	0.1 (0.0)	0.0 (0.0)	0.1 (0.1)	0.4 (0.2)	0.3 (0.1)	0.0 (0.0)	0.1 (0.1)	0.1 (0.1)	0.1 (0.1)

Disorder														
Affective disorders	4.4 (0.5)	6.4 (0.4)	5.2 (0.4)	2.5 (0.3)	3.5 (0.3)	6.6 (0.3)	1.0 (0.5)	1.2 (0.2)	0.5 (0.2)	0.7 (0.2)	2.5 (0.8)	0.7 (0.2)+	7.8 (0.9)	11.0 (1.6)
Manic episode	0.6 (0.2)	0.6 (0.1)	0.2 (0.1)	0.0 (0.0)	0.3 (0.1)	0.4 (0.1)							0.3 (0.2)	1.0 (0.3)
Major depressive episode	2.2 (0.4)	3.0 (0.3)	2.0 (0.3)	0.7 (0.1)	1.6 (0.2)	2.9 (0.2)	5.7 (1.5)	6.8 (0.5)	3.7 (0.7)	3.8 (0.4)	4.9 (0.8)	5.7 (0.7)	4.9 (0.7)	8.4 (0.8)
Dysthymia#	2.2 (0.4)	4.0 (0.3)	3.8 (0.3)	1.8 (0.2)	2.2 (0.3)	4.2 (0.3)	3.3 (1.1)	3.2 (0.4)	1.8 (0.5)	2.3 (0.3)	3.6 (0.7)	3.9 (0.5)	4.8 (0.8)	4.1 (0.6)
Anxiety disorders	7.7 (0.7)	8.3 (0.4)	6.6 (0.5)	5.5 (0.4)	4.7 (0.3)	9.7 (0.4)							14.5 (1.1)	13.6 (1.2)
Phobia	6.4 (0.6)	6.9 (0.4)	6.0 (0.4)	4.8 (0.3)	3.8 (0.3)	8.4 (0.3)	1.3 (0.6)	1.5 (0.2)	1.6 (0.4)	1.3 (0.2)	1.1 (0.3)	1.6 (0.4)	13.5 (1.2)	10.7 (1.0)
Panic	0.4 (0.2)	0.7 (0.1)	0.6 (0.2)	0.1 (0.1)	0.3 (0.1)	0.7 (0.1)	2.7 (0.8)	2.6 (0.3)	2.7 (0.5)	3.1 (0.4)	1.5 (0.4)	2.0 (0.4)	1.2 (0.3)	1.8 (0.4)
Obsessive-compulsive	1.8 (0.4)	1.6 (0.2)	0.9 (0.2)	0.8 (0.2)	1.1 (0.1)	1.5 (0.2)							1.8 (0.4)	3.0 (0.5)
Somatization	0.1 (0.0)	0.1 (0.0)	0.1 (0.0)	0.1 (0.0)	0.0 (0.0)	0.2 (0.0)	0.7 (0.4)	0.1 (0.0)	0.1 (0.1)	0.1 (0.1)	0.4 (0.2)	0.1 (0.1)		
Antisocial personality	0.9 (0.3)	0.8 (0.1)	0.1 (0.1)	0.0 (0.0)	0.8 (0.1)	0.2 (0.1)	1.7 (0.6)	2.1 (0.3)	2.3 (0.5)	2.7 (0.4)	3.9 (0.9)	3.1 (0.5)	3.6 (0.5)	3.0 (0.5)
Severe cognitive impairment	0.6 (0.2)	0.4 (0.1)	1.2 (0.2)	0.1 (0.1)	1.3 (0.1)	1.4 (0.1)	1.9 (0.6)	1.3 (0.2)	1.8 (0.3)	1.1 (0.2)	2.2 (0.3)	0.7 (0.2)++		

*DIS/DSM-III refers to the Diagnostic Interview Schedule, based on American Psychiatric Association, Committee on Nomenclature and Statistics, Diagnostic and Statistical Manual of Mental Disorders (1980).

†"Any DIS disorder" for race (New Haven, Baltimore, and St. Louis) includes phobia and anorexia nervosa, though individual estimates are not reported for these diagnoses.

‡"Any DIS disorder" for race (Los Angeles) includes cognitive impairment, anorexia nervosa, and somatization, though individual estimates are not reported for these diagnoses.

§Rates are standardized to the age, sex, and race distribution of the 1980 noninstitutionalized population of the United States ages eighteen and older.

||Numbers in parentheses refer to the standard errors of the estimates.

#Was asked about only as a lifetime disorder. The one-month rate is, therefore, considered to be the same.

+ $p < .05$

++ $p < .001$

Source: Table 5 (pp. 982–983) in Regier et al. (1988). One-month prevalence of mental disorders in the United States. Archives of General Psychiatry, 45, 977–986. Copyright 1988, American Medical Association. Table 7 in Robins et al. (1984). Lifetime prevalence of specific psychiatric disorders in three sites. Archives of General Psychiatry, 41, 949–958. Copyright 1984, American Medical Association. Table 1 in Karno et al. (1987). Lifetime prevalence of specific psychiatric disorders among Mexican Americans and non-Hispanic whites in Los Angeles. Archives of General Psychiatry, 44, 695–701. Copyright 1987, American Medical Association.

Adults under forty-five years of age had the highest rates of alcohol and drug abuse, schizophrenic disorders, manic episodes, panic disorders, and antisocial personality disorders. The percentage with affective disorder was higher for adults under sixty-five years of age, while the percentage with severe cognitive impairment was highest for those sixty-five or older (4.9 percent).

Women had somewhat higher rates of mental disorders in general. However, men had significantly higher rates of alcohol abuse, drug abuse, and antisocial personality disorders compared to women, while women had higher rates of affective, anxiety, and somatization disorders. A study of cohorts of male veterans showed that the prevalence of substance abuse and antisocial disorders was even higher among young, post–Vietnam era veterans compared to nonveterans (Norquist, Hough, Golding, & Escobar, 1990).

Epidemiological studies of ethnic variations in mental illness have been criticized for their failures to represent high-risk groups (such as those who are incarcerated or homeless), as well as to account for cultural variations in the meanings of questions or concepts (Roberts & Vernon, 1984; Williams, 1986). Data from the ECA surveys showed little or no differences between blacks and whites, except for the higher one-month prevalence of phobia among blacks in the St. Louis and Baltimore sites (Brown, Eaton, & Sussman, 1990). They also showed a somewhat higher six-month prevalence of depression among white men compared to black men, and for black women eighteen to twenty-four years of age compared to white women of the same age, across all five sites (Somervell, Leaf, Weissman, Blazer, & Bruce, 1989).

The differences in the overall lifetime prevalence rates (or the percentage ever having mental illness) for Mexican Americans (34.6 percent) and non-Hispanic whites (35.2 percent) in the Los Angeles ECA survey were not statistically significant. However, drug abuse/dependence was over three times more prevalent among non-Hispanic whites (13.2 percent versus 3.7 percent), and whites were almost twice as likely to have experienced a major episode of depression (8.4 percent versus 4.9 percent). Native Mexican Americans also reported higher lifetime prevalence rates of phobias than did immigrant Mexican Americans or native non-Hispanic whites (Karno et al., 1989).

Systematic epidemiological data are not available on the prevalence of mental illness among Native Americans. An OTA report synthesizing existing research on the mental health of Native American adolescents indicated that they have more serious psychological and behavioral problems than all other racial groups in the following areas: developmental disabilities, depression, suicide, anxiety, alcohol and substance abuse, self-esteem, running away, and school dropout rates (OTA, 1990b).

Based on analyses aggregating the ECA data for all five sites, Holzer and others (1986) found that the six-month prevalence of schizophrenia, alcohol abuse and dependence, and major depression (to a lesser extent) were inversely related to socioeconomic status, using a composite of income, educational, and occupational ranks.

Treated Rates — Inpatient Psychiatric Services. As Table 3.5 indicates, adults twenty-five to forty-four years of age had the highest rates of being under inpatient psychiatric care (102.9 per 100,000) and children less than eighteen the lowest (25.6). Adults were most likely to be under care in state and county mental hospitals, while children had the highest rates of care in private psychiatric hospitals. Men were more likely to be in state and county hospitals and the VA. (Gender differences in rates of VA use are largely due to the fact that the veteran population is predominantly male.)

Nonwhites, compared to whites, were much more likely to be under care in state and county mental hospitals (89.7 versus 30.4) and nonfederal general hospitals (20.9 versus 12.1). Inpatient psychiatric admission rates as a whole were highest at nonfederal general hospitals (331.7).

Treated Rates — Outpatient Psychiatric Services. Table 3.6 shows that children and the elderly had lower rates of being under outpatient psychiatric care (350.2 and 307.2, respectively) than did adults eighteen to sixty-four years of age (473.1 to 851.2). The elderly were much less likely to be seen in freestanding outpatient clinics, compared to other age groups. Males and females had similar rates of care, as did whites and nonwhites. However, whites were more likely to receive care at private psychiatric hospitals (21.3) compared to nonwhites (10.1), while nonwhites (50.1) were much more likely to be seen at state and county mental hospital outpatient departments than were whites (18.4).

Children's admission rates to outpatient services (872.3) were high compared to older adults forty-five to sixty-four years of age (567.4) and the elderly (229.6), in contrast to the rates for these groups currently under care. Men were somewhat more likely to be admitted (964.8) than women (817.3) — particularly to state and county mental hospitals and multiservice mental health organizations. Nonwhites' greater use of state and mental hospitals is borne out for admission rates as well. Admission rates to VA outpatient services were also higher for nonwhites compared to whites.

Treated Rates — Nursing Homes. Around three-fourths (75.8 percent) of nursing home residents less than sixty-five years of age had a mental impairment compared to 63.9 percent of the elderly. (See Table 3.7.) Among those less than sixty-five, schizophrenia (31.2 percent), mental retardation (25.7 percent), and organic brain syndrome (19.5 percent) were the major psychiatric diagnoses. Among the elderly, half (50.3 percent) had organic brain syndrome (OBS). Around two-thirds of both men and women residents had a mental problem. Men were more likely to have a diagnosis of mental retardation or alcohol and drug abuse, while women more often had OBS. Three-fourths (75.4 percent) of Hispanic residents had a mental dis-

Table 3.5. Indicators of Mentally Ill and Disabled by Demographic Subgroups: Treated Rates—Inpatient Psychiatric Services.

Indicators[1]	Age					Sex		Race		Total
	<18	18–24	25–44	45–64	65+	Male	Female	White	Other	
Rate per 100,000 Civilian Population, 1986										
Under care										
Total, all inpatient services	25.6	69.7	102.9	68.5	61.4	82.2	53.1	56.5	126.8	67.2
State and county mental hospitals	10.8	41.1	62.2	41.1	38.7	48.7	30.7	30.4	89.7	39.4
Private psychiatric hospitals	10.6	7.4	6.0	3.8	4.9	6.8	6.9	7.1	5.3	6.9
VA medical centers		0.9	9.6	9.4	5.3	11.1	0.3	5.0	8.6	5.5
Nonfederal general hospitals	2.9	18.0	22.0	12.8	11.4	13.3	13.6	12.1	20.9	13.5
Multiservice mental health organizations	1.2	2.3	3.2	1.4	1.0	2.3	1.7	1.9	2.4	2.0
Admissions										
Total, all inpatient services	177.3	802.5	1,118.9	663.3	447.2	790.4	550.9	593.6	1,074.5	666.8
State and county mental hospitals	25.2	215.5	251.9	107.0	50.9	176.6	98.1	106.7	299.8	136.1
Private psychiatric hospitals	67.1	81.3	121.6	75.2	61.9	92.1	81.5	87.3	83.1	86.7
VA medical centers		17.5	141.7	125.9	39.8	149.3	5.1	65.0	129.5	74.8
Nonfederal general hospitals	72.0	443.7	540.4	314.9	281.5	327.6	335.5	299.0	514.3	331.7
Multiservice mental health organizations	12.9	44.5	63.3	40.3	13.1	44.7	30.6	35.6	47.8	37.4

Source: Rosenstein, Milazzo-Sayre, & Manderscheid, 1990; see Resource B for further detail.

Table 3.6. Indicators of Mentally Ill and Disabled by Demographic Subgroups: Treated Rates—Outpatient Psychiatric Services.

Indicators[1]	Age					Sex		Race		Total
	<18	18-24	25-44	45-64	65+	Male	Female	White	Other	
Rate per 100,000 Civilian Population, 1986										
Under care										
Total, all outpatient services*	350.2	473.1	851.2	682.4	307.2	580.3	576.0	576.2	588.5	578.1
State and county mental hospitals	10.3	21.1	31.9	28.1	23.2	23.2	23.1	18.4	50.1	23.2
Private psychiatric hospitals	18.9	20.6	29.5	9.3	10.6	16.5	22.5	21.3	10.1	19.6
VA medical centers		2.3	45.2	60.4	39.3	59.7	3.2	30.9	28.9	30.6
Nonfederal general hospitals	55.6	43.5	99.3	112.3	63.3	61.9	96.0	78.6	84.5	79.5
Multiservice mental health organizations	169.9	299.3	499.8	361.0	137.2	316.8	322.4	316.8	335.7	319.7
Freestanding outpatient clinics	89.5	83.4	140.4	109.8	30.8	98.6	104.1	106.0	75.6	101.4
Admissions										
Total, all outpatient services*	872.3	1,098.9	1,276.2	567.4	229.6	964.8	817.3	889.2	885.5	888.6
State and county mental hospitals	15.0	40.2	40.0	15.4	2.5	30.0	18.8	22.5	33.8	24.2
Private psychiatric hospitals	49.7	40.6	40.3	22.5	12.3	34.6	37.4	41.6	5.3	36.1
VA medical centers		3.9	44.0	42.7	22.1	50.1	1.4	22.1	41.0	25.0
Nonfederal general hospitals	103.9	124.2	198.0	107.6	68.5	118.9	144.4	126.7	161.8	132.0
Multiservice mental health organizations	496.2	655.9	697.0	285.0	99.1	557.9	424.4	493.3	464.6	489.0
Freestanding outpatient clinics	190.6	222.3	249.3	91.1	24.9	164.1	182.6	174.4	169.4	173.7

*Includes residential treatment centers for emotionally disturbed children.

[1]Includes residential treatment centers for emotionally disturbed children.

Source: Rosenstein, Milazzo-Sayre, & Manderscheid, 1990; see Resource B for further detail.

Table 3.7. Indicators of Mentally Ill and Disabled by Demographic Subgroups: Treated Rates—Nursing Homes.

Indicators[1]	Age		Sex		Race		
	<65	65+	Male	Female	White	Black	Hispanic
Mental Disorders, 1985							
Percent of all residents with mental misorders†							
Total	75.8	63.9	65.2	65.4	65.4	63.9	75.4
Mental retardation	25.7	2.9	8.9	4.3	5.6	4.5*	5.4*
Alcohol and drug abuse	10.5	3.1	8.9	2.0	3.8	5.9	5.2
Organic brain syndromes (including Alzheimer's disease)	19.5	50.3	40.3	49.3	46.7	48.2	58.3
Depressive disorders	14.4	10.8	9.6	11.8	11.3	8.2	11.9*
Schizophrenia and other psychoses	31.2	10.7	15.3	12.2	12.9	15.3	18.8
Anxiety disorders	13.0	10.7	10.5	11.2	11.0	10.1	12.0*
Other mental illnesses	3.2	0.9	2.0	0.9	1.2	0.9	2.0*

*Estimate does not meet standards of reliability or precision.
†Figures may not add to totals because of rounding.
Source: Strahan, 1990; see Resource B for further detail.

order compared to around two-thirds of whites (65.4 percent) and blacks (63.9 percent). Hispanics were more likely to have OBS (58.3 percent) compared to either whites (46.7 percent) or blacks (48.2 percent).

Alcohol or Substance Abusers

Young adults in their late teens and early twenties, particularly men, are more likely to smoke, drink, and use illicit drugs than their younger or older counterparts. Native American youth are much more apt to use alcohol, drugs, and cigarettes than are either white or other minority youth. Minority users are also more likely to develop life-threatening patterns of abuse, as evidenced by higher rates of addiction-related deaths. Death rates for cirrhosis or other alcohol-related causes are greater among Native Americans. Minorities (particularly African Americans) constitute a disproportionate number of medical emergencies and deaths due to cocaine abuse. (See Tables 2.8 and 3.8.)

Household Population, 12 + Years. The prevalence of illicit drug use has declined for all age groups over the past decade. However, rates of use have been and continue to be greater for eighteen- to twenty-five-year olds compared to either younger or older age groups. In 1991, among youth twelve to seventeen years of age, 14.8 percent had used an illicit drug in the past year and 6.8 percent had done so at least once in the past month. Comparable rates for young adults (eighteen to twenty-five) were 29.2 percent and 15.4 percent, respectively, and for adults twenty-six years of age or older, they were 9.6 percent and 4.5 percent. (See Table 2.8.)

The rates of alcohol and tobacco use also remain highest for those eighteen to twenty-five years of age. In 1991, 40 percent of youths twelve to seventeen had used alcohol in the past year, which reflected a steady decline from a high of 53.6 percent in 1979. In 1991, around one in five twelve- to seventeen-year-olds (down from the 1990 prevalence rate of 24.5 percent) had used alcohol in the past month. Alcoholic beverage use was much higher among young adults eighteen to twenty-five: 82.8 percent had used alcohol in the past year, and 63.6 percent had done so in the past month. These rates were, however, significantly lower than the highs of 87.1 percent who had used it in the past year in 1982 and 75.9 percent who had used it in the past month in 1979. Current cigarette use was highest for eighteen- to twenty-five-year-olds (32.2 percent), compared to those twenty-six or older (28.2 percent) and twelve to seventeen (10.8 percent). Three percent of youths and 6 percent of young adults used smokeless tobacco during the past month—reflecting little change since 1988 (NIDA, 1991c, 1991d, 1991e, 1991f).

In 1990, the rates of illicit drug use were higher for men compared to women—both over the past year (15.5 percent versus 11.4 percent) and past month (7.9 percent versus 5.1 percent). (See Table 3.8.) The prevalence

Table 3.8. Indicators of Alcohol or Substance Abusers by Demographic Subgroups.

Indicators[1]	Sex		Race			Adult Education			
	Male	Female	White	Black	Hispanic	Less than high school	High school graduate	Some college	College graduate
Household Population 12+ Years									
(%)[1] Drug use									
Marijuana and hashish									
Past year									
1985	19.5	11.5	15.4	17.9	11.5	9.9	15.2	19.0	15.8
1990	12.1	8.4	10.1	11.2	10.9	8.8	11.0	11.6	8.1
Past month									
1985	12.3	6.8	9.1	13.1	7.4	6.4	9.9	11.3	8.9
1990	6.4	3.9	5.0	6.7	4.7	5.2	5.1	6.6	3.2
Hallucinogens									
Past year									
1985	2.6	0.8	1.9	0.5	1.0	1.5	1.0	2.5	1.7
1990	1.7	0.6	1.3	0.3	1.1	1.3	0.8	1.4	0.6
Past month									
1985	1.1	*	0.9	*	0.5	0.7	0.6	1.2	0.5
1990	0.4	0.2	0.3	†	†				
Cocaine (Crack)[+]									
Past year									
1985	8.4	4.4	6.4	6.2	5.1	3.7	6.6	9.8	6.9
1990	4.3 (0.8)	2.0 (0.3)	2.8 (0.4)	4.0 (1.7)	5.2 (†)	3.0 (0.7)	3.3 (0.5)	4.2 (0.6)	2.3 (†)
Past month									
1985	3.9	2.0	3.0	3.2	2.4	2.1	3.4	4.3	2.4
1990	1.1 (0.4)	0.5 (0.1)	0.6 (0.2)	1.7 (0.9)	1.9 (†)	0.8 (–)	0.9 (–)	1.2 (–)	0.4 (–)

Any illicit drug use									
Past year									
1985	15.5	11.4	13.1	14.9	14.8	11.2	13.6	15.7	11.5
1990									
Past month									
1985	7.9	5.1	6.2	8.6	6.6				
1990									
Alcohol use									
Past year									
1985	78.6	68.8	76.3	59.0	64.0	57.1	78.7	85.9	86.2
1990	71.0	61.5	68.3	55.6	64.5	52.4	67.7	80.1	79.1
Past month									
1985	67.8	51.1	61.8	47.5	50.5	41.5	64.2	73.2	76.4
1990	58.9	44.1	53.1	43.7	47.1	39.5	51.2	64.5	66.3
Cigarette use									
Past year									
1985	40.5	32.3	36.3	38.1	34.7	39.7	41.2	39.3	26.1
1990	35.3	29.0	32.5	32.4	28.7	38.6	38.0	33.3	17.7
Past month									
1985	35.3	28.0	31.5	34.0	29.3	37.3	37.0	32.6	23.0
1990	29.4	24.2	27.4	26.7	20.8	34.7	33.2	27.2	12.9

Table 3.8. Indicators of Alcohol or Substance Abusers by Demographic Subgroups, Cont'd.

| | Sex by Race | | | | | | | | | | | | | |
| | Male | | | | | | | Female | | | | | | |
Indicators	White	Black	Mexican American	Puerto Rican/ Latin American	Native American	Asian	Other	White	Black	Mexican American	Puerto Rican/ Latin American	Native American	Asian	Other
High School Seniors (%)² Drug use														
Marijuana and hashish														
Past year														
1976–1979	54.7	48.0	54.5	48.0	61.4	42.8	53.7	44.5	31.2	37.7	30.3	57.3	30.7	44.4
1985–1989	40.2	29.8	37.3	30.6	42.0	19.6	37.8	36.0	18.4	26.0	21.3	44.0	17.1	28.6
Past month														
1976–1979	41.1	37.2	38.7	37.2	50.1	30.2	41.5	30.9	22.5	25.5	20.7	43.6	20.3	32.5
1985–1989	25.0	18.5	22.0	18.9	27.6	9.7	24.4	19.8	9.9	13.6	9.6	23.9	8.1	17.5
Inhalants														
Past year														
1976–1979	5.6	2.7	4.3	2.9	11.5	2.5	6.1	3.2	1.1	2.4	0.7	4.6	2.9	2.6
1985–1989	8.8	2.6	6.0	5.1	9.6	4.8	8.5	5.2	2.2	4.3	2.9	4.4	3.2	3.8
Past month														
1976–1979	1.9	1.1	1.2	1.0	4.6	1.4	3.2	0.9	0.6	1.0	0.0	2.0	1.4	0.6
1985–1989	3.4	1.4	2.3	2.0	5.2	1.3	4.5	2.0	1.4	2.1	0.8	0.9	0.8	2.5
Hallucinogens														
Past year														
1976–1979	12.3	3.4	9.0	12.0	14.6	8.1	14.2	8.0	1.2	5.3	3.9	9.8	6.6	9.9
1985–1989	8.3	1.9	5.9	6.5	10.0	3.0	10.0	5.0	0.6	2.2	2.1	9.0	2.2	4.6
Past month														
1976–1979	5.2	1.4	4.9	4.1	8.1	3.5	5.9	2.9	0.6	1.5	0.9	4.0	3.0	4.2
1985–1989	3.5	0.9	2.4	3.0	3.6	1.5	5.1	1.7	0.3	0.7	0.4	2.7	0.3	1.3
Cocaine														
Past year														
1976–1979	11.1	6.4	9.7	14.9	15.7	8.6	12.0	6.7	3.5	4.7	3.8	8.0	5.9	10.2
1985–1989	11.9	6.1	14.7	15.6	14.2	5.8	14.6	9.3	2.6	7.6	8.2	15.5	5.7	10.4
Past month														
1976–1979	4.7	2.4	4.6	8.2	8.4	2.8	6.2	2.7	1.6	2.1	1.1	3.8	3.7	3.7
1985–1989	5.6	2.6	8.2	8.1	7.3	1.8	9.1	4.1	1.3	3.0	2.9	9.2	2.6	5.0

Alcohol use
Past year

1976–1979	90.7	80.1	87.5	85.3	94.3	77.9	87.3	87.7	68.6	79.0	81.4	89.0	67.4	84.2
1985–1989	88.3	72.5	82.4	80.6	82.0	69.3	84.0	88.6	63.9	73.6	77.2	81.3	67.5	77.7

Past month

1976–1979	78.9	58.6	72.5	66.2	85.3	55.0	74.9	69.4	40.9	58.4	52.5	65.6	43.5	64.8
1985–1989	72.3	49.2	65.0	55.4	69.0	43.7	65.4	66.6	32.8	50.5	43.0	60.2	34.2	50.1

Cigarette use
Past month

1976–1979	35.0	33.1	30.6	29.7	50.3	20.7	41.6	39.1	33.6	30.1	33.9	55.3	24.4	43.6
1985–1989	29.8	15.6	23.8	22.0	36.8	16.8	31.5	34.0	13.3	18.7	24.7	43.6	14.3	30.5

Daily use

1976–1979	25.8	23.6	19.5	21.2	40.9	13.3	33.7	29.7	22.3	16.3	20.5	50.3	15.4	34.6
1985–1989	18.8	8.6	11.6	13.3	26.0	9.0	23.2	22.5	7.1	8.1	13.3	33.8	9.4	21.1

Indicators	Age								Race	
	15–24	25–34	35–44	45–54	55–64	65–74	75–84	85+	Native American	All races
Alcohol-Related Mortality Rates, 1986–1988‡ Age-adjusted rate per 100,000	0.1	2.3	8.5	15.8	20.5	16.0	8.9	3.2	33.9	6.3

Indicators	Age							Sex		Race			
	6–17	18–19	20–29	30–39	40–49	50–59	60+	Male	Female	White	Black	Hispanic	Other
Emergency Room Drug Abuse Reports, 1990 (Percent)*§													
Total episodes	13.5	7.2	31.5	29.6	12.2	3.2	2.6	46.6	52.3	58.5	23.8	8.0	1.0
Cocaine mentions	2.3	3.6	40.5	40.9	10.6	1.6	0.3	65.0	33.8	30.0	53.5	8.2	0.4

*Less than one-half of 1 percent.
+Numbers in parentheses refer to crack cocaine use.
†Low precision; no estimates reported.
‡Breakdowns by race are age-adjusted.
-Breakdowns by adult education are not available.
§Percentages reflect distributions of reports across the respective demographic (age, sex, race) subgroups. The percentages may not sum to 100 percent due to missing data on these demographic variables.
Source: NIDA and IHS reports; Bachman, Wallace, Kurth, Johnston, & O'Malley, 1991. See Resource B for specific references.

of current cocaine use among men (1.1 percent) was twice that of women (0.5 percent). Larger percentages of men (58.9 percent) had used alcohol in the past month compared to women (44.1 percent). Though the differences were not as dramatic, more men (29.4 percent) than women (24.2 percent) had also smoked cigarettes during that period.

In 1990, the current prevalence of illicit drug use overall was similar for blacks (14.9 percent) and Hispanics (14.8 percent)—somewhat higher than the white rate of 13.1 percent. Marijuana use was slightly higher among blacks than Hispanics, while the opposite was the case for cocaine. Current alcohol use was higher among whites (53.1 percent), compared to either Hispanics (47.1 percent) or blacks (43.7 percent). The percent who had smoked in the past month was higher for both whites (27.4 percent) and blacks (26.7 percent) compared to Hispanics (20.8 percent). The prevalence of illicit drug use was, in general, greatest for those who attended but did not graduate from college. The highest percentages of current smokers were among those with a high school education (33.2 percent) or less (34.7 percent), while the lowest percentage (12.9 percent) was for those with a college education.

High School Seniors. Based on combined data from 1985 to 1989 on U.S. high school seniors, females generally were less likely to have used drugs than males, though the patterns varied across racial/ethnic groups. Native Americans reported the highest rates of drug, alcohol, and cigarette use of any group, while Asian Americans had the lowest. Black youth consistently reported lower rates of use than whites, while Hispanic youths tended to have intermediate rates between those of blacks and whites, except for higher rates of cocaine use among Hispanic males (Bachman, Wallace, Kurth, Johnston, & O'Malley, 1991).

Comparisons between combined data from 1976–1979 and 1985–1989 show diminished rates of use in general for most forms of drug use. Cigarette use did, however, decline more sharply for black compared to white seniors over that period. The rates of white male (18.8 percent) and female (22.5 percent) students who smoked daily were much higher than the corresponding rates for black males (8.6 percent) and females (7.1 percent).

Alcohol-Related Mortality Rates. The number of deaths due to alcohol-related causes per 100,000 deaths was highest for adults fifty-five to sixty-four (20.5). The overall rate for Native Americans (33.9) was more than five times that of the other races (6.3).

Emergency Room Drug Abuse Reports. The vast majority of people seen in an emergency room for drug-related problems were twenty to thirty-nine years of age (61.1 percent). Somewhat more women (52.3 percent) than men (46.6 percent), and more whites (58.5 percent) than blacks (23.8 percent), were seen. However, many more men (65.0 percent) than women (33.8 percent), and more blacks (53.5 percent) than whites (30.0 percent), were seen for cocaine-related emergencies. (These estimates here and in Table 3.8 do not add up to 100 percent because of missing data on these variables.)

Suicide- or Homicide Prone

Of those who die from intentional acts of violence, elderly white men and young Native American men are most likely to kill themselves, and young African-American, Native American, and Hispanic men are most likely to be killed at the hand of others. The violence-related death rates for these groups have increased dramatically in recent years, primarily due to the greater use of deadly weapons, particularly firearms, in these encounters (Table 3.9).

Suicide. Although the overall suicide rate did not change significantly from 1950 to 1980, suicide rates among young persons—particularly young white men—increased dramatically. From 1950 to 1980, the rates among white males fifteen to twenty-four years of age increased 324 percent, from 6.6 per 100,000 to 21.4 per 100,000. The number of suicides among white males and females fifteen to nineteen years of age in which firearms were used doubled between 1968 and 1980 (Fingerhut & Kleinman, 1989; NCHS, 1991c).

Based on 1989 data, death rates due to suicide were much higher for white males (19.6), compared to black males (12.5), white females (4.8), or black females (2.4). Rates were dramatically higher for elderly white males seventy-five to eighty-four years of age (55.3) and eighty-five or older (71.9). Further, the percent increase from 1980 to 1989 in the suicide rate for white males seventy-five to eighty-four (21 percent) and eighty-five or older (36 percent) was two to four times the rate of increase (8 percent) for young white males fifteen to twenty-four—from 21.4 in 1980 to 23.2 in 1989 (NCHS, 1992b).

Compared to rates of whites as a whole, suicide rates tend to be lower for Hispanics and higher for Native Americans. As with whites, males are most at risk of committing suicide. The five-year (1976–1980) rate of suicide for Hispanics (9.0) in the five Southwestern states, in which the majority of Mexican Americans reside, was less than half that of white Anglos (19.2) in the area. The rates for Hispanic males were highest among men twenty to twenty-four and over seventy years of age (Smith, Mercy, & Rosenberg, 1986). The suicide rate for Native Americans in 1988 (14.5) was higher than the national average (11.4). The death rates for Native American males fifteen to twenty-four (40.7) and twenty-five to thirty-four (49.6) were particularly dramatic (IHS, 1991, p. 46).

Year 2000 Objectives for lowering suicide rates are targeted toward at-risk age, sex, and race/ethnicity groups: youth aged fifteen to nineteen (8.2), men aged twenty to thirty-four (21.4), white men aged sixty-five and older (39.2), and American Indians and Alaskan Natives (12.8) (PHS, 1990). The 1988 and 1989 rates for all of these groups, particularly elderly males, fell short of these objectives.

Table 3.9. Indicators of Suicide- or Homicide-Prone by Demographic Subgroups.

| Indicators | Age[1] | | | | | | | | | | | Race by Sex[1] | | | | |
| | | | | | | | | | | | | White | | Black | | Native |
	<1	1-4	5-14	15-24	25-34	35-44	45-54	55-64	65-74	75-84	85+	Male	Female	Male	Female	American[2]
Age-Adjusted Death Rates per 100,000 Resident Population																
Suicide																
1980			0.4	12.3	16.0	15.4	15.9	15.9	16.9	19.1	19.2	18.9	5.7	11.1	2.4	14.1
1989			0.7	13.3	15.0	14.6	14.6	15.5	18.0	23.1	22.8	19.6	4.8	12.5	2.4	14.5*
Homicide and legal intervention																
1980	5.9	2.5	1.2	15.6	19.6	15.1	11.1	7.0	5.7	5.2	5.3	10.9	3.2	71.9	13.7	18.1
1989	8.5	2.7	1.5	16.9	16.3	11.0	7.6	5.0	4.1	4.2	4.3	8.1	2.8	61.5	12.5	14.1*

*The 1989 estimates for Native Americans are based on 1988 data.
Source: NCHS and IHS reports; see Resource B for specific references.

Based on the Epidemiological Catchment Area Survey, 2.9 percent of adults reported they had attempted suicide at some time in their life. Those groups with the highest risk of attempted suicide included those who had a lifetime diagnosis of a psychiatric disorder, females, were separated or divorced, in the lowest socioeconomic status group, and white (Moscicki et al., 1988). In general, those people who die from suicide attempts use more lethal weapons (such as firearms) than those who survive such attempts (drug overdoses, for example).

Homicide and Legal Intervention. While white males are most at risk of death due to suicide, black males are most at risk of a homicide-related death. Findings from the 1979–1987 National Crime Surveys showed that as a group, young black urban males were most likely to be victimized by an offender armed with a handgun. Urban black men aged sixteen to twenty-four were likely to be attacked at more than twice the rate of urban white men or urban black women of similar ages (Rand, 1990).

From 1978 through 1987, the annual death rates due to homicide for young black males fifteen to twenty-four years of age was four to five times that of young black females, five to eight times that of young white males, and sixteen to twenty-two times that of young white females. From 1984 to 1987, the differences between these rates for young black men increased even more dramatically. The percent increase in homicides from 1984 to 1987 was particularly high for adolescent black males aged fifteen to nineteen (55 percent) compared to those twenty to twenty-four years of age (33 percent). Firearm-associated homicides accounted for 78 percent of homicides among young black males from 1978 to 1987 and 96 percent of the increase in the homicide rate for this group from 1984 to 1987 (CDC, 1990f).

Based on 1989 data, the disparity between homicide rates per 100,000 for black males (61.5) compared to black females (12.5), white males (8.1), and white females (2.8) continued. The annual rate of increase in previous years was greatest for black males fifteen to twenty-four years of age (NCHS, 1991c). A particularly alarming trend is the increase in gun-related deaths (due to homicides, suicides, and accidental deaths) among teenagers. One out of five deaths of teens and young adults in 1988 was gun related. In that year, for the first time, deaths due to firearms for both white and black male teenagers exceeded the mortality from all other natural causes of death (Fingerhut, Kleinman, Godfrey, & Rosenberg, 1991).

Rates of homicide are higher for both Hispanics and Native Americans than for whites. Based on data from the five major Southwestern states with large concentrations of Mexican Americans, the homicide rate for Hispanics (20.5) was more than twice that of white Anglos (7.9). The homicide rate for young Hispanic males twenty to twenty-four (83.3) was exceptionally high (Smith, Mercy, & Rosenberg, 1986). The 1988 homicide rate for Native Americans (14.1) was about 1.6 times that of the national average (9.0) that year. This disparity has declined over time—from a high of five times the deaths due to homicide among Native Americans compared to whites in 1955. As with suicide rates, the rates of homicide-related deaths are highest for Native American males fifteen to twenty-four (32.1) and twenty-five to thirty-four years of age (44.7) (IHS, 1991, p. 48).

The 1989 homicide rates exceeded the Year 2000 Objectives for American Indians/Alaskan Natives (11.3), young Hispanic men fifteen to thirty-four (42.5), and particularly at-risk young black men fifteen to thirty-four (72.4) (PHS, 1990).

Abusing Families

Unemployment and associated economic hardship play a major role in cases of maltreatment, and particularly neglect, within families. Though minority children are disproportionately reported to authorities as being victims of abuse or neglect, it is not apparent that maltreatment in general is more prevalent in minority families (Table 3.10).

Child Abuse and Neglect Reports. The age distribution of children for which maltreatment was reported in 1986 was as follows: zero to five years (43 percent), six to eleven years (33 percent), twelve to seventeen years (24 percent). The mean age was 7.2 years. From 1976 to 1983, there was a gradual decline in the average age, from 7.8 to 7.1. Since 1983, the mean age has been fairly stable. The percent of maltreated children who were female increased from 50.0 percent in 1976 to 52.5 percent in 1986.

In 1986, the racial/ethnic distribution of maltreated children was as follows: white (66 percent), black (20 percent), Hispanic (11 percent), other (3 percent). A larger percentage of maltreated children reported were minority (34 percent), compared to the population of U.S. children as a whole (19 percent). They were also younger on average (7.2 versus 8.6 years of age) (American Humane Association, 1988).

The profile of families of children referred to Child Protective Services (CPS) differed for different types of maltreatment. In general, however, there is evidence of considerable economic hardship—particularly among neglect cases. Almost half (48.9 percent) of all families reported for maltreatment in 1986 received public assistance (American Humane Association, 1988). Black families were more prone to be involved in neglect situations, were more often on public assistance, and had younger single, female caretakers. Children who were sexually abused experienced little maltreatment of other kinds, the victims were mostly white females, and the family had two caretakers who were less likely to be on public assistance (American Humane Association, 1984).

Child Abuse and Neglect Incidence Rates. Due to weighting problems with the original estimates generated from the 1986 Study of National Incidence and Prevalence of Child Abuse and Neglect, the estimates by child and family

Table 3.10. Indicators of Abusing Families by Demographic Subgroups.

| | Age | | | Sex | | Race | | | | Unemployed |
Indicators[1]	<5	6–11	12–17	Male	Female	White	Black	Hispanic	Other	Caretaker
Characteristics of Child Abuse and Neglect Reports, 1986*										
Percent distribution	43	33	24	48	52	66	20	11	3	35

*Characteristics are available only in the twenty-eight states for which case-specific data were obtained.
Source: American Humane Association, 1988; see Resource B for further detail.

characteristics were reanalyzed. Between-group differences found in the original analyses were largely reconfirmed, however. This includes the findings that older children, those in larger families or ones earning less than $15,000, and girls, primarily due to their greater vulnerability to sexual abuse, were most subject to maltreatment. Black children had marginally (but not statistically significant) higher rates of physical abuse and neglect (National Center on Child Abuse and Neglect, 1988; Sedlak, 1991).

Domestic Elder Abuse. In FY 1988, the rates of domestic elder abuse were higher in urban (3.77 reports per 1,000 elders) compared to rural states (2.60), and in those states with mandatory (3.96) compared to voluntary (2.23) reporting systems. Older women were much more likely to be victims of elder abuse than were men, relative to their distribution in the population: the ratio of female to male elderly victims was 1.79, compared to the ratio of female to male elderly in the population of 1.33. The major perpetrators of domestic elder abuse were adult children (30.0 percent), spouse (14.8 percent), grandchildren (1.9 percent), sibling (1.7 percent), other relatives (17.8 percent), service provider (12.8 percent), friend/neighbor (10.0 percent), and all others or unknown perpetrators (10.9 percent) (Tatara, 1990).

Family Violence. Findings from the National Surveys of Family Violence confirm that "economic adversity and worries about money pervade the typical violent home" (Gelles & Straus, 1988, p. 84). According to these investigators, the prototypical abusive parent was single, under thirty, married less than ten years, had his or her first child before the age of eighteen, and was unemployed or, if employed, worked part time in a manual labor job. There were no differences between blacks and whites in the rates of abusive violence toward children.

The typical "wife beater," according to that study, experienced status inconsistency—that is, a man's educational background was higher than his occupational attainment, or his neighbor's or wife's attainments were greater than his own. He was young (eighteen to twenty-four), married less than ten years, employed part time or not at all, and was dissatisfied about his economic security—though many individual abusers were also quite affluent. The authors concluded, "Perhaps the most telling of all attributes of the battering man is that he feels inadequate and sees violence as a culturally acceptable way to be both dominant and powerful" (Gelles & Straus, 1988, p. 89). Though the rate of wives battering husbands was also high, three-fourths of the violence committed by women was estimated to be in self-defense (Gelles & Straus, 1988, p. 90).

Homeless

The precise composition of the homeless varies in different cities and localities. Nonetheless, a profile of the homeless appears to be emerging from the array of national and local studies done in recent years (Table 3.11).

Table 3.11. Indicators of Homeless by Demographic Subgroups.

Indicators	Family Type					Race				
	Children	Single men	Families with children	Single women	Unaccompanied youth	White	Black	Hispanic	Native American	Asian
Characteristics of Homeless, 1991 (Percent Distribution)										
U.S. Conference of Mayors	24	50	35	12	3	34	48	15	3	1

Source: U.S. Conference of Mayors, 1991.

A twenty-eight-city survey conducted in 1991 by the U.S. Conference of Mayors showed the following characteristics of the homeless population in the cities studied: single men (50 percent), families with children (35 percent), single women (12 percent), unaccompanied youth (3 percent). Around a fourth (24 percent) of the homeless were children. Data from this and other sources demonstrated a decline from 1985 to 1991 in the proportion of the homeless who were single men (from 60 to 50 percent) and an increase in the proportion that were families with children (27 to 35 percent). The racial/ethnic composition of the homeless was 48 percent black, 34 percent white, 15 percent Hispanic, 3 percent Native American, and 1 percent Asian. The U.S. Conference of Mayors study also documented that only 18 percent of the homeless were employed in full- or part-time jobs, 23 percent were veterans, 29 percent were mentally ill, 40 percent were alcohol or substance abusers, and 7 percent had AIDS (U.S. Conference of Mayors, 1991).

These findings bear out the profile of the homeless found in other studies. In general, they are relatively young adults: the median age is between the late twenties and late thirties. The average age of homeless women is generally younger than that of men, and a relatively small percent are sixty-five or over, compared to the general U.S. population. Traditionally, more men than women have been homeless, though the proportion of women among the homeless has increased in recent years to an estimated 20 to 35 percent. Minorities are overrepresented among the homeless in most cities. Adults are much less likely to have a high school education and to be employed full or part time compared to the U.S. population as a whole. The homeless have extremely low incomes — generally much lower than the U.S. poverty level. The majority have physical health problems, an estimated 25 percent to a third have mental health problems, and a comparable proportion have alcohol or substance abuse problems.

Around one out of five homeless has been homeless for several years. However, families with children are much more likely to have been homeless for relatively short periods of time (several months). Contrary to stereotypes, many of the homeless have lived in their communities a number of years prior to becoming homeless (Burt & Cohen, 1989; OM, 1988c; National Alliance to End Homelessness, 1988; Partnership for the Homeless, 1989; Reyes & Waxman, 1989; U.S. Commission on Security and Cooperation in Europe, 1990; U.S. Conference of Mayors, 1991).

Approximately 12.5 percent of the homeless are estimated to reside in nonmetropolitan areas (CDF, 1991b). Based on the limited data available, the rural homeless, compared to the urban homeless, are more likely to be younger and female, less likely to be members of minority groups, more likely to be doubled up or living with other family members, and fewer have been homeless for long periods of time (several years) (National Alliance to End Homelessness, 1988; Roth, Bean, Lust, & Saveanu, 1985).

Immigrants and Refugees

During the 1960s, the largest number of immigrants came from Europe and North America—particularly Mexico. In the 1980s, most came from Asia, reflecting the out-migration subsequent to the Vietnam War. Refugees were a particularly substantial proportion (27 percent) of the Asian immigrants during this period. The estimated number of illegal aliens from Central and South America that have fled in response to the warfare in those areas but who do not have official refugee status has also increased substantially over the last decade. The demographic and socioeconomic profiles of different immigrant and refugee groups vary a great deal (Table 3.12).

Table 3.12. Indicators of Immigrants and Refugees by Demographic Subgroups.

Indicators[1]	Continent of Birth					
	Europe	Asia	North America	South America	Africa	Other
Total Number						
Immigrants						
1961–1970	1,238,600	445,300	1,351,100	228,300	39,300	19,100
1971–1980	801,300	1,633,800	1,645,000	284,400	91,500	37,300
1981–1989	593,200	2,478,800	2,167,400	370,100	156,400	35,600
Refugees						
1961–1970	55,235	19,895	132,068	123	5,486	36
1971–1980	71,858	210,683	252,633	1,244	2,991	38
1981–1989	122,401	660,225	111,930	1,712	19,937	51

Source: U.S. Bureau of the Census, 1991c; see Resource B for further detail.

Compared to documented Mexican immigrants, undocumented Mexican aliens are likely to be younger, have been in the United States a shorter period of time, have fewer years of education, are less likely to read and write English, and have lower incomes (Chavez, Cornelius, & Jones, 1985; Rumbaut, Chavez, Moser, Pickwell, & Wishik, 1988).

The characteristics of different subgroups of Indochinese refugees (such as Chinese, Vietnamese, Hmong, Khmer, and Lao) also differ. The fertility of Hmong women (number of children under five years of age per 1,000 women of childbearing age) has been found to be much higher than that of the other Asian subgroups, for example. The literacy rates in general and in terms of the ability to read or speak English are low—particularly for Indochinese refugee women. The vast majority of Indochinese refugees have incomes below the poverty level. Those most disadvantaged, however, have been in the United States the shortest period of time.

Those who have been here the longest—particularly the Vietnamese refugees—appear to have fared better than the other groups in terms of finding employment and earning incomes sufficient to elevate them above the poverty level. The first wave of refugees (almost all Vietnamese) admitted to the

United States during 1975–1976 were, in general, better educated and came under more favorable economic conditions than did later and larger waves of refugees who arrived after 1979 (Haines, 1989; Rumbaut, Chavez, Moser, Pickwell, & Wishik, 1988).

The earlier waves of refugees from Cuba in the late 1950s and 1960s were of a much higher socioeconomic status than those who came later — particularly the approximately 125,000 people who were admitted to the United States as a part of the Mariel boat lift of 1980. A number of former prisoners and others deemed "undesirable" by the Cuban regime entered the United States under this arrangement.

The Central American population, many of whom do not have official legal status in the United States, tend to be comprised of a larger proportion of males, particularly young males. Literacy rates and rates of employment are low. As with many of the Indochinese refugee population, those who do work are employed in very low-paying service jobs (Urrutia-Rojas & Aday, 1991).

The 1980s was a harmful, not a kind and gentle, decade for many vulnerable Americans. The next chapter explores the deep social, political, and economic conditions that give rise to the disproportionate risk of poor physical, psychological, or social health.

4

Why Are They Vulnerable?

This chapter addresses the question of why some groups are more vulnerable than others. We will consider whether some groups are more at risk of poor physical, psychological, and/or social health as a result of the increasingly limited availability of community and associated individual resources (social status, social capital, and human capital). (See Figures 1.1 and 1.2 and Table 1.1.)

National Profile and Trends

The current and changing profile of the American people, the ties between them, and the neighborhoods in which they live will be examined.

The People

As the United States approaches the twenty-first century, older Americans are living longer and families are having fewer children. As a result of these and other demographic changes, such as the aging of the baby-boom generation, the number of elderly is increasing and the number of children is declining in proportion to the rest of the U.S. population.

The number of Americans sixty-five and over nearly doubled between 1960 and 1990—from 16.7 million to 31.2 million or from 9.2 to 12.6 percent of the population. The number of elderly is expected to increase to nearly forty million or 14 percent by the year 2010, and a growing proportion of the elderly will be among the oldest old (eighty-five years of age or older).

On the other hand, although the number of children under age eighteen in 1990 (around 64 million) is similar to that in 1960, the proportion children represent of the U.S. population has declined sharply over that same period—from 36 percent in 1960 to 26 percent in 1990. By 2010, the proportion of children is expected to be around 23 percent (National Commission on Children, 1991; U.S. Bureau of the Census, 1991a, 1991b, 1991c).

Minorities — including African Americans, Hispanics, Native Americans, and Asian Americans — make up a larger proportion of the U.S. population than they did in the past. Over the last decade (from 1980 to 1990), the Asian and Pacific Islander population almost doubled — from approximately 3.7 million (1.6 percent) to 7.2 million (2.9 percent). The Hispanic population increased around 53 percent — from 14.6 million (6.4 percent) to 22.3 million (9.0 percent), and the Alaskan Indian, Eskimo, and Aleut population increased over 40 percent — from 1.4 million (0.6 percent) to 2.0 million (0.8 percent). The growth of the Hispanic population has been due both to immigration and natural increase, while the rapid growth of the Asian population has been due largely to immigration. Around four out of ten of the legal immigrants to the U.S. since 1980 were from Asia (U.S. Bureau of the Census, 1991a, 1991b, 1991c).

The number and percent blacks represent of the U.S. population also increased from 26.5 million (11.7 percent) in 1980 to 30.0 million (12.1 percent) in 1990. Though the actual number of whites increased from 1980 (188.4 million) to 1990 (199.7 million), the percent they represented of the total U.S. population declined (from 83.1 to 80.3 percent) (U.S. Bureau of the Census, 1991a, 1991b).

The rate of growth in the number of minority children in particular has been and is expected to continue to be greater than for nonminority children over the coming decade. The number of white children under five years of age is projected to decline around 11 percent, compared to a 2 percent decline for blacks and an 18 percent increase for children of other races (U.S. Bureau of the Census, 1991c).

Overall, U.S. baby-boomer adults and the elderly are an increasingly graying population, while new and newborn Americans increasingly reflect a rainbow of racial and ethnic diversity.

Ties Between People

The number of people who live together in the same household has diminished steadily over time. The average number of people per household was 2.63 in 1990, down from 3.14 in 1970. Around twenty-three million people — or one-quarter of U.S. households — live alone. This represents an increase of almost five million people since 1980 and more than a doubling of those living by themselves since 1970. This increase in the number living alone reflects a combination of major social trends, including more elderly widows, more young people delaying marriage, and lower overall birth rates.

In 1990, only 55 percent of U.S. households consisted of married-couple families, down from 61 percent in 1980 and 74 percent in 1960. The number and proportion of children living in single-parent families has also increased dramatically. In 1970, about 12 percent of (or eight million) children lived with only one parent; in 1989, the number had doubled to around 24 percent (or about sixteen million) children under eighteen years of age.

Divorce and separation are the major causes of single parenthood. About half of all U.S. marriages can be expected to end in divorce, and the majority involve children. The other major cause of single parenthood is out-of-wedlock births. In 1970, approximately 11 percent of all births in the United States were to unmarried mothers. By 1988, more than 25 percent were.

Though African-American children are more likely to live with one parent than are white or other minority children, the growth in single parenthood was substantial for all racial and ethnic groups during the 1970s and 1980s. Further, though for whites the increase in the number of children living with their mother is primarily due to divorce and separation, the number of births among young unmarried white teens has also increased substantially over this period. Taken together, these trends suggest that more than half of all white children and three-fourths of African-American children born in the 1970s and 1980s are likely to live some portion of their childhood in single-parent (largely female-headed) families (National Commission on Children, 1991; U.S. Bureau of the Census, 1991a, 1991b, 1991c).

Around three out of ten of the elderly live by themselves. The likelihood of living alone increases with age. Among those living in the community, almost half (45 percent) of the oldest old (eighty-five years of age or older) live by themselves. Women outnumber men among all age categories of the elderly and account for the vast majority (around 80 percent) of the elderly living alone. Men, regardless of age, are much more likely to be living with a spouse. Most elderly women living by themselves are widows. African-American elderly people are more likely to live alone than are whites, while a smaller percentage of Hispanics do so (Commonwealth Fund Commission on Elderly People Living Alone, 1988).

In summary, then, an increasing number of young as well as elderly U.S. adults are living by themselves, and more and more U.S. children are growing up in families with one, rather than two, parents at home to care for them.

The Neighborhood

Social and economic trends indicate a declining level of material and nonmaterial investments in U.S. neighborhoods and associated human capital resources (schools, jobs, family incomes, and housing).

The federal commitment to providing funds for education has declined over the previous decade. The percent of all federal outlays allocated to education and related programs declined from 5.8 percent in 1980 to 4.2 percent in 1990. The proportion of total expenditures for elementary and secondary education provided by the federal government was 7.4 percent in 1970, rose to 9.1 percent in 1980, and then declined to 5.9 percent by 1987. During this same period, state governments assumed a greater role in funding education—from 34.6 percent in 1970 to 45.5 percent in 1987. The

Children's Defense Fund reported that though state spending on schools rose substantially during this period, the growth of state investments in prisons was still twice that for education. Further, considerable disparities exist within and across states in the level of investments in primary and secondary education. Equity in the financing of schools across well-to-do and poor districts has been a major political and legal controversy in many states and localities (Children's Defense Fund, 1990; U.S. Bureau of the Census, 1991c).

During the 1980s, the number of high-paying jobs in manufacturing decreased, and it is expected to continue to decline during the coming decade. The new jobs that have been and that are likely to be created are primarily in the lower-paying service sector, such as the fast-food industry and building and hotel maintenance and housekeeping sectors. Further, despite generally more favorable economic trends subsequent to a deep recession in the early part of the decade, wages in the service sector have not increased as much as have those of managerial, professional, or technical workers. A contributor to the increasing disparity in wages between the lowest- and highest-paying sectors is the fact that for the decade from 1981 to 1990, the federal minimum wage remained constant at $3.35 per hour until 1990. It was increased to $3.80 in 1990 and then to $4.25 in 1991. Even with the increase in the federal minimum wage, a parent working full time throughout the year at the minimum wage would still earn less than 90 percent of the poverty-level income for a family of three (Children's Defense Fund, 1991a; U.S. Bureau of the Census, 1991c).

Trends in employment and associated wages during the previous decade, as well as changes in the tax laws during this same period, have contributed to increasing disparities in the distribution of family income in the United States. In 1980, 15.3 percent of the aggregate money income was received by the U.S. families that were in the top 5 percent of the income categories, while by 1989, their share had increased to 17.9 percent. A similar trend was observed for those who were in the top 20 percent of income categories, whose share of income increased from 41.6 to 44.6 percent over the same period. For all other income tiers, the percentage share of income declined—and at progressively *higher* rates, the *lower* their family incomes. The number and percent of Americans who have incomes below federal poverty-level standards declined substantially from 1960 (39.9 million, 22.2 percent) to 1979 (26.1 million, 11.7 percent), and then began to climb during the decade of the 1980s. In 1989, 12.8 percent or 31.5 million Americans were below the poverty level (U.S. Bureau of the Census, 1991c).

The number of affordable housing units for low-income families and individuals has sharply diminished since the late 1970s. Overall, assistance provided by the Department of Housing and Urban Development to add new units to the stock of low-income housing declined from about $32 billion in 1978 to about $10 billion in 1989—a reduction of over 80 percent adjusted for inflation. While spending for low-income housing has sharply declined, the federal government provides around $50 billion annually in indirect tax subsidies to homeowners through allowing them to deduct mortgage interest and property taxes. In 1989, about three-fourths of the tax deductions benefited homeowners with the highest 15 percent of incomes (Levitan, 1990).

The impacts of these economic and social trends have been greatest for particularly vulnerable subgroups of the U.S. population.

Despite the overall growth in the economy that began in 1983, the number of children in poverty increased by more than 2.2 million from 1979 to 1989. In 1989, around twelve million, or one out of five (19.6 percent of) children, were in poverty. For very young children (younger than six), the proportion was even higher (22.5 percent). The percent of poor children was much greater for African-American (43.7 percent) and Hispanic (36.2 percent) compared to white (14.8 percent) children. The rates of increase in child poverty were particularly high among Hispanics. Nonetheless, the vast majority (7.6 million or 63 percent) of poor children in 1989 were white (Children's Defense Fund, 1991a).

The Children's Defense Fund estimated that only one in fifty-six poor children fit the popular stereotype of child poverty: poor black children in female-headed families in the central city, on AFDC, born to teenage mothers who did not work during the previous year. Nearly two out of three poor families with children in 1989 had at least one worker. The total earned income for these families was more than twice as great as the income they received through means-tested public assistance programs. About one in five poor families with children had a household head who worked full time but still did not earn enough to lift the family out of poverty. Nearly five million of the twelve million poor children lived in married-couple families.

Families headed by women, high school dropouts, or persons younger than age twenty-five still face the greatest risks of living in poverty, however. Employment opportunities and earning potential during the previous decade have been most sharply reduced for young workers, particularly males, those with less than a high school education, and minorities. Young men between the ages of twenty and twenty-nine who cannot earn enough to support a family are three to four times less likely to marry than those with adequate earnings. Among those who are married, at the time of divorce the man's economic status is generally enhanced and the woman's diminished. An Urban Institute study, for example, found that whereas the living standards for women and children fell to two-thirds of their former levels, the average man was slightly better off after a divorce (Burkhauser & Duncan, 1988).

Though a much greater proportion of women, and particularly women who are single parents, have entered the labor force in recent years, women continue to earn lower average incomes than do men. For female heads of families who are on public assistance, the level of benefits has not kept pace with inflation. The real value of the median state's maximum monthly AFDC payment declined some 37 percent between 1970 and 1989, to $360 for a

family of three (or only 46 percent of the 1988 poverty threshold). Though
social security has greatly reduced the rates of poverty among the elderly,
older women — and particularly minority women living alone — are much
more likely to have incomes below the poverty level than are majority males
and/or those living with others (Children's Defense Fund, 1990, 1991a; Commonwealth Fund Commission on Elderly People Living Alone, 1988; Levitan, 1990).

　　　This review of the profile and trends in the characteristics of the U.S.
population has highlighted increasing social and economic vulnerability in
general and for certain subgroups of Americans in particular.

Cross-Cutting Issues

An assessment of the impact of social status, social capital, and human capital resources on the risks of poor physical, psychological, and/or social health
confirms that these factors have played an important role in exacerbating
the vulnerability of many subgroups of U.S. society.

Social Status

Infants and children whose mothers are in economically and socially impoverished circumstances are at a particularly high risk of having poor health
(including cognitive or physical impairments, AIDS, or perinatal addiction)
or being homeless. Adolescents in general are vulnerable because they are
at a critical natural juncture in their own physical, emotional, and social
development, which could, however, be made more problematic if they are
in chaotic, addictive, or abusive family situations.

　　　The elderly often suffer a variety of losses, including economic self-
sufficiency, physical or cognitive function, or the support and care of loved
ones due to death or serious illness. These losses put many elderly in a position of particular vulnerability as they look to others for help and find that
it is not forthcoming or is more hurtful than helpful, or, in some cases, feel
that the significance of these losses leads them to consider taking their own lives.

　　　Both men and women are made vulnerable by social sex-role expectations. Single mothers are particularly vulnerable because child-care responsibilities may make it difficult for them to work full time. Even if they are
working, they are very likely to earn less than a male breadwinner would;
the child's father is likely to be providing little if any support; and, if the
mother does qualify for AFDC, the actual benefits are very limited. Family
abuse and violence is directly rooted in the traditional economic and power-
dependence relationships assumed between men, women, and children. Acts
of violence within families often represent attempts on the part of those whom
society sanctions as having power over others (husbands, parents of children, adult children of the elderly) to reinforce this position of dominance.

　　　Drinking, smoking, and using drugs is the "macho" thing to do in many adolescent and young adult male subcultures. Elderly white males and young minority males may experience either diminished or blocked opportunities, respectively, to the job-related rewards of money, prestige, or accompanying sense of power or self-esteem. A consequence for many is a violent death—either at their own hand or as a result of violent encounters with others, many of whom are from within their own circle of acquaintances.

The roots of minorities' economic and social disadvantage lie deep in the soil of American social and political history. Less than two generations of African Americans have been born since the civil rights activities of the 1960s and early 1970s led to removing many racial barriers to jobs, schools, and housing that had evolved over ten generations of overt racial discrimination.

Similarly, Native Americans residing on reservations have been in a status of mandated dependency on federal prerogatives for generations, following the successes of the U.S. domestic policy of winning the West for Anglo homesteaders and immigrants. Ironically, many twentieth-century immigrants to the United States (a large number of whom are Hispanic or Asian minorities) have also come in search of a home, in response to the economic adversities and political conflict in their own countries, which U.S. foreign policy often helped to exacerbate, if not create.

These historical and political occurrences have had significant social, economic, physical, and psychological impacts on many foreign-born and racial/ethnic communities. U.S. domestic and foreign policies over the past two decades have displayed vacillating levels of commitment and correspondingly mixed results in narrowing the associated racial and ethnic disparities in physical, psychological, and social health and well-being.

Social Capital

The absence of caring others in people's lives makes them especially vulnerable. Pregnant women who lack emotional or material support from the child's father, other family members, or friends are less likely to be in a position to readily care for themselves and their child. Many chronically ill and disabled children and adults would not be able to live in their own homes without the support of family members and friends. Persons with AIDS are particularly likely to experience the rejection or death of affected loved ones.

The prospect of mental illness, substance abuse, and violent behavior is strongly influenced by the nature and quality of connections one has with other people. Individuals who are in chaotic, addictive, or abusive family or social environments are much more likely to manifest these problems and have much less support to draw on to deal with them.

The wounds of broken relationships are particularly deep among abusing families, the homeless, and immigrant and refugee populations. These individuals are especially likely to be bereft of a caring network of family and friends because of emotional estrangement, permanent physical separation, or death.

Human Capital

The investments communities make in good jobs, schools, and housing, and the corollary payoffs to individuals and families in terms of working, getting a good education, and having an adequate place to live, also directly affect vulnerability.

The diminished numbers of well-paying jobs in manufacturing and the movement of businesses and industry out of the core of major U.S. cities have resulted in a substantial loss of employment opportunities and a declining tax base for the support of public education in inner-city neighborhoods. Urban gentrification and U.S. federal housing policy have sharply reduced the availability of affordable housing for low-income individuals and families in these same areas. The result of these and other changes has been the emergence of a hard-core extremely socially and economically disadvantaged underclass, many of whom are very likely to be numbered among the categories of vulnerable populations studied here. These include high-risk mothers and infants; people with chronic physical or mental illness or AIDS; alcohol and drug abusers; victims of suicidal, homicidal, or family violence; and the homeless from within our own country, as well as outside it, who either sought or were forced to leave their homeland (Chicago Tribune Staff, 1986; Ellwood, 1988; Jencks & Peterson, 1991; Katz, 1989; Lynn & McGeary, 1990; Palmer, Smeeding, & Torrey, 1988; Phillips, 1990; Wilson, 1980, 1989, 1990).

The discussion that follows reviews the effects of these social and economic changes on specific groups of the vulnerable. (See Table 4.1.)

Population-Specific Overview

High-Risk Mothers and Infants

The most vulnerable mothers and infants are those in a disadvantaged socioeconomic position, who experience the corollary environmental and behavioral risks associated with poverty (such as unsafe or unsupportive living situations or substance abuse).

Social Status. The relative risks of inadequate prenatal care and adverse pregnancy outcomes were noted earlier (Chapter Three) to be considerably greater for African-American compared to white mothers and infants. Recent research has examined the relative importance of social, biological, and medical factors in accounting for these differences. Substantial evidence exists that both the contemporary and historical effects of poverty and related risks (sanitation, crowding, nutrition, injury, smoking, and substance abuse) and resource disparities (income, insurance coverage) have played a major role in contributing to low-birthweight and infant mortality differentials for African Americans compared to whites (Behrman, 1987; Boone, 1989; Collins

Table 4.1. Principal Community Correlates of Vulnerability.

Vulnerable Populations	Community Correlates		
	Social status	Social capital	Human capital
High-risk mothers and infants	Minorities Adolescent and young women	Unmarried female-head of family	<High school education Poor
Chronically ill and disabled	Minority children Elderly women	Female-headed families Living alone	<High school education Blue-collar job Poor Substandard housing
Persons with AIDS	Minority men, women, children	Weak social networks	<High school education Unemployed Poor
Mentally ill and disabled	Minorities Adolescents, elderly	Separated, divorced, widowed	Unemployed Poor Substandard housing
Alcohol or substance abusers	Minorities Adolescent and young men	Single, separated, divorced	<High school education Unemployed Poor
Suicide- or homicide-prone	*Suicide* Adolescent and elderly white men *Homicide* Adolescent and young minority men	Single, separated, divorced, widowed Single	Unemployed Unemployed Poor
Abusing families	Infants, children, adolescents, elderly Girls and women	Weak social networks Not member of voluntary organizations	<High school education (especially women) Unemployed
Homeless	Infants, children, adolescents Women Minorities	Living alone Female-headed families Single, separated, divorced Weak social networks Not member of voluntary organizations	Unemployed Poor Substandard housing
Immigrants and refugees	Infants, children Women Minorities	Single, widowed Weak social networks Not member of voluntary organizations	<High school education Unemployed Poor Substandard housing

& David, 1990; Davis, 1988; Geronimus & Bound, 1990; Kessel, Kleinman, Koontz, Hogue, & Berendes, 1988; Kleinman & Kessel, 1987; Mayberry & Lewis, 1990; Yankauer, 1990).

The higher postneonatal mortality rates observed for Native Americans relative to whites are similarly related to the poorer socioeconomic conditions and associated problems experienced by Native American populations (unsafe environments, unemployment, family disorganization, and alcoholism) (Honigfeld & Kaplan, 1987).

The fact that Hispanics have lower rates of prenatal care utilization, in tandem with lower infant mortality rates, is hypothesized to be due to cultural factors that inhibit the operation of certain other risk factors associated with high-risk pregnancies (such as out-of-wedlock births and maternal smoking and alcohol use) (Scribner & Dwyer, 1989; Smith, 1986).

Social Capital. Well-developed social networks help to mediate stress in general and provide resources to cope with the fact of being pregnant in particular. Such networks can, however, either encourage or discourage a woman from seeking prenatal care—depending on the particular attitudes or beliefs of network members. Inner-city African-American women are more likely to be unmarried, to rely on female relatives or friends, and to feel a lack of social, emotional, and material support during their pregnancy. The presence (or absence) of strong social networks can directly affect whether they receive encouragement or support (child care, for example) to seek prenatal care (Boone, 1985, 1989; St. Clair, Smeriglio, Alexander, & Celentano, 1989; Turner, Grindstaff, & Phillips, 1990).

Human Capital. Mothers with less than a high school education are much more likely to have inadequate prenatal care and poor pregnancy outcomes (IOM, 1985, 1988d). The impact of the mother's education has been variously attributed to its correlation with the father's education, family income, a higher probability of being employed, a greater awareness of preventive health practices, and/or more coping resources (Cleland & van Ginneken, 1988; Cramer, 1987). Based on analyses of data from United Nations-sponsored surveys in over thirty countries, Cleland and van Ginneken (1988) estimated that the economic advantages associated with the mother's education (such as having adequate income and housing) accounted for about half of education-related differentials observed in infant and child mortality rates.

Chronically Ill and Disabled

The availability of social, economic, and community resources directly affects the prospects for physical, psychological, and social functioning among the chronically ill and disabled of all ages.

Social Status. Chronically ill children have recently been characterized as "children with special needs" (Palfrey, Singer, Walker, & Butler, 1987) or "special health care needs" (Shelton, Jeppson, & Johnson, 1989). These include the traditional categories of children who are crippled or handicapped, as well as an increasingly prevalent number of those with "new morbidities," such as developmental, learning, and behavioral problems, eating disorders, allergies, and asthma—conditions thought to have large psychosocial components attributed to the growing proportion of children who experience parental divorce, are born to single-parent families, or are raised in low-income, low-education households (Newacheck, Budetti, & McManus, 1984; Newacheck, Budetti, & Halfon, 1986; Zill & Schoenborn, 1990).

The risks of death or disability from injury are much greater for poor and minority (particularly African-American and Native American) children compared to white, nonpoor children (Centers for Disease Control, 1990b). The risks of having no or inadequate prenatal care, less than an optimum birthweight, or congenital or birth-associated disabilities are greater for minority and economically disadvantaged mothers and infants. Some disability (such as ventilator dependency) is, in fact, created by the high-technology interventions employed to save high-risk newborns (OTA, 1987b).

The probability of being disabled increases substantially with age. However, an emerging emphasis in public health and health care research emphasizes the causes and correlates of functional disability among the elderly and the interventions most likely to "compress morbidity" (Olshansky & Ault, 1986), enhance "successful aging" (Roos & Havens, 1991), and/or increase "quality-adjusted life years (QALYs)" (Rothenberg & Koplan, 1990).

Nonetheless, the increasing feminization of poverty, particularly among the elderly, as well as the growing proportion of elderly women living alone, compounds the prospect of poor health and associated functional dependence for women as they age (Commonwealth Fund Commission on Elderly People Living Alone, 1987, 1988; Stone, 1989).

Social Capital. A great deal of research has focused on the impact of caregiving and social support available to the elderly from family or friends for enhancing the prospect of maximum functioning and particularly for reducing the need for institutionalized care. The physiological and psychological benefits appear to be greatest when this care maximizes the individual's own perceived goals and capacity for independence (Gibson & Jackson, 1987; Krause, 1987; Magaziner & Cadigan, 1988; Manton, 1989; Stoller, 1984; Ward, 1985).

Human Capital. The jobs working-age adults assume affect the likelihood of their being injured and subsequently unable to work. Griss (1988) pointed out that among all persons eighteen to sixty-four with a work disability, 87.7 percent were disabled during their working-age years, while only 12.3 percent were disabled at birth or during childhood. The majority (63.1 percent) were employed at the onset of disability. Among those for whom their disability resulted from an injury, about half of these injuries (45.6 percent) occurred on the job. The working-age disabled are more likely to have less than a high school education, to be poor, and to have been employed in blue-collar jobs than are their nondisabled counterparts (International Center for the Disabled, 1986; Office of Assistant Secretary for Planning and Evaluation, 1989). The incidence of injury tends to be highest for laborers—particularly those involved in the construction and mining industries (NCHS, 1989b). Increases in the reported prevalence of work-related disability have been attributed to the increased availability of benefits as well as a greater tendency on the part of the disabled to file for them (Chirikos, 1986; Wolfe & Haveman, 1990; Yelin, 1986).

Fear of being victimized by crime prevents many elderly disabled, in particular, from continuing to live in their own homes and communities (International Center for the Disabled, 1986). Adaptations to their "built environment" (housing) are also often required to maximize the ability of disabled elderly and others to function on their own (Manton, 1989).

Persons with AIDS

A complex profile of social and economic disadvantage has contributed to the spread of AIDS—particularly among minority men, women, and children.

Social Status. The growing impoverishment of nonwhite women and those who are single parents has contributed to increased stress, the corollary use of alcohol or drugs, and—in an increasing number of cases—prostitution or drug-related activity to earn money. High rates of unemployment and associated increases in drug-related activity among minority males have correspondingly increased their risk of contracting AIDS. The sharing of needles for illicit drug injections or even sharing sewing needles for cosmetic purposes, such as do-it-yourself tattoos or ear piercing, is also more likely to occur among the poor (OMH, 1990; Primm, 1990).

Social Capital. The advent of AIDS has called into question the traditional concepts of family and social supports available to mediate the stress that leads to high-risk behavior, as well as to assist in caring for those with the illness. Infants and children with AIDS face the prospect of being abandoned by their families. This is because the parents, who are themselves likely to be infected with AIDS, either have died or are physically, financially, or otherwise not able to take on the burden of caring for the infant (Division of Maternal and Child Health, 1987). The emergence from the closet of a well-kept family secret when a young homosexual male contracts the disease has challenged the capacity of many families and communities to deal openly with the issue. The resulting discrimination and fear of reprisal has tended to drive many at-risk individuals underground, instead of encouraging them to seek appropriate information or counsel (Fox, 1986; Levine, 1990; Macklin, 1989; van Steijn, 1989).

Effective social networks among the gay community in San Francisco seem to have facilitated the sharing of information requisite to reducing the prevalence of high-risk sexual practices (Ekstrand & Coates, 1990). Much less understanding exists of the social organization of the high-risk population of HIV drug users and their sexual partners, to assess how these networks might be used in developing or targeting educational or behavioral interventions.

Human Capital. African-American and Hispanic teenagers have less accurate knowledge of how AIDS can be transmitted than do white teenagers (DiClemente, Boyer, & Morales, 1988). The dropout rates for minority adolescents are also higher than those of whites, so that they are less likely to have the benefit of school-based sex or AIDS education programs. Community-based educational efforts also often fail to orient their messages to the unique language, literacy, or cultural aspects of high-risk racial/ethnic communities. There is also a resistance to such educational programs, as well as to the attendance of HIV-infected children, in many public school systems — as in the case of Ryan White of Kokomo, Indiana, who contracted AIDS through a hemophilia-related transfusion (Kirp et al., 1989).

In the early stages of the epidemic, persons with AIDS were often dismissed from their jobs, with a resultant loss in income and insurance benefits required to obtain adequate medical care. In 1989, amendments to the civil rights bill barred dismissals from employment due to having AIDS and levied fines on companies that did so (APHA, 1989). Yelin, Greenblatt, Hollander, & McMaster (1991) found, in a study in San Francisco, that nonetheless half of those with HIV-related illness were physically unable to continue working two years after the onset of symptoms.

Mentally Ill and Disabled

The dominant model in the study of the psychosocial causes of mental illness emphasizes the role that stressful life events play in producing mental illness. This applies particularly to events that require a great deal of change by adaptation — positive events such as marriage as well as negative ones such as the loss of a spouse. Both social resources (such as social support) and personal resources (such as a sense of personal control or mastery) can mediate the effects of these stresses (Rosenfield, 1989). The stresses and the resources for dealing with them are, however, differentially distributed by age and sex, minority status, poverty level, family structure, and employment status.

Social Status. Data from the ECA study showed that adolescence and young adulthood are important periods for the onset of major mental illness, such as unipolar major depression, bipolar illness, phobias, and drug and alcohol abuse/dependence (K. C. Burke, J. D. Burke, Regier, & Rae, 1990). The major stressors associated with the onset of mental illness in children include poverty, minority-group status, having parents who were mentally ill or alcoholic, living in divorced or single-parent families, having been phys-ically or sexually abused, or having a major chronic illness (OTA, 1986).

The prevalence of most mental illnesses, except for cognitive impair-ment, has been found to be greater among noninstitutionalized younger adults than among the elderly. Those elderly who were in good health, were better educated, and had higher incomes were in particular less likely to experi-ence mental illness (Blazer, 1989; Feinson, 1989; Haug, Belgrave, & Grat-ton, 1984; Weissman et al., 1985).

Research has focused on trying to explain the findings that married women appear to have more mental illness than unmarried women, while the reverse is true for married men. Explanations have emphasized both the greater likelihood that men who are mentally ill will not be selected for marriage, as well as the traditional role expectations in marriage that tend to limit women's opportunities and increase the stress associated with filling multiple roles (housework, child care, and outside employment) (Dean & Ensel, 1983; Kessler & McRae, 1984). On the other hand, there is evidence that poor single female heads of households experience particularly high levels of stress and mental illness, as a result of both diminished social sup-port and the increased environmental stressors associated with poverty (Ben-nett, 1988).

The effects of minority status on mental health are associated with the influence of socioeconomic disadvantage. Baker (1987) has pointed out that the mental health of African Americans at all stages of the life cycle is affected by their membership in a "victim system," which includes histori-cal and existing barriers to equivalent educational and job opportunities. These in turn limit educational and economic attainment, which in turn lead to poverty and exacerbate the stress on both individuals and families. A num-ber of studies comparing minorities (particularly African Americans and Hispanics) and whites have found that, after controlling for age, sex, edu-cation, and income, differences in mental health status observed between racial or ethnic groups tend to diminish or disappear (Golding & Lipton, 1990; Roberts & Vernon, 1984; Vega, Kolody, Hough, & Figueroa, 1987).

The major stressors that have been found to be associated with greater mental illness among Native Americans, particularly children, include recur-rent otitis media (middle ear infections) and the consequences for learning disabilities and psychosocial deficits, fetal alcohol syndrome, physical and sexual abuse and neglect, parental alcoholism, family disruption, and poor school environments (McShane, 1988; OTA, 1990b).

Social Capital. Family disruption (through death or divorce, for example) has been found to be associated with a greater prevalence of both adult and childhood mental disorders. Based on the Duke ECA study, the six-month prevalence of panic attacks was found to be significantly higher among those who experienced the death of their mother or parental separation/divorce early in childhood (Tweed, Schoenbach, George, & Blazer, 1989). Individuals who lack social support, either from family or other sources, have been found to experience more stress and hence greater mental illness than those who did not have this stress-buffering resource available to them. This was particularly the case for individuals who lacked personal coping resources as well (such as feelings of self-esteem and personal mastery) (Rosenfield, 1989).

Human Capital. Two major theoretical explanations — social stress and social selection — have traditionally been used to account for the greater prevalence of mental illness among lower–socioeconomic status (SES) individuals. The social stress explanation suggests that rates of some types of disorders are higher in lower-SES groups because of the greater environmental adversity they experience (such as unemployment, inadequate housing, crime). The social selection explanation argues, particularly with respect to rates of schizophrenia, that persons with these disorders or characteristics predisposing them to these disorders (probably genetic in origin) drift down or fail to rise out of the lower-SES groups.

Dohrenwend (1990) has pointed out that contemporary psychiatric epidemiology has tended to focus on the micro-level individual/psychological correlates of stress, rather than macro-level environmental/societal correlates, such as SES. He argues, however, for a more in-depth, analytical look in understanding both the structural and psychological dynamics of socioeconomic status that could account for the persistent differences by SES. For example, unemployment, particularly chronic unemployment as well as the lowered self-esteem resulting, have been found to be associated with poorer mental health status.

Alcohol or Substance Abusers

The origins of substance abuse have been examined from both developmental and cultural perspectives. That is, they have been considered from the point of view of the contributions of particular events in an individual's normal life course (adolescence, aging) as well as the values and norms derived from families, peers, and/or the larger social environment (drinking attitudes and practices) (Lawson & Lawson, 1989).

Social Status. Adolescence is a period in which a high probability exists for initiating drinking, smoking, and/or the use of drugs. This stage of development is characterized by more risk taking in general in the context of the normal developmental task of transition to the independence of adulthood, as well as a heightened susceptibility to the influence of peers on behavior. The initiation of the use of certain substances during the teen years (such as alcohol, smokeless tobacco, or marijuana) appears to increase the propensity, or serve as a "gateway," for the use of more serious or addictive drugs (such as cigarettes or cocaine) later. Excessive use of these gateway substances and/or progression to more serious substance abuse or dependence is often associated with a complex of other problem behaviors (such as poor school performance, truancy, or delinquent criminal behavior) (Archambault, 1989; Bailey & Hubbard, 1990; Barrett, Simpson, & Lehman, 1988; Cleary, Hitchcock, Semmer, Flinchbaugh, & Pinney, 1988; Dent, Sussman, Johnson, Hansen, & Flay, 1987; Henderson & Anderson, 1989; Jones & Battjes, 1990b; Lettieri & Ludford, 1981; Macdonald, 1987; Maddahian, Newcomb, & Bentler, 1986; Robinson et al., 1987).

Adolescence is also a period of transition toward separation from family. Research suggests that at other stages of the life course as well, separation, loss, or isolation from family or caring others—through divorce or death—can give rise to the onset of serious substance abuse problems. The elderly frequently suffer from excessive use of prescribed, as well as over-the-counter, drugs. Though the elderly have lower rates of use of alcohol in general, around 2 to 10 percent of the elderly are estimated to have problems with alcohol abuse or dependence. For some elderly, late-onset alcoholism may be a response to serious losses of physical, psychological, and/or social functioning (Glantz, Peterson, & Whittington, 1983; Lawson & Lawson, 1989).

The pattern of distribution of mental health and related substance abuse disorders by sex is also influenced by varying gender and family roles. Underlying affective disorders are more often manifested in substance abuse (alcoholism and drug abuse) among men and in clinical depression among women (Regier et al., 1990; Robbins, 1989). Some data suggest that women who work may have higher rates of alcohol use than those who do not—perhaps due to the role conflicts and strains associated with trying to fulfill traditional family or child-care responsibilities, as well as make it in a "man's world" (Beschner & Thompson, 1981; Fellios, 1989; Glynn, Pearson, & Sayers, 1983).

Cultural factors play a large role in influencing the patterns of substance use and abuse for different racial/ethnic groups. The use of certain drugs (such as peyote) has been a component of traditional religious and spiritual practices in some Hispanic and Native American subcultures. The role of alcohol in the social life of different racial/ethnic subgroups (such as the Irish, Italian, Muslim, and Jewish cultures) also influences the levels and patterns of consumption across these groups. Both advertising and cultural norms attribute desired sex-role characteristics (such as the image of being "macho" for males or "liberated" for women) to smoking or the use of smokeless tobacco. Excessive consumption of alcohol or other drugs has also been viewed as a means for minority groups, which have historically been subject to social, economic, and political discrimination by the dominant culture, to cope with the resultant powerlessness, dependency, and destruction of community identity (Austin, Johnson, Carroll, & Lettieri, 1977; Babor & Mendelson, 1986; Beauvais, Oetting, Wolf, & Edwards, 1989; Brown & Tooley, 1989; Caetano, 1988; Davis, 1987; Eden & Aguilar, 1989; Fiore et al., 1989; Hill, 1989; Krug, 1989; Lindenthal & Miller, 1989; Moncher, Holden, & Trimble, 1990; Schinke, Moncher, Palleja, Zayer, & Schilling, 1988; Spiegler, Tate, Aitken, & Christian, 1989; Trimble, Padilla, & Bell, 1987; Westermeyer & Neider, 1986).

Social Capital. Families play a significant role in the development and transmission of substance use and abuse practices. Research has demonstrated a genetic link with alcohol and, to some extent, drug use. The impact of biological vulnerability on alcohol and drug abuse is, however, intertwined with the corollary influences of the family and larger social and cultural environment of which the individual is a part (Glynn, 1980; Gordis, 1987–88; Kress, 1989; Moore, 1986; Pickens & Svikis, 1988; Plant, Orford, & Grant, 1989; Reich, Cloninger, Van Eerdewegh, Rice, & Mullaney, 1988; Zucker & Gomberg, 1986).

Substantial evidence exists that both the presence and quality of family ties and the attitudes and practices of the families themselves are correlated with individuals members' propensity to drink, smoke, or use drugs. Rates of alcoholism, smoking, and drug use are higher among adults and children in families in which the parents are divorced or separated or in which there is considerable family dysfunction or disorganization. Substance abuse may, however, be either a cause or a consequence of family dysfunction and dissolution (Beschner & Thompson, 1981; Fellios, 1989; Glynn, Pearson, & Sayers, 1983; Selnow, 1987; Waldron & Lye, 1989). An analysis of data from the CDC Behavioral Risk Factor Surveys in twenty-six states showed that, overall, unmarried women were considerably more likely to smoke during their pregnancy than were their married counterparts (Williamson, Serdula, Kendrick, & Binkin, 1989).

Human Capital. The patterns of substance use and abuse by income and education vary for different substances. The prevalence of smoking is less among those with higher levels of education and income, while the opposite is the case for the use of alcohol. Cocaine was traditionally a drug of the rich and heroin that of the poor. The availability of crack and other cheaper forms of cocaine has resulted in its wider use among low-income populations (Escobedo, Anda, Smith, Remington, & Mast, 1990; Lawson & Lawson, 1989).

Unemployment and underemployment are both correlates and consequences of substance (particularly alcohol and drug) abuse. Rates of substance abuse are higher among the unemployed. Lost earnings potential is also substantial for those who are unable to work regularly because of problems with alcoholism, drugs, or smoking-related illnesses (Mullahy & Sindelar, 1989). On the other hand, being employed can present a double hazard for smokers who work in occupations for which there is also a high risk of exposure to dust, fumes, and/or toxic chemicals (Sterling & Weinkam, 1989).

Suicide- or Homicide-Prone

Biological, psychological, and sociological explanations have been offered for intentional acts of violence that culminate in suicides or homicides. A number of biochemical indicators have been found to be correlated with suicidal intentions or acts (Hendin, 1987; Holinger & Offer, 1981; Maris, 1986; Nordlicht, 1986). Biopsychiatric models have examined the role of aggression in human development and behavior. Psychiatrically or psychologically oriented explanations of suicide and/or homicide have explored the role of losses or of separation from significant love objects, poor self-esteem, mental illness, and substance abuse (Dukes & Lorch, 1989; Holinger & Offer, 1981; Kreitman, 1988; Rudd, 1990; Stark, 1990). Nonetheless, strong support exists for sociological explanations of violence—which emphasize the impact of social status (age, sex, race), social integration (or support), and ecological (labor market) factors.

Social Status. Based on 1978–1984 vital statistics data from the National Center for Health Statistics, suicide clusters (unusually high numbers of suicides occurring in a small area in a brief time period) were found to be two to four times more common among adolescents and young adults than among other age groups (Gould, Wallenstein, Kleinman, O'Carroll, & Mercy, 1990).

Some investigators have pointed directly to the effects of poverty, sexism, and racism and the resultant differentials in wealth and power as predictors of violence (Gibbs, 1988; McDowall, 1986; Rosenberg, Gelles, et al., 1987; Sanborn, 1990; Stark, 1990; Williams, 1984).

Stark (1990) argued that interpersonal violence is basically a "friendly affair" rooted in patterns of male-female and related power dominance and abuse. Children who are abused or grow up in environments in which they witness substantial violence are more likely to perpetuate these patterns in their own adult lives (Sadoff, 1986; Straus, 1986). More than half of all homicide victims are killed by someone they know (CDC, 1990f).

As with other groups, among Hispanics, suicidal tendencies have been found to be higher among those with psychiatric diagnoses, those with alcohol and drug abuse, and/or those who were divorced or separated (Fernandez-Pol, 1986; Kraus, Sorenson, & Juarez, 1988; Sorenson & Golding, 1988). However, cultural factors such as families (a strong orientation toward the authority and ties of family) and fatalism (attribution of circumstances to factors that humans are powerless to change) have been credited with moderating suicide rates for Hispanics as a whole (Hoppe & Martin, 1986).

The risk factors associated with higher rates of suicide among Native Americans similarly include a history of mental health problems, having another family member or friend who committed suicide, alcohol problems, and a history of sexual or physical abuse (Grossman, Milligan, & Deyo, 1991). The collapse of traditional Native American ways of life and religion, high unemployment, and sending children to boarding schools have been credited with exacerbating chaotic family structures and associated substance abuse that give rise to higher rates of suicide and interpersonal violence (Berlin, 1985, 1987).

Social Capital. Durkheim posited the role of social integration (or ties) with others (through families, friendships, neighborhoods, work or voluntary associations, for example), as predictors of suicidal behavior. He identified three types of suicide that could result from (1) isolation from a human community (egoistic), (2) total identification with such a community to the extent that one's own self-interests are denied (altruistic), or (3) ambiguity and uncertainty regarding one's roles in or contributions to such a community as a result of major political or economic changes (anomic) (Gibbs, 1988; Kreitman, 1988).

Homicide and suicide rates are higher among individuals in chaotic or abusive family environments (Asarnow & Carlson, 1988; Heath, Kruttschnitt, & Ward, 1986; Rudd, 1990; Tolan, 1988). The high suicide rates among the elderly have been attributed to illness, economic insecurity, and the "losses" and associated loneliness, isolation, and depression that result from the death of a spouse or adult children moving away during this stage of life (Achté, 1988; Osgood & McIntosh, 1986).

Human Capital. Ecological explanations have focused on the role of broad economic or demographic trends, such as the unemployment or competition resulting from downturns in the economy and/or a large age cohort seeking access to limited employment or educational opportunities (Araki & Murata, 1986, 1987; Dooley, Catalano, Rook, & Serxner, 1989a, 1989b). The availability and ownership of firearms have also been found to be highly associated with violent death rates (Lester, 1988; Markush & Bartolucci, 1984; Mercy & Houk, 1988; Sloan et al., 1988).

The increased rates of male (particularly young white male) suicides in recent years have been attributed to the increased ambiguity and loss of power associated with changing sex roles. Other factors include the increasing difficulties in general, given shifts in the U.S. economy, in finding and retaining well-paying jobs (Holinger & Offer, 1981; Sanborn, 1990). Increased rates of violence turned inward (suicide) have resulted because white males tend to blame themselves for perceived personal, educational, and/or professional failures, since societal expectations and objective opportunities for success have traditionally been greater for them (Osgood & McIntosh, 1986).

The increased rates of violence turned outward (homicide) among black males have been attributed to responses to blocked opportunities, exacerbated and sustained by a poor economy, continuing racial and socioeconomic discrimination, diminished levels of investments in inner-city schools and institutions, and the growth of the drug economy in many minority neighborhoods. Approximately one in four young African-American males in their twenties is in jail or otherwise under the control of the criminal court, for example (Gurr, 1989; Savage, 1990).

Abusing Families

Victims of family abuse are especially "vulnerable," according to the concept of vulnerability developed here (Figure 1.1): "regardless of age, victims of family violence often share a dependence for their very survival upon someone who harms them" (Straus, 1988, p. 3). Further, the principal correlates of family violence are rooted in the differential availability of personal, social, and human resources (Figure 1.2): the social inequality associated with the statuses of age, gender, race, and income, among others, and the social isolation of families and individuals reinforced by norms of privacy and patriarchal dominance that have traditionally governed family life in our and other societies (Gelles & Cornell, 1990; Pagelow, 1984; Quinn & Tomita, 1986; Scheper-Hughes, 1987; Straus, 1988).

Social Status. Initially, child abuse was identified and defined as a medical problem based on the evidence gathered by physicians in the early 1960s and 1970s of childhood injuries that clearly resulted from externally imposed trauma. This early characterization led to the medical/clinical identification of the "battered child syndrome." It also led to the exploration of the causes of this and other forms of violence among intimates from individually oriented psychiatric and psychopathological perspectives on the mental health of the batterer (Helfer & Kempe, 1987). In recent years, with the availability of more empirical evidence on the perpetrators as well as the victims of intimate violence, theory development in this area has shifted from micro- (individual) to more macro- (societal) levels of explanations and analysis. These include perspectives that emphasize patterns of abuse or neglect as learned behaviors that lead to intergenerational cycles of violence (social learning theory). They also take into account the fact that there are rewards (such as control and dominance) as well as costs (risk of arrest) associated with such behaviors (exchange theory). Finally, these approaches proceed from the assumption that fundamental social inequalities, such as those associated with men's and women's sex roles and differential access to wealth in our society, help to empower and sanction a culture of intrafamily and interpersonal violence (social-situational or social systems theory).

Typically, wide power differentials exist between the subject and object of maltreatment, linked to the social statuses they occupy respectively. Further, maltreatment most often occurs at the interstices where the relative power differentials between groups tends to be the greatest (parent-to-child, husband-to-wife, and caretaker–to–dependent elderly). Patterned modes of interaction between these groups that lead to violence are clearly rooted in long-standing historical, sociocultural, and/or social-structural norms. Tenets such as "spare the rod and spoil the child" and related child-rearing practices have been and continue to be endorsed in many U.S. families. The "rule of thumb" refers to eighteenth-century law that a husband had the right to physically chastise his wife, as long as the stick or strap for doing so was no wider than his thumb. Patriarchal systems of family organization have traditionally assumed that the male is the head of the family, that boys must be trained to be manly and dominant and that girls learn to be feminine and submissive.

Social Capital. Social isolation is also a defining characteristic of many abusing families. The families in which child or spousal abuse occurs are much less likely to participate in organized community or religious activities or to have informal social ties with neighbors or other friendship networks. The abused elderly are particularly likely to be invisible, since they may have been relocated from their own homes to be cared for by a child or other relative and are less likely to participate in external activities, such as going to work regularly, that would carry them into contact with other people. Further, the perpetrators of maltreatment often use force or intimidation to insulate their victims from social contact and thereby avoid detection.

Human Capital. Empirical evidence regarding the perpetrators and victims of maltreatment points clearly to the socioeconomic origins of the problem. The profile of abusive families outlined in Chapter Three highlighted the fact that rates of abuse were highest in those families in which poverty and related unemployment or underemployment and inadequate housing were problematic. They were also highest where the male head of the household experienced considerable status insecurity or inconsistency relative to his desired goals and expectations. The risk of intrafamilial violence is also exacerbated when the women involved have less education or occupational skills for achieving economic self-sufficiency and thus lack the means for removing themselves from the abusive situation (Gelles, 1987a, 1987b; Hotaling, Finkelhor, Kirkpatrick, & Straus, 1988a, 1988b).

The dependence of elderly on others resulting from the loss of physical or cognitive functioning, and the corollary loss of power and control over personal or financial resources, has been found to be associated with caregivers' propensity to abuse or neglect their dependent charges (Johnson, O'Brien, & Hudson, 1985; Quinn & Tomita, 1986; Steinmetz, 1988).

These and a variety of other reported correlates of intrafamilial abuse or neglect (such as alcoholism or the intergenerational transmission of learned behaviors) are not singularly determinant of these outcomes. Further, a substantial proportion of families that possess all of a series of characteristics still do *not* evidence these behaviors.

We need to mediate the harm to some of the most vulnerable in our society—those who are dependent for their very survival on intimate others who injure or neglect them. A logical first step is to examine the elements of the social structure that promote and sanction the power and dominance of certain individuals over others and reinforce the isolation, rather than the ties, between people.

Homeless

The major reason for the increase in homeless men, women, and children in the 1980s and 1990s is the diminished availability of affordable housing. This problem disproportionately affects people who are poor and/or at risk due to other limitations in physical, psychological, or social functioning (such as mental illness, substance abuse, or family violence).

Social Status. Social, political, and economic trends have made it increasingly difficult for low-income people to afford a roof over their heads, and a diminished stock of low-income housing has increased the price of remaining units (Bingham, Green, & White, 1987; Caton, 1990; CDF, 1991c; IOM, 1988c; Momeni, 1989, 1990; Ropers, 1988; Rossi, 1989, 1990; U.S. Congress, Senate Committee on Labor and Human Resources, 1990).

Children and youth are an increasingly visible and vulnerable component of the homeless population. An estimated 68,000 to 100,000 children are thought to be homeless at any given point in time. Homeless children are much more likely to experience physical, mental, emotional, educational, developmental, and behavioral problems, and they are less likely to have obtained basic preventive health care services, such as immunizations, compared to children who are not homeless (Alperstein & Arnstein, 1988; Alperstein, Rappaport, & Flanigan, 1988; American Academy of Pediatrics, Committee on Community Health Services, 1988; Bassuk & Rubin, 1987; CDF, 1991c; GAO, 1989d, 1989f; Hu, Covell, Morgan, & Arcia, 1989; Miller & Lin, 1988; National Resource Center on Homelessness and Mental Illness, 1990; Shulsinger, 1990; Wood, Valdez, Hayashi, & Shen, 1990).

Very young children are likely to be accompanied by their mothers. However, there are an increasing number of "runaway," "throwaway," or "homeless" youth (older children and teenagers) as well, living on their own with little or no contact with kin. Many such youth literally deem themselves homeless, rather than runaway, since their families have forcibly expelled them from their homes. These families are often ones in which there were problems of physical, sexual, substance, or other abuse (Adams, Gullotta, & Clancy, 1985; AMA, 1989; GAO, 1989d, 1989f; Hermann, 1988; Pennbridge, Yates, David, & Mackenzie, 1990; U.S. Congress, House Select Committee on Children, Youth, and Families, 1990; U.S. Congress, Senate Subcommittee on Children, Family, Drugs, and Alcoholism, 1990).

Women and minorities are also particularly vulnerable groups of homeless. The prevalence of mental illness appears to be greater among homeless women, while alcohol and substance abuse are more prevalent among homeless men—as is the case in the general population. Homeless women are, on the other hand, uniquely vulnerable to unwanted pregnancies, adverse birth outcomes, and sexual and physical assault. The traditional social and economic inequities by race and gender, reinforced by the increasing proportion of women, children, and minorities among the poor, also contribute to the increasing number of these groups among the homeless (Anderson, Boe, & Smith, 1988; Bachrach, 1987; First, Roth, & Arewa, 1988; Hagen & Ivanoff, 1988).

Social Capital. A unique and particularly important characteristic across all categories of the homeless is their social isolation. They are much less likely to have regular or strong social ties with family, friends, or other social networks, which further increases their vulnerability to other disabilities or deprivations. For example, Rossi, Wright, Fisher, & Willis (1987, p. 1339) conclude that "the implication of widespread social isolation is that the literal homeless lack access to extended social networks and are therefore especially vulnerable to the vagaries of fortune occasioned by changes in employment, income, or physical or mental health."

Human Capital. All but two of the cities in the twenty-eight-city 1991 U.S. Conference of Mayors survey cited the lack of affordable housing by low-income persons as a central cause of homelessness in their community (U.S. Conference of Mayors, 1991). Rossi (1990), in contrasting the "old" homeless in the decades from 1950 to 1970 with the "new" homeless, concluded that, although inadequate by any standards, most of the homeless in previous decades had some shelter (flophouses, single-room occupancy hotels, or mission shelters). Very few were literally sleeping on the streets, as do many of the contemporary homeless.

A direct relationship exists between the reduced availability of low-cost housing and the increased number of homeless. Since 1980, the supply of low-income housing has declined by approximately 2.5 million units. Each year, approximately half a million housing units are lost through conversion, abandonment, fire, or demolition. The extremely low rate of replacement of low-income housing has not kept pace with this natural attrition. The reduction of low-income housing stock was in particular accelerated during the 1950s and 1960s. The policy of urban renewal and associated gentrification during that period resulted in the widespread demolition of flophouses and single-room occupancy hotels traditionally occupied by skid row residents. These units were replaced with middle- and upper-class housing (such as condominiums and townhouses) and with shopping or other business complexes (Bingham, Green, & White, 1987; Caton, 1990; Hope & Young, 1986; IOM, 1988c; Momeni, 1989, 1990; Ropers, 1988; Rossi, 1989, 1990; Rossi & Wright, 1987; U.S. Commission on Security and Cooperation in Europe, 1990).

A corollary policy development exacerbating the decline in affordable housing for the poor was the withdrawal of a federal role in subsidizing low-income housing alternatives. From the Depression years until 1980, the federal government was the primary source of low-income housing subsidies. Since 1980, federal support has been reduced over 80 percent, and most of the remaining subsidies represent commitments made prior to 1980. An

IOM report on homelessness concluded, "Federal support for development of new low-income housing has essentially disappeared" (IOM, 1988c, p. 25; Levitan, 1990).

Other factors that have been cited as major contributors to the growing number of homeless are the deinstitutionalization of the chronically mentally ill population, the expanding prevalence of substance abuse, and the increased social isolation resulting from marital dissolution, mobility, and family violence. In his analysis of the old and new homeless, Rossi (1990) pointed out that in some sense these were problems for the old as well as the new homeless. Both the former and current generations of homeless were extremely poor, had tenuous or no ties with families or friends, and suffered from disabilities associated with physical handicaps, alcohol or drug abuse, and mental illness. To the extent that these deprivations and disabilities are becoming more prevalent—particularly for certain subgroups in our society—the likelihood of their being homeless will also increase. However, deinstitutionalization particularly exacerbated the problem of homelessness because of the failure, in implementing this policy, to develop a system of housing and other supportive services before releasing vulnerable mentally ill and disabled individuals into the community (Bingham, Green, & White, 1987; Caton, 1990; Dear & Wolch, 1987; Francis, 1987; IOM, 1988c; Momeni, 1989, 1990; Ropers, 1988; Rossi, 1989, 1990; Rossi & Wright, 1987; Wright, 1988).

Immigrants and Refugees

Refugees and undocumented aliens are particularly vulnerable categories of in-migrants to the United States because of their fewer economic and social resources and ties.

Social Status. Many refugees experience substantial problems in adjusting to life in the United States because of the vast cultural differences with their home countries, as well as the traumatic and violent circumstances often associated with their exodus. For example, the Khmer refugees, many of whom were from rural areas of Cambodia, and the Hmong refugees, who were predominantly subsistence farmers from the mountains of Northern Laos, experience many problems in adjusting to urban life in the United States—many in the most impoverished core of U.S. cities.

In some refugee groups, women are much less likely to have formal education, and therefore are unable to read or write their own language, much less English. The roles traditionally assumed by such women in their own societies are often brutally disrupted by the death of a spouse or other significant family members or by the experiences of rape or sexual assault. The prevalence of depression and posttraumatic stress syndrome is great among certain refugee populations, and particularly refugee women and children, as a result (Ahearn & Athey, 1991; Baughan, White-Baughan, Pickwell, Bartlome, & Wong, 1990; Kulig, 1990; Rodriguez & Urrutia-Rojas, 1990; Westermeyer, 1987; Westermeyer, Callies, & Neider, 1990).

In some groups of immigrants, such as Southeast Asians, bipolar groupings often occur that reflect more socially and economically advantaged versus disadvantaged statuses, based on socioeconomic level, migration cohort, and/or refugee status. The most disadvantaged subgroups are least likely to have had routine preventive care (such as childhood immunizations and dental and prenatal care) and are likely to have the most numerous and most serious health problems, such as gastrointestinal disorders, parasitic infections, respiratory disease, flu, pneumonia, tuberculosis, injuries, or, in the instance of Asian immigrants in particular, sudden unexplained death syndrome (SUDS) and hepatitis (CDC, 1987b, 1987c, 1988d; Fitzpatrick, Johnson, Shragg, & Felice, 1987; Franks et al., 1989; Lin-Fu, 1988; Magar, 1990; Munger, 1987; Rumbaut, Chavez, Moser, Pickwell, & Wishik, 1988; Stehr-Green & Schantz, 1986; Wilk, 1986).

Social Capital. Some subgroups have lost their families in military or guerilla warfare in their home countries. Others are unable to bring family members with them because they are seeking entry illegally or because they lack a means of supporting them once they are in the United States. U.S. immigration policy has contributed to the separation of refugee families, once in the United States, by "scattering" or making sure such populations are broadly dispersed throughout the country (Westermeyer, 1987). They are, as a result, often socially isolated — an isolation that is reinforced by language barriers and, in the instance of undocumented aliens, fear of being discovered by Immigration and Naturalization Service officials.

Immigrants who can enter the United States as refugees from those countries for which such a status is formally granted under U.S. law have greater legal access to systems of support and services than is the case for illegal aliens. As will be seen in Chapter Seven, there are nonetheless many restraints and holes in the safety net of support provided for this group as well.

Human Capital. Many immigrant groups, such as Mexican nationals who migrate to the United States, are pulled by the lure of better jobs and higher wages than are possible in their country of birth. Refugees, such as those from Cuba and Southeast Asia, are pushed out of their home countries because of oppressive domestic or foreign policies and the military conflicts often associated with them. Some groups of undocumented (or illegal) aliens, such as Mexican nationals, leave their country primarily for economic reasons, and others, such as Central American refugees, primarily to escape political or military conflicts. They have, however, not sought permanent legal residence status in the United States — often because of federal immigration policies that preclude their doing so. The groups for which there has been the largest influx of immigrants and refugees during the past two decades (Cuba, Southeast Asia, and Central America) are directly related to U.S. foreign policy and/or military intervention in those areas (Guttmacher, 1984; Lundgren & Lang, 1989; Nicaragua Health Study Collaborative at Harvard, CIES, and UNAN, 1989; Rumbaut, Chavez, Moser, Pickwell, & Wishik, 1988).

Immigrants with an official refugee status have been termed "over-documented," because of the paperwork and screening required to certify their health and prospect for economic self-sufficiency. "Undocumented" aliens obviously have none of these credentials. "Documented" immigrants fall somewhere in between in terms of status and entitlements. They have an official legal status that assures them greater access to better-paying jobs and benefits, such as welfare or Medicaid, than is the case for undocumented immigrants. However, they are forced to earn their way to a greater extent than those with official refugee status. On the other hand, they are more likely to have been pulled from their homeland in search of economic opportunities, rather than pushed out by military or political persecution. Therefore, they may not experience the same magnitude of cultural, social, and psychological disruption and trauma as political refugees would face.

Undocumented aliens have the most tenuous legal and social status, networks of family or community support, and financial or other resources for sustaining themselves in U.S. society. For example, "feet people" (political immigrants from Central America) or "wetbacks" (Mexican nationals who cross the Rio Grande border illegally) — often enter the United States with no possessions other than what they can carry with them. The Immigration Reform and Control Act of 1986 attempted to reduce the flow of undocumented aliens to the United States by imposing sanctions on employers who knowingly hired them (Bean, Vernez, & Keely, 1989).

An undetermined number of illegal aliens continue to work in the United States. They are, however, likely to be employed in the least desirable, lowest-paying jobs — as agricultural day laborers, dish washers, and janitors, or in the garment industry "sweat shops" of big cities, for example. They generally have no job security, health benefits, or salaries that even approximate the minimum wage. They live in crowded, substandard, unsanitary housing in the impoverished areas of large cities, or in Third World–like rural poverty in the colonias along the U.S.-Mexico border (Gibney, 1987; Guttmacher, 1984; Rumbaut, Chavez, Moser, Pickwell, & Wishik, 1988).

The next chapter reviews the programs and services that have been developed to mitigate the vulnerability of these and other subgroups of U.S. society.

5

What Programs Are There
to Address Their Needs?

This chapter identifies the major programs and services that have been developed or proposed to address the health and health care needs of vulnerable populations, in the context of an underlying continuum of care for the vulnerable. This continuum emphasizes that efforts to prevent poor health are just as important as, if not more important than, those to restore maximum functioning for people who already have serious physical, psychological, and social health problems. (See Figure 5.1.)

Figure 5.1. Continuum of Care for Vulnerable Populations.

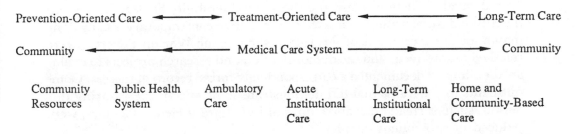

Such a continuum would encompass programs and services to (1) inhibit the onset of problems initially (prevention-oriented care); (2) restore a person who is already affected to maximum functioning (treatment-oriented care); and (3) minimize the deterioration of function for people with problems that are essentially not curable (long-term care). The major assumption underlying this continuum is that people can be made less vulnerable if the objective of maximizing physical, psychological, or social capacity undergirds each stage of the caregiving process.

The programs and services currently available to support this continuum of care for the vulnerable include (1) primary prevention-oriented community resource development and public health programs, (2) treatment-oriented care delivered primarily through the medical care and related professional service delivery systems, and (3) long-term care institutional and community-based programs and services. However, existing programs and services, particularly in the treatment and long-term care sectors, have not necessarily had this broader concept of maximizing patient functioning as either an explicit or an implicit focus. Further, the organization and integration (more often lack of integration) of these programs do not typically acknowledge the development of vulnerability over the life course of individuals. They also neglect the essential roots of vulnerability in the communities from which people emerge and to which they return after being treated by the formal professional service delivery systems.

The discussion of programs in this chapter is, of necessity, illustrative rather than exhaustive. This overview is intended to set the stage for a more evaluative look in the chapters that follow regarding the adequacy, cost, and quality of existing programs and services for mitigating, if not eliminating, the vulnerability of those most at risk.

Cross-Cutting Issues

The current profile of programs and services to address the health and health care needs of vulnerable populations falls far short of an integrated continuum of care.

Prevention-Oriented Care

As indicated in Chapter Four, the roots of vulnerability lie deep in the sentiments and social arrangements that characterize contemporary society. The major social experiments of the 1960s, such as the War on Poverty, were relatively short lived, and the demonstration and research projects to evaluate their impact documented a correspondingly mixed record of success. Commitments to programs that did demonstrate some effectiveness during this period, such as Head Start and Community/Migrant Health Centers, were reduced in subsequent decades.

In the 1970s and 1980s, U.S. domestic policy promulgated a diminished and decentralized federal role, along with a free-market orientation, to solving domestic social and economic problems. These policies, along with major shifts in the U.S. economy during this same period (including inflation, recession, and loss of jobs in manufacturing and industry and a corresponding growth in the service economy), have conspired to exacerbate, rather than eliminate, the socioeconomic origins of vulnerability.

The social and economic roots of public health problems, such as those of high-risk mothers and infants, the mentally ill, and homeless, among others examined here, are well documented. Nonetheless, contemporary public health and medical care interventions focus primarily on the behavioral, environmental, and clinical correlates and consequences of socioeconomic disadvantage, rather than on sociopolitical prescriptions to remedy it.

The Public Health Service Year 2000 Objectives for the nation provide a philosophical basis as well as a concrete set of means and ends for improving the health and well-being of many of the vulnerable populations examined here. However, a major Institute of Medicine report on public health concluded that the infrastructure for delivering public health messages and programs is poorly organized and managed and underfunded (IOM, 1988b).

The life-style- or individual-change-oriented bases of many interventions (such as how to stop smoking or drinking or say no to drugs) often fail to take into account the larger social milieu of the family or neighborhood in which the individual lives, which can have a major influence on the success of these initiatives. In addition to not being well researched in terms of their effectiveness, legally oriented interventions, such as mandatory testing for drugs or HIV antibodies or issuing restraining orders on abusing husbands or fathers, raise serious ethical questions regarding the rights of the affected individuals.

The medical care system plays a limited role in delivering prevention-oriented services. Many front-line medical providers have either not been trained or have not had any particular incentive (due to lack of reimbursement, for example) to include prevention-oriented procedures in their practices (such as AIDS, injury, mental illness, or family abuse risk assessment). As will be discussed further in Chapter Seven, organizational or financial barriers may also preclude some particularly at-risk groups (such as high-risk mothers and children or elderly minorities) from getting even traditional prevention-oriented medical services, such as prenatal care, immunizations, or regular high blood pressure screening.

Treatment-Oriented Care

A complex, costly, highly technology-oriented and specialized system of medical care has evolved in this country—the primary focus of which is treating or curing disease. Many people, however, may present with problems in physical, psychological, or social functioning that medical care providers have not necessarily been trained to identify or treat (such as mental illness, substance abuse, and child maltreatment). The complex origins of many of these problems lie outside the domain that medical providers traditionally address, and they are not readily fixed (or cured) by high-technology medical silver bullets. Further, the individuals themselves may also return directly to environments (such as abusing homes or living on the streets) that exacerbate the problem they presented initially or make it harder to carry out medically prescribed follow-up care.

The acute medical care system has, in effect, become a very expensive place of last resort for many of the vulnerable. These are the individuals who have not reaped the benefits of earlier, more fundamental, investments in their health and well-being—through good schools, jobs, or housing, or knowing about good health maintenance practices, or having access to preventive health care services. This is manifested in the expensive and technology-intensive hospital care needed by high-risk newborns that could have been avoided with adequate prenatal care, or the child with cognitive impairments that could have been prevented by early case identification and treatment for lead poisoning, for example.

Long-Term Care

The deinstitutionalization movement has focused on moving people out of depersonalized and bureaucratic institutional environments into less restrictive home or community settings. One of the problems with deinstitutionalization is that it encouraged or pushed individuals (particularly the mentally ill) to leave institutions, often with no arrangements having been made for those who had serious limitations in physical, psychological, or social functioning to have another supportive place to go.

There is some evidence that a reinstitutionalization movement is occurring. Local jails and prisons are being increasingly filled with people who are mentally ill, homeless, drug dependent, HIV infected, or perpetrators (as well as victims) of violence. Nursing homes house a substantial proportion of young and old people with cognitive or mental impairments. Intensive care units of major inner-city hospitals are feeling the strain and costs of increasing numbers of HIV-positive or crack-dependent infants or ventilator-dependent children and adults, who have no home or family to go home to.

A parallel and equally important trend is the development of more community-based options as treatment and support alternatives for many categories of the vulnerable. These options include meals on wheels to the homebound elderly, friendly visitor volunteers to persons with AIDS, street outreach to homeless runaway youth, and alcohol or drug user peer support groups, among a multitude of others. Families continue to bear a large part of this caregiving burden for many of the vulnerable. Others have no one from a close circle of family or friends to help.

The focus of community-based, long-term care programs and services is to directly provide, or to support others in providing, the complex array of services required to care for people who have serious, long-term limitations in physical, psychological, and/or social function. Because of the fragmentation and poor coordination of these services across many medical and social service sectors, case managers are often employed to create a system of care for an individual, where no such service exists in the community.

The final chapter will address the process for developing a more integrated, community-oriented, continuum of care for vulnerable populations.

Population-Specific Overview

High-Risk Mothers and Infants

The issues of preventing low birthweight and reducing infant mortality have recently been the focus of a number of national expert panels. Since 1985, three National Academy of Science Committees have published major reports regarding this issue: *Preventing Low Birthweight* (IOM, 1985), *Risking the Future: Adolescent Sexuality, Pregnancy, and Childbearing* (Hayes, 1987), and *Prenatal Care: Reaching Mothers, Reaching Infants* (IOM, 1988d). A 1988 report prepared by the Office of Technology Assessment Advisory Panel on Technology and Children's Health examined the access, cost, and quality of prenatal care services (OTA, 1988b). In 1989, a Public Health Service Expert Panel on the Content of Prenatal Care released its report detailing the recommended content of prenatal care visits (PHS, 1989). Similarly, the National Commission to Prevent Infant Mortality (1988a) and the Southern Regional Project on Infant Mortality (1989) issued recommendations regarding national and regional strategies, respectively, to reduce the high rates of infant deaths.

All of these groups highlight the importance of a comprehensive, coordinated system of care to serve high-risk mothers and infants. (See Table 5.1.)

Prevention-Oriented Care. Public health programs provide a variety of prevention-oriented maternal and child health services. Title V of the Social Security Act authorized the establishment of the Maternal and Child Health (MCH) and Crippled Children Services (CCS) programs (now the Program for Children with Special Health Care Needs), and Title X of the Public Health Service Act provided federal funding for family planning services. The U.S. Department of Agriculture has supported the Special Supplemental Food Program for Women, Infants, and Children (WIC), as well as the Food Stamp Program for welfare-eligible mothers, to enhance the availability of adequate nutrition for poor pregnant women and their children. Maternity and Infant Care Projects, Community and Migrant Health Centers, and National Health Services Corps physicians have also been major providers of care to women in many low-income neighborhoods.

The funding levels for all of these programs were, however, considerably diminished during the Reagan administration, due to the increased use of block-grant funding to states and political pressures to reduce support for social services programs in general and family planning and abortion-related services in particular (Wallace, Ryan, & Oglesby, 1988). The Bush administration sought to prohibit providing information about abortion services in counseling clients seen at federally funded family planning clinics.

In fiscal years 1988 and 1989, the Comprehensive Perinatal Care Program awarded $40 million in grants to over 268 Community or Migrant Health Centers (C/MHCs) to fund comprehensive perinatal delivery systems stressing case finding and coordinated case management services (DSPPD, 1990a). President Bush endorsed a Healthy Start program to target services to cities with excessively high infant mortality rates, though considerable controversy surrounded the fact that the funds for this initiative would be drawn from other MCH programs and services (Mason, 1991).

Family life (sex) education and related behavioral risk education programs (relating to AIDS, smoking and substance abuse, and childhood injury)

Table 5.1. Principal Programs and Services for High-Risk Mothers and Infants.

	Prevention-Oriented Care	Treatment-Oriented Care			Long-Term Care
	Ambulatory	*Ambulatory*	*Institutional*		
Public health system	*Prevention-oriented*	*Treatment-oriented*	*Acute care*	*Long-term care*	*Home and community-based care*
Family planning	Prenatal care	High-risk mother and infant services	Level I or II delivery	Neonatal intensive care	Child protective services
Community outreach and case finding	Pre- and postpregnancy counseling	Abortion services	Birth centers		Home visiting
Nutritional services	Well-baby care	Smoking and substance abuse cessation programs			School-based clinics
Sex education					Case management
AIDS education					
Smoking and substance abuse prevention					

are available in some schools. Many at-risk teenagers are not reached by these programs, however (Dryfoos, 1990).

Prenatal care is the major medically oriented primary prevention intervention to enhance positive pregnancy outcomes (IOM, 1988d; PHS, 1989). Physicians are also encouraged to counsel their patients regarding family planning and the risks associated with pregnancy, and to encourage well-baby checkups and immunizations.

The Early and Periodic Screening, Diagnosis, and Treatment (EPSDT) program provides Medicaid-eligible children nutrition, vision, dental, and hearing screening; a physical history and exam; and immunizations. In 1988, only 20 to 30 percent of eligible children were estimated to have received this service. The Omnibus Reconciliation Act of 1989, however, included provisions to expand the number of participating providers and allow more flexibility in scheduling screenings, to enhance Medicaid-eligible children's access to the program (Yudkowsy & Fleming, 1990).

The Head Start Program, first funded under Title V of the Economic Opportunity Act of 1964 and currently authorized under Title I of the Human Services Reauthorization Act, provides education, social services, and health programs to disadvantaged preschoolers—most of whom are minority children. This program also provides well-child screening and immunizations. Fewer than 20 percent of eligible low-income children are actually enrolled (Stubbs, 1988).

Infant stimulation and early childhood intervention programs help reduce the risk of cognitive and physical impairments among low-birthweight, premature, or otherwise at-risk infants and children (Infant Health and Development Program, 1990).

Treatment-Oriented Care. The relationship of adverse pregnancy outcomes to maternal smoking and alcohol use, as well as the increased incidence of drug-exposed infants, has resulted in an expanded interest in smoking and substance abuse cessation programs for pregnant women. Such programs are not widely available, however, and their effectiveness—particularly for drug abusing mothers—has not been well established.

The vast majority of women deliver in hospitals. The growth of free-standing birthing centers (Rooks et al., 1989) and reemergence of nurse practitioner– or lay-midwife-assisted deliveries (Butter & Kay, 1988) attest to women's increasing interest in delivering children at home or in homelike settings.

A particular focus of perinatal care demonstration and research projects in recent years has been the development of regionalized systems of perinatal care services, including the integration of services among hospitals having differing levels of capacity to handle high-risk newborns. Level III hospitals serve as regional centers and have the capacity for providing long-term newborn intensive care. Level II can provide short-term respiratory support, and Level I hospitals provide newborn care and have no special units for seriously ill infants.

Long-Term Care. Major regionalized perinatal network demonstration projects include the federally supported Maternity and Infant Care Program—Improved Pregnancy Outcome Program (IPOP) (McNellis, 1988) and the Robert Wood Johnson Foundation's Perinatal Program (RWJF, 1985) and Rural Infant Care Program (Gortmaker, Clark, Graven, Sobol, & Geronimus, 1989; RWJF, 1986). The results of the evaluations of these programs and regionalized perinatal service systems in general demonstrate that the availability of Level III hospitals and the appropriate integration of a system of referrals among the different levels of institutions result in improved perinatal outcomes—particularly the reduction of the birthweight-specific death rates for very-low-birthweight infants. Neonatal intensive care for high-risk newborns is very expensive to provide. Further, these hospital-based regionalized systems of service have not been successful in reducing the overall incidence of low-birthweight infants in the populations they serve (OTA, 1987b; Paneth et al., 1982).

The risks for high-risk infants and their families remain high once they leave the hospital. Programs and services to reduce child abuse and neglect—including parenting skills training, social support, and child care—may be important to ensure the infant's health and well-being after discharge (Cohn & Lee, 1988). School-based clinics and/or day-care arrangements provide needed support for teenage mothers at risk of dropping out of school prior to graduation (Dryfoos, 1990; Flinn Foundation, 1989).

Many mothers may need case management assistance to effectively apply for and negotiate the fragmented and poorly integrated set of services for which they are potentially eligible. Case management is an important component of the C/MHC Comprehensive Perinatal Care Program described earlier (DSPPD, 1990a).

Home visiting of families with special needs has long been a component of public health nursing and social work practice. With the increased fragmentation of families, systems of social support, and care systems, home visiting offers promise as both a primary and tertiary intervention strategy for high-risk mothers and their infants (Combs-Orme, Reis, & Ward, 1985; GAO, 1990d; National Commission to Prevent Infant Mortality, 1989).

Several resource directories provide additional information on programs and agencies to serve high-risk mothers and infants: *Healthy Mothers, Healthy Babies: A Compendium of Program Ideas for Serving Low-Income Women* (HRSA, 1986), *Prevent Infant Mortality: A Resource Directory* (National Commission to Prevent Infant Mortality, 1988c), and *Starting Early: A Guide to Federal Resources in Maternal and Child Health* (National Center for Education in Maternal and Child Health, 1988).

Chronically Ill and Disabled

As with the issue of high-risk mothers and infants, in recent years major national commissions have studied the prevalence of disability, the factors that lead to it, and the interventions that could be designated for the primary, secondary, and tertiary prevention of functional incapacity. Since 1985, a number of major reports have been published, dealing in particular with the causes, consequences, and costs of injury: *Injury in America: A Continuing Public Health Problem* (National Research Council, 1985), *Injury Control: A Review of the Status and Progress of the Injury Control Program at the Centers for Disease Control* (CDC, 1988b), *Cost of Injury in the United States: A Report to Congress, 1987* (Rice, MacKenzie, & Associates, 1989), and *Injury Prevention: Meeting the Challenge* (National Committee for Injury Prevention and Control, 1989). A 1991 study by the IOM Committee on a National Agenda for the Prevention of Disabilities—*Disability in America: Toward a National Agenda for Prevention*—focused on developmental disabilities, chronic disease, injury, and secondary interventions to limit the impact of these conditions (IOM, 1991b). (See Table 5.2.)

Prevention-Oriented Care. The Public Health Service Year 2000 Objectives for primary prevention interventions include educational programs on nutrition, smoking, and substance abuse and on how to prevent injuries in the home and workplace. They also encourage increased participation in a regular program of exercise—for all ages. In addition to these individual-oriented public health interventions, there are recommendations to reduce environmental risks of injury through safety regulations governing the use of lead paint, motor vehicles, firearms, and other products (PHS, 1990).

Prenatal care is an important medical care–oriented intervention to detect and avert the risks of infant and early childhood disability (IOM, 1988d). Newborn screening can help detect phenylketonuria (PKU) or congenital hypothyroidism, for example. Vision and hearing screening can help identify and lead to the correction of impairments for both children and the elderly. Screening for lead paint poisoning, cancer, hypertension, and diabetes permits the early detection and management of these problems (Beers, Fink, & Beck, 1991; Houk & Thacker, 1989; IOM, 1991b; Needleman, 1991).

There has been increasing emphasis on prevention-oriented interventions for the elderly, including the 1988 report *The Aging Population in the Twenty-First Century: Statistics for Health Policy* (National Research Council, 1988), the 1991 IOM report *The Second Fifty Years: Promoting Health and Preventing Disability* (IOM, 1991c), an OTA study on *The Use of Preventive Services by the Elderly* (OTA, 1989), demonstrations by the Health Care Financing Administration to enroll Medicare-eligible elderly in a package of preventive-related services, and health promotion initiatives on the part of Kaiser and other private foundations (Fries, 1989; IOM, 1991b; Kane, Kane, & Arnold, 1985).

Collaborative arrangements between the Bureau of Health Care Delivery and Assistance and the Agency on Aging have encouraged Community and Migrant Health Centers to develop educational programs for the elderly

Table 5.2. Principal Programs and Services for Chronically Ill and Disabled.

Prevention-Oriented Care		Treatment-Oriented Care		Long-Term Care	
	Ambulatory		Institutional		
Public health system	Prevention-oriented	Treatment-oriented	Acute care	Long-term care	Home and community-based care
Nutritional services	Prenatal care	Chronic disease management	Acute hospital care	Nursing homes	Home health care
Smoking and substance abuse prevention	Screening Newborn Lead Cancer Hypertension Diabetes Vision Hearing	Medications management	Intensive care	Hospices	Caregiver respite
Injury prevention programs Childhood Home Work		Rehabilitation therapies		Social HMOs	Day care Child Adult
Exercise programs		Durable medical equipment			Home-delivered meals
Environmental risk abatement programs Lead Product safety Motor vehicle safety Gun control		Emergency medical services			Home visiting
		Smoking and substance abuse cessation programs			Housekeeping services
Education Infant stimulation Early childhood intervention					Transportation services
					Case management
					Independent living centers
					Board-and-care homes
					Lifecare communities
					Education Special education Vocational training Rehabilitation

emphasizing home safety, nutrition, physical fitness, and medications management (DSPPD, 1990c). In 1988, the Centers for Disease Control instituted a Disabilities Prevention Program to increase the state and local capacities to prevent the primary onset and secondary consequences of developmental, as well as injury- and chronic illness–related, disability (Houk & Thacker, 1989; Viano, 1990).

Treatment-Oriented Care. Smoking is a significant risk factor for major chronic illnesses such as cancer, heart disease, and chronic obstructive pulmonary disease, and alcohol is an important risk factor for cirrhosis. Programs to reduce the prevalence of these risk factors are important in enhancing both the primary and secondary prevention of serious chronic illness and associated functional limitations.

Care for long-term chronic disease often requires continuous, comprehensive medical management over an extended period of time. The onset of secondary disabilities (such as impaired vision) resulting from chronic illness (diabetes) can be delayed or prevented if the appropriate medical regimens (insulin) are introduced and followed by the patient. A particular problem, however, in the care of chronically ill, particularly elderly, patients is the medical management of multiple prescriptions. Many elderly experience serious physical or emotional side effects as a result of overmedication. The chronically ill and disabled may also have extensive needs for rehabilitation therapies, such as occupational, physical, and speech therapy, among others, as well as durable medical equipment or assistive devices (such as prostheses or wheelchairs) (Albrecht, 1976; IOM, 1991b; Stein, 1989).

Adequate regionalized emergency medical and trauma center services are important in reducing the risk of death or long-term disability of intentional or unintentional injury (Champion et al., 1989). Chronically ill and disabled adults and children often face long and expensive hospital stays or long-term stays in hospital intensive care units. The expenditures for these services under Medicare are greatest during the last year of life (Eggert & Friedman, 1988).

Long-Term Care. A focus on community-based options to institutionalized care and on forging more effective linkages between acute and long-term care services for chronically ill and disabled children and adults has emerged in recent years (Bowlyow, 1990; Firman, 1983; Knight & Walker, 1985; Koff, 1988; Patrick & Peach, 1989; Stein, 1989; Strauss & Corbin, 1988; Traxler & Dunaye, 1987; Weissert, Cready, & Pawelak, 1988). The Bureau of Maternal and Child Health and Resources Development has encouraged the development of models of comprehensive, coordinated family-centered care for children with special health care needs (BMCHRD, 1988; Perrin & Ireys, 1984; Shelton, Jeppson, & Johnson, 1989; Stein, 1989).

Nursing homes are the primary providers of institutionalized long-term care. Based on the 1985 nursing home survey, 4.4 percent (or 1.3

million) of the elderly lived in nursing homes (NCHS, 1989d). Recent projections estimate that at least 43 percent of Americans who turned sixty-five in 1990 will enter a nursing home at least once before they die (Kemper & Murtaugh, 1991; Murtaugh, Kemper, & Spillman, 1990). Physical dependency, cognitive impairment, and living alone are some of the major predictors of nursing home admission (Roy, Ford, & Folmar, 1990; Shapiro & Tate, 1988; Weissert & Cready, 1989b). Hospices provide an alternative for palliative care for terminally ill patients (Torrens, 1985).

Social health maintenance organizations (S/HMOs) are designed to cover long-term as well as acute, primary, and preventive health care on a prepaid basis. The S/HMO model emphasizes continuous care management, home care, and social services as alternatives to institutionalization (Harrington & Newcomer, 1983, 1991; Newcomer, Harrington, & Friedlob, 1990).

The home care industry has burgeoned in recent years in an effort to respond to the growing number of adults and children who could live in the community, if required medical and social support services are provided (Commonwealth Fund Commission on Elderly People Living Alone, 1989; DSPPD, 1990d; Spohn, Bergthold, & Estes, 1988; U.S. Congress, House Select Committee on Aging, 1983). However, the majority of the care for the community-dwelling disabled is still provided by family or friends. About 75 percent of disabled older persons living in the community rely on these informal support systems. About 72 percent of informal caregivers are women — either wives or daughters of the elderly person (Stone & Kemper, 1989; Stone, Cafferata, & Sangl, 1987; U.S. Congress, House Select Committee on Aging, 1987).

Programs to support the caregivers are essential if they are to continue to assume these roles. An important component of caring for the caregivers is to provide respite or homemaker services to reduce the day-to-day stress associated with taking care of a seriously ill or impaired family member (GAO, 1989h; Montgomery, 1988). Social day-care programs for both the elderly and disabled children provide options for more independent living, as well as respite for family caregivers (Harder, Gornick, & Burt, 1986; Hedrick et al., 1991; RWJF, 1990a; U.S. Congress, Senate Special Committee on Aging, 1988).

Under Title III of the Older Americans Act, Area Agencies on Aging have home-delivered meals, as well as providing a number of other support and referral services, for homebound elderly (AARP, 1991b). In 1987, approximately two million (36 percent) of the 5.6 million noninstitutionalized Americans sixty-five and over with functional limitations used formal home-based care services, such as homemaker services and home-delivered meals, as well as care provided by home health aides, nurses, and physicians (Short & Leon, 1990). The Robert Wood Johnson Foundation Interfaith Volunteer Caregivers and Family Friends Projects provide examples of using volunteers to provide needed social support for the homebound elderly and disabled children and their families, respectively (RWJF, 1989, 1990a).

Case management is being increasingly promulgated as a means for coordinating the complex array of medical and social services required by the elderly and disabled, though the organization and objectives (patient care, cost containment, and/or service coordination) of various case management models differ substantially (Capitman, 1988; Carcagno & Kemper, 1988; MacAdam et al., 1989; Shaughnessy & Kramer, 1990).

Lifecare communities, independent living centers, and board-and-care homes provide options for individuals who either elect not to or cannot continue to live in their own homes because of mental or physical limitations (Moon, Gaberlavage, & Newman, 1989; Mor, Sherwood, & Gutkin, 1986; Tell, Wallack, & Cohen, 1987). Based on a 1987 survey, there were estimated to be 41,381 licensed board-and-care homes, with 526,837 beds. About 10,000 homes served the elderly only and the balance mentally ill, mentally retarded, or mixed populations (GAO, 1989c).

The U.S. Department of Education, Office of Special Education and Rehabilitative Services, supports state efforts in providing special education and related services to handicapped children from birth to age twenty-one. The Basic Vocational Rehabilitation Service Program supports the states in assisting physically and mentally handicapped individuals to become gainfully employed, regardless of age (GAO, 1986; Office of Assistant Secretary for Planning and Evaluation, 1990).

Persons with AIDS

The National Academy of Sciences has generated several reports in recent years that deal with the design and evaluation of interventions to prevent the onset and spread of AIDS: *Confronting AIDS: Directions for Public Health, Health Care, and Research* (IOM, 1986), *Confronting AIDS: Update 1988* (IOM, 1988a), *AIDS: Sexual Behavior and Intravenous Drug Use* (Turner, Miller, & Moses, 1989), *AIDS: The Second Decade* (Miller, Turner, & Moses, 1990), and *Evaluating AIDS Prevention Programs* (Coyle, Boruch, & Turner, 1991). Programs have, in particular, focused on the need for AIDS prevention and risk reduction through a variety of public information and health education efforts. (See Table 5.3.)

Prevention-Oriented Care. Prevention-oriented programs are directed to three principal audiences: the general public, target populations in particular communities, and individuals.

Mass media campaigns have been a major focus of the Public Health Service and Centers for Disease Control initiatives to increase generalized public awareness of AIDS risks. These have included, among others, the mass mailing of the pamphlet *Understanding AIDS,* with a message from Surgeon General C. Everett Koop, to every residential address in the United States in the summer of 1988; the preparation and airing of public service announcements (PSAs); dissemination of educational videos; the National AIDS Hotline; the National AIDS Information Clearinghouse; outreach to

Table 5.3. Principal Programs and Services for Persons with AIDS.

| | Prevention-Oriented Care | Treatment-Oriented Care | | Long-Term Care | |
| | Ambulatory | Ambulatory | Institutional | Institutional | Home and community-based care |
Public health system	Prevention-oriented	Treatment-oriented	Acute care	Long-term care	Home and community-based care
Media campaigns	Sexual and drug history-taking	Posttest counseling	Acute hospital care	Nursing homes	Home health care
Health education and risk reduction projects	Pretest counseling	AIDS treatment therapies	Intensive care	Hospices	Caregiver respite
Community-based	Testing				Family/partner support or therapy
School-based					
Testing and counseling	Substance abuse cessation programs				Volunteer services
Safe-sex education					Case management
Substance abuse prevention					
Street outreach for high-risk populations					

the entertainment community; and public health communication assistance to state AIDS programs (Coyle, Boruch, & Turner, 1991; Public Health Reports, 1990a).

Health education and risk reduction projects have focused on community-based organizations (CBOs), including schools, to target AIDS prevention education and behavioral change interventions. In addition to Centers for Disease Control programs in this area, in 1988 the Robert Wood Johnson Foundation initiated its AIDS Prevention and Services Program to assist community groups (such as churches, schools, labor unions, and PTAs, among others) in developing local initiatives to respond to the spread of AIDS (RWJF, 1990b). CDC's efforts have also included accumulating and disseminating adolescent and school health curriculum resources on HIV and AIDS (CDC, 1990c).

Individual testing and counseling for AIDS has been a particularly sensitive topic, because of the issues of whether testing should be mandatory or voluntary as well as whether and/or how the results should be made available to public health officials (Goedert, 1987; Rhame & Maki, 1989; Weiss & Thier, 1988). According to a 1989 survey conducted by the Intergovernmental Health Policy Project, anonymous testing for AIDS was available in around 80 percent of the states ("Survey Shows," 1989).

As indicated in Chapter Two, an increasing mode of AIDS transmission — particularly among women and newborns — is through intravenous drug use. The National Research Council has recommended that rigorous efforts in sex and substance abuse education, in addition to a variety of other interventions, be undertaken focusing on populations at greatest risk (Turner, Miller, & Moses, 1989). Homeless and runaway youth, many of whom resort to prostitution or drug-related activity, have been the focus of street outreach efforts to diminish the spread of AIDS in this population (GAO, 1990a).

Front-line providers of care need to be trained to take detailed sexual and drug use histories and to do pretest counseling for patients who present themselves as being, or who the provider judges to be, at risk of AIDS (HRSA, 1988).

Treatment-Oriented Care. Posttest counseling by medical providers is also necessary to advise patients of the outcome of the test and to advise patients regarding the importance of risk reduction behaviors or, should the test be positive, the probable course of the disease and subsequent care needs. No pharmacological or clinical intervention exists to cure AIDS. However, there is evidence that the drug AZT has met with some success in prolonging the lives of persons with AIDS. One of the dilemmas both providers and patients face is assessing the probable risk and benefits of more experimental drugs for arresting the progress of the disease.

Many AIDS patients are in and out of the hospital with the immune deficiency–related morbidities associated with AIDS (such as pneumonia or neurological impairment). Demonstration projects funded by the Health Resources and Services Administration, as well as private initiatives, such as Robert Wood Johnson Foundation AIDS Health Services Programs, among others, have attempted to integrate early intervention and intensive case management services in community-based health care delivery organizations for persons with AIDS (Benjamin, Lee, & Solkowitz, 1988; DSPPD, 1990e; HRSA, 1989, 1990; Mor, Piette, & Fleishman, 1989; RWJF, 1990b).

Long-Term Care. Substantial parallels exist between the long-term care needs of persons with AIDS and the elderly and chronically ill and disabled. Both populations are heavily dependent on formal or informal systems of care over prolonged periods of time, which requires the availability and coordination of an array of personal, medical, and social support services.

Nursing homes are the primary institutionalized long-term care option available to the infirm elderly. Many of these institutions are, however, not geared to serving younger populations or those with alternative (gay or drug use) life-styles, for example. AIDS hospices—which have sprung up in many communities, principally through volunteer efforts—provide a palliative, more humane, and generally lower-cost alternative, as a place to die, than hospitals or nursing homes for persons with AIDS (Benjamin, 1988; Mechanic & Aiken, 1989a).

The availability of home health care services to AIDS patients is largely a function of the extent to which they have third-party coverage. Because of the rejection experienced from families as a result of their homosexuality, or the absence of stable systems of family support in many cases among IV drug users, many persons with AIDS lack traditional family-based systems of care. Gay friendship networks do, however, provide much of the informal social, emotional, and material support for persons with AIDS and their lovers or other caregivers (Macklin, 1989; Riley, Ory, & Zablotsky, 1989).

An array of community-based volunteer services programs has emerged to provide services to persons with AIDS (PWAs) similar to those available to the elderly through the Office of Aging—such as home-delivered meals, home visiting, housekeeping, and transportation (Shelp, DuBose, & Sunderland, 1990; United Hospital Fund, 1991; Velentgas, Bynum, & Zierler, 1990). Publicly and privately supported AIDS health services delivery demonstration projects mentioned earlier have included case management as a key component—to better coordinate the array of services required for PWAs to remain in the community. Private insurers are increasingly interested in case management services for PWAs as a cost-containment mechanism (Fleishman, Mor, & Piette, 1991; HIAA, 1989a).

Mentally Ill and Disabled

Early in the century, seriously mentally ill patients were institutionalized in state and county mental hospitals. During and after World War II, a greater awareness of the poor conditions in these institutions and a theoretical reorientation toward the role of the environment in influencing mental health led to the emergence of a community mental health movement and an impetus for the "deinstitutionalization" of mental patients.

This new community-based care perspective received considerable support from the Kennedy administration, culminating in the Community Mental Health Center Act of 1963. This act and a series of amendments that followed encouraged the states to devote matching funds to community-based centers providing an array of mental health services. The number and growth of these centers was less than expected due to lack of state financial support. In 1970, the Nixon administration dramatically curtailed federal funding for the program. President Jimmy Carter provided strong political endorsement for the continuance of this program during his administration through the formation of the President's Commission on Mental Health in 1977, the issuance of a major report on the U.S. mental health care system by that commission (President's Commission on Mental Health, 1978a, 1978b, 1978c), and the enactment of the 1980 Mental Health Systems Act. In 1981, President Ronald Reagan effectively repealed that act and eliminated categoric support for Community Mental Health Centers (CMHCs) through the creation of a block grant for alcohol, drug abuse, and mental health (ADAMH) to the states.

The community mental health movement nonetheless catalyzed the large-scale deinstitutionalization (or discharge) of the mentally ill from public and private hospitals. Other factors that provided an impetus for deinstitutionalization, in addition to the ideological and political underpinnings just summarized, included the wider availability of psychotropic drugs that could be used to control or modify patient behavior on an outpatient basis, the belief that community care would be a less expensive alternative, and court decisions guaranteeing institutionalized patients rights to treatment that many states deemed too expensive to continue to assure (Bachrach, 1976; Cameron, 1989; Dowell & Ciarlo, 1989; Grob, 1987; Lieberman, 1975; Premo & Wiseman, 1981; Reamer, 1989; Wagenfeld, Lemkau, & Justice, 1982). (See Table 5.4.)

Prevention-Oriented Care. Primary prevention strategies to reduce the onset of learning, developmental, behavioral, and related mental disorders in children include adequate prenatal care, newborn (particularly phenylketonuria or PKU) screening, infant stimulation, and early childhood intervention programs for high-risk children (premature infants, minority and poor children), as well as parenting skills programs for their parents (IOM, 1989d). Good maternal and child nutrition is also essential to ensure the developing infant and child's cognitive and physical development. Family planning, particularly for adolescent women and their sexual partners, will help to reduce the risk of pregnancy among teenage women—for whom the likelihood of stresses and poor outcomes of pregnancy are apt to be the greatest.

Table 5.4. Principal Programs and Services for Mentally Ill and Disabled.

Prevention-Oriented Care		Treatment-Oriented Care			Long-Term Care
Ambulatory		Ambulatory	Institutional		
Public health system	Prevention-oriented	Treatment-oriented	Acute care	Long-term care	Home and community-based care
Education	Prenatal care	Outpatient mental health services	Short-term inpatient mental health services	Long-term inpatient mental health services	Family/caregiver support or therapy
Parenting skills	Screening	Crisis response services			Home visiting
Infant stimulation	Newborn	Substance abuse cessation programs			Child/adult protective services
Early childhood intervention	Lead				Education
Nutritional services	Psychological				Developmental
Substance abuse prevention					Special education
Family planning					Vocational
Stress reduction programs					Skills training
Consultation and education					Rehabilitation
Environmental risk abatement programs					Community residential care
Lead					Family care homes
Motor vehicle safety					Halfway houses/ psychosocial rehabilitation
Injury prevention programs					Board-and-care homes
Childhood					Satellite housing
Home					Day treatment or partial care
Work					Psychiatric rehabilitation
					Educational
					Vocational
					Residential
					Case management
					Protection and advocacy

Other important areas of primary prevention include programs to reduce unintentional injuries for children due to lead paint or other poisoning, or from motor vehicle or other accidents or injuries for adults and children that are likely to lead to serious cognitive impairment. Screening for lead paint poisoning or the psychological testing of at-risk children and adults through schools or clinic settings can also assist in the early identification of those who have or are most likely to develop cognitive or mental health impairments (Bachrach, 1985; Lorion & Allen, 1989).

Programs to reduce stress in families and at the worksite are an important focus of the Year 2000 nation's Health Objectives. The relationship of substance abuse and mental impairment has also been recognized in encouraging programs to prevent alcohol and drug use — particularly among adolescents and pregnant women. Federal funding for substance abuse prevention and treatment has often been linked to mental health services provision through, for example, the 1970 Drug Abuse Prevention and Control Act, and more recently the combined ADAMH block grant.

A primary focus of prevention efforts in CMHCs was the provision of "Consultation and Education" (C & E) services to clients. Evaluations suggest that the centers in fact devoted a small proportion of staff time and resources to these activities. They also failed to implement a number of recommendations emanating from an American Psychiatric Association Task Force review of successful mental illness prevention programs (Dowell & Ciarlo, 1989).

More research is needed to identify the most efficacious strategies to prevent the onset of mental disorders. Since 1982, the National Institute of Mental Health has funded a core of Prevention Intervention Research Centers (PIRC) throughout the country, as well as a Center for Prevention Research and specialized research centers within the agency, which could provide insights into what interventions might be most effective (GAO, 1989g; Lorion & Allen, 1989).

Treatment-Oriented Care. Outpatient psychiatric services are delivered both through the specialty mental health and general medical care sectors. The principal providers of outpatient specialty mental health services, in order of numbers of admissions, are multiservice mental health organizations (which provide at least two of three services — inpatient, outpatient, or partial care), freestanding outpatient clinics, nonfederal general hospitals, private psychiatric hospitals, VA medical centers, and state and country hospitals (Rosenstein, Milazzo-Sayre, & Manderscheid, 1990, p. 164). The number of new outpatients seen primarily in ambulatory mental health organizations (multiservice and freestanding clinics) almost tripled from a low of 761,572 in 1969 to 2.2 million in 1979. Since then, the number has leveled off to 1.8 to 1.9 million per year (Witkin, Atay, Fell, & Manderscheid, 1990, p. 24).

Data from the ECA survey indicate that the highest proportions of visits to specialty mental health care, compared to general medical care, providers are for schizophrenia, substance abuse, and antisocial personality disorder, with lower proportions for affective and anxiety disorders. This is consistent with the literature in general medical practice, which suggests that depression and anxiety are major reasons for seeking primary medical care (Mechanic, 1990). Depression, anxiety, and related mental disorders are estimated to be present in approximately 25 percent of the patients seen on an ambulatory basis by primary care physicians (Hankin & Oktay, 1979; Schulberg & Burns, 1988; Schurman, Kramer, & Mitchell, 1985). Emergency and crisis response services, as well as substance abuse cessation programs, are also components of treatment-oriented outpatient mental health services.

The percentage of inpatients treated in mental health organizations dropped from 42 percent in 1971 to around 27 percent in 1975, and has stayed in the range of 26 to 27 percent since that time (Witkin, Atay, Fell, & Manderscheid, 1990, p. 3). The largest number of short-term admissions for specialty mental health care is to nonfederal general hospitals with psychiatric services (Rosenstein, Milazzo-Sayre, & Manderscheid, 1990).

Long-Term Care. Prior to the advent of the community mental health movement, state and county mental hospitals were the major providers of long-term institutional care. From 1950 to 1985, the number of these hospitals dropped from 322 to 279, and the number of patients in residence in these institutions declined from 512,501 to 116,136 (Morrissey, 1989, p. 317). Over that same period, there has, however, been a substantial growth in the number of private psychiatric hospitals, nonfederal general hospitals with psychiatric services, and residential treatment centers (RTC) for emotionally disturbed children. In 1969, for example, there were 7,596 RTCs, compared to 24,511 in 1986 (Witkin, Atay, Fell, & Manderscheid, 1990, p. 32).

Nursing homes are now the main institutional providers of long-term care for the mentally ill (Freiman, Arons, Goldman, & Burns, 1990; Linn & Stein, 1989). In 1985, 974,300 nursing home residents were diagnosed as having a mental disorder (Strahan, 1990, p. 228). This is more than ten times the number of persons under inpatient care in 1986 in the largest provider of inpatient psychiatric services—state and county mental hospitals (94,353) (Rosenstein, Milazzo-Sayre, & Manderscheid, 1990, p. 154).

Many mentally retarded and mentally ill children and adults are still being cared for by their families. The provision of family and caregiver respite and therapy services is important for continuing to support and strengthen their ability to sustain their caregiving role. Home visiting and child and elder abuse and neglect services also serve to monitor and enhance the capacities of at-risk families to provide for a disabled family member (Knitzer & Olson, 1982; OTA, 1986).

Though fragmented and poorly developed in many communities, the community mental health movement has given rise to a number of home and community-based long-term care options (Craig, 1988a). Support for educational services to mentally retarded and mentally ill adults and children is provided through developmental disabilities, special education, and vocational rehabilitation and training programs (Ciardiello & Bell, 1988; Knitzer & Olson, 1982).

Since the advent of deinstitutionalization, housing has been one of the most pressing community care needs for persons with cognitive or mental impairments. Major options include family care arrangements (including foster family care); psychosocial rehabilitation facilities, such as halfway houses or other transitional care facilities; board-and-care homes; and satellite housing dispersed throughout the community (Segal & Kotler, 1989). With the limited availability of these specific housing options and the diminished availability of low-income housing in general, the number of mentally ill who are homeless has increased as well. At least 25 percent of the current homeless population is estimated to be mentally ill (Levine & Haggard, 1989).

The Robert Wood Johnson Foundation Mental Health Services Development Program and the jointly sponsored RWJF–Housing and Urban Development Program for the Chronically Mentally Ill have funded local programs to develop community housing, social service, educational, and related service capacity for serving the chronically mentally ill and homeless.

Partial care services provide another option to traditional inpatient and outpatient mental health services. With these arrangements, patients can be admitted to day treatment programs, or stay overnight, but be free to go to a job or other community activities during the day (Witkin, Atay, Fell, & Manderscheid, 1990).

The NIMH Community Support Program (CSP) for the chronically mentally ill and the comparable Child and Adolescent Service System Program (CASSP) are charged with ensuring the availability of a comprehensive, coordinated system of care for these populations (Jaskulski & Robinson, 1990; Knitzer & Olson, 1982). The Robert Wood Johnson Foundation Mental Health Services Program for Youth was intended to build state and local financial and organizational capacity to provide services to at-risk youth (Beachler, 1990).

Public Law 99-660 mandated that state mental health authorities provide case management services to every person identified with serious and persistent mental illness. A range of case management models has been developed to serve the mentally ill, which vary in their relative emphasis on program personnel's versus the client's assessment of needs, and in linking the client to services versus trying to enhance the client's own strengths and capacities for obtaining what he or she needs (Dill, 1987; Robinson & Toff-Bergman, 1990).

The psychiatric rehabilitation model emphasizes the importance of the individual's own needs assessment and decision-making processes for maximizing functioning in "working, living, and learning" in the community (Farkas & Anthony, 1989). The Fairweather Lodge Experiment, for example, created a community-based residential facility to train discharged hospital patients to (1) live together in a supportive, familylike environment, and (2) seek jobs in the community. The rates of rehospitalization were lower and sustained employment higher for patients who participated in these arrangements compared to those who were trained in the hospital and then simply discharged into the community (Segal & Kotler, 1989).

State mental health protection and advocacy programs oversee placement decisions made by agents acting on behalf of the mentally ill and disabled through guardianship, protective order, or community commitment procedures (Crystal & Dejowski, 1987; Scallet, Marvelle, & Davidson, 1990).

Alcohol or Substance Abusers

The Institute of Medicine has issued several major reports on the prevention and treatment of drug and alcohol problems in recent years: *Causes and Consequences of Alcohol Problems: An Agenda for Research* (IOM, 1987), *Prevention and Treatment of Alcohol Problems: Research Opportunities* (IOM, 1989c), *Broadening the Base of Treatment for Alcohol Problems* (IOM, 1990), and *Treating Drug Problems* (Gerstein & Harwood, 1990). These reports acknowledge alcohol, drug, and other substance abuse as long-term problems associated with an array of physical, psychological, and social correlates and consequences. A broad-based, multifaceted approach to prevention, treatment, and long-term care is required to address the onset and progression of these problems through the complex and interactive stages of use, abuse, dependence, abstinence, recovery, and relapse. (See Table 5.5.)

Prevention-Oriented Care. Considerable debate surrounds whether prevention efforts should focus more on restrictive legal means for limiting the supply or availability of alcohol, drugs, or other addictive substances versus community- or individual-oriented educational programs to diminish individuals' interest in or susceptibility to initiating the use of these substances (DuPont, 1989; Goplerud, 1990; Jarvik, 1990; Reuter, 1991).

A variety of legal means have been used to restrict the availability and use of drugs, alcohol, and tobacco. State and federal laws impose criminal penalties on those who have been found to be supplying or using certain substances (such as cocaine or heroin). Federal law enforcement agencies (such as the FBI, CIA, and Border Patrol) have assumed major roles in halting (interdicting) shipments of designated substances to the United States.

State and local laws impose restrictions on where and to whom alcoholic beverages or cigarettes are to be sold (Office of the Attorney General, 1989; Office of National Drug Control Policy, 1989; Office of the Surgeon General, 1989; OTA, 1987a; White House Conference for a Drug Free America, 1988). Dram Shop Laws in a number of states assign liability to owners of establishments that sell alcoholic beverages to obviously intoxicated customers, and drunk driving laws impose fines or penalties on indi-

Table 5.5. Principal Programs and Services for Alcohol or Substance Abusers.

Prevention-Oriented Care		Treatment-Oriented Care			Long-Term Care
	Ambulatory	*Ambulatory*	*Institutional*	*Institutional*	
Public health system	*Prevention-oriented*	*Treatment-oriented*	*Acute care*	*Long-term care*	*Home and community-based care*
Legal deterrence	Counseling	Pharmacological	Hospital-based treatment programs	Therapeutic communities	Skills development
Criminalization	Individual	Agonist		Rehabilitation units	Social
Interdiction	Family	Antagonist			Vocational
Restricted access		Symptomatic			Stress management
Screening		Behavioral			Peer support self-help
Media campaigns		Verbal therapy			Alcoholics Anonymous
		Contingency management			Narcotics Anonymous
Substance abuse prevention programs		Conditioning therapy			Halfway houses
Affective education					Aftercare programs
Social influence					Worksite/EAPs
Social skills training					Correctional facilities

viduals who are deemed to be legally intoxicated—in efforts to both deter and punish such behaviors (Graitcer, 1989; Mosher & Colman, 1986; Worden, Flynn, Merrill, Waller, & Haugh, 1989).

Mandatory, as well as voluntary, testing or screening (particularly for drugs) is a controversial intervention that has been used by employers, insurers, the military, and criminal justice officials to deter potential users or detect, punish, and/or refer those who are found to be using or abusing such substances (Gust & Walsh, 1989).

Major public and private mass media campaigns about the dangers of drug, alcohol, tobacco, and/or other substance abuse have been undertaken in recent years in an effort to diminish individuals' propensity to use or abuse these substances. These campaigns are viewed as antidotes to the massive advertising conducted by the alcohol and tobacco industries to sell their products, which are often directed to particular market segments, such as women, adolescents, or minorities (Bauman, LaPrelle, Brown, Koch, & Padgett, 1991; Davis, 1987; DeJong & Winsten, 1990).

Some forty-seven states have Coalitions for the Prevention and Control of Tobacco Use, which engage in a variety of public education, lobbying, and research and development efforts to diminish the use of tobacco products (CDC, 1990h). A variety of private advocacy groups have also launched major media or public education campaigns to encourage safer practices (including the use of designated drivers) or the development or enforcement of stricter antisubstance abuse legislation (OSAP, 1990a). These groups include Mothers Against Drunk Driving (MADD) and Students Against Drunk Driving (SADD).

A number of primary prevention-oriented programs, rooted in psychosocial theories of the etiologies of drug and related substance abuse, have been developed to target particularly at-risk groups such as adolescents (Bell & Battjes, 1990; Goplerud, 1990; Jones & Battjes, 1990a; NIDA, 1987, 1991b). These initiatives may be broadly classified as more traditional versus psychosocial prevention methods.

The traditional approaches are either mainly informational or affective. Informational methods have emphasized potential dangers and efforts to arouse fears as a deterrence to use. Affective or humanistic education methods were designed to enhance overall self-esteem and encourage responsible decision making. Available research on these approaches has shown little demonstrable impact on reducing the use of drugs or other addictive substances.

The two major psychosocial approaches—social influence and personal and social skills training—are rooted in somewhat different theories of causality. The social influence approach recognizes the role that the social influence of family and peers has on adolescents in particular in engaging in high-risk behaviors. Programs based on this approach have attempted to make participants aware of these influences, teach specific coping skills ("Just Say No"), and correct misperceptions of social norms regarding those behaviors (such as acquainting students with the fact that most people do *not* smoke).

Personal and social skills training builds on the social influence approach but emphasizes that these behaviors are basically learned through modeling and reinforcement. Programs based on these assumptions focus on learning other skills (such as self-control, assertiveness, or tension reduction) that may be useful in resisting the temptation or invitation to engage in these behaviors. Evaluations of programs based on these models have demonstrated greater success in preventing adolescent drug use (Bangert-Drowns, 1988; Ellickson & Bell, 1990a, 1990b; Graham, Johnson, Hansen, Flay, & Gee, 1990; NIDA, 1987, 1991b; Tobler, 1986).

Private physicians and therapists are often in a position of counseling high-risk patients or families about the prevention or treatment of substance abuse.

Treatment-Oriented Care. The treatment of substance abuse disorders is multifaceted and involves an array of providers and interventions, often based on competing theoretical conceptions of underlying causes. Treatment has been variously characterized according to the mode of intervention used (pharmacological or psychological), as well as the location at which services are provided (outpatient, inpatient, residential, community-based) (Friedman & Beschner, 1985; Gerstein & Harwood, 1990; IOM, 1990; NIDA, 1987, 1991b).

Major pharmacological interventions involving the use of prescribed medications include the substitution of a medication that has actions that are similar to the abused drug but that are much less physically or psychologically harmful, such as methadone treatment for heroin addiction or the use of nicotine chewing gum by smokers — either on a long-term or short-term basis to suppress withdrawal symptoms during detoxification. These interventions also include treatment with a medication that blocks the effects of the abused drug, such as naltrexone treatment for heroin addiction. Another alternative is treatment with medications to relieve some of the symptoms associated with using the addictive drug, such as the insomnia and anxiety associated with opiate withdrawal.

Psychologically oriented therapies include the following:

1. Individual, family, or group counseling and psychotherapy (verbal therapy)
2. Systematic scheduling of positive or negative consequences as incentives for behavioral change, based on Skinner's principles of operant conditioning (contingency management)
3. Systematic exposure to drug-related stimuli in the absence of abuse behavior to reduce or eliminate feelings of drug craving, based on Pavlov's principles of classical conditioning (conditioning therapy)
4. Long-term treatment in a closed residential setting, emphasizing abstinence and learning new attitudes and behaviors (therapeutic community)
5. Teaching skills in areas (such as the social or vocational) where deficits are thought to contribute to abuse (skills development)

6. Groups (such as Alcoholics or Narcotics Anonymous) in which recovering abusers share their experiences and support one another in remaining free of the substance (peer support self-help groups) (NIDA, 1991b)

The National Drug and Alcoholism Treatment Utilization Survey (NDATUS) collects data on the characteristics of facilities providing drug and alcohol abuse treatment. The major types of facilities serving alcohol and drug abuse clients (and the percentage of all clients served by each type of facility) in 1989, based on the NDATUS client data, were as follows: outpatient facility (46.5 percent), community mental health centers (22.1 percent), hospital inpatient (13.8 percent), correctional facility (2.0 percent), halfway house (2.5 percent), other residential facility (6.3 percent), and other (6.8 percent) (NIDA, 1990b, p. 18).

Long-Term Care. The regimens and facilities in which alcohol and substance abuse–related services are rendered reflect a varied mix of both treatment and long-term care–oriented services. The five major types of care provided at the facilities identified through the NDATUS data were classified as follows:

1. Detoxification (medical) — use of medication under treatment of medical personnel to reduce or eliminate the effect of the drug in hospital or other twenty-four-hour care facility
2. Detoxification (social) — systematic reduction or elimination of the effects of the drug in a specialized nonmedical facility by trained personnel with a physician on call
3. Rehabilitation/recovery — planned program of professionally directed evaluation, care, and treatment for the restoration of functioning
4. Custodial/domiciliary — provision of food, shelter, and assistance on a long-term basis
5. Outpatient/nonresidential — treatment/recovery/aftercare or rehabilitation services in unit in which the person does not reside, with or without medication, but including counseling and supportive services (IOM, 1990; NIDA, 1990b)

Sustained abstinence or the long-term maintenance of other desired treatment outcomes is difficult for individuals who are attempting to recover from prolonged substance abuse. Relapse (or a return) to these behaviors — either on an intermittent or irreversible basis — is frequently an outcome for many "in recovery." Aftercare or continuing care programs are intended to facilitate the development or maintenance of the requisite skills, as well as to effect changes in their family, work, or social environments, to facilitate the long-term maintenance of positive treatment outcomes (Tims & Leukefeld, 1988).

A variety of custodial as well as community-based self-help options are components of this continuing care process. Employee Assistance Programs (EAP) are major worksite-based initiatives that have been employed in facilitating the diagnosis and treatment, as well as the continuing care, of substance abusing employees (Brody, 1988; Gust & Walsh, 1989; Trice & Beyer, 1984). Further, a plethora of self-help groups (such as Alcoholics Anonymous and Narcotics Anonymous, among a multitude of others) are available to those who are in long-term recovery from chemical dependency (OSAP, 1990a).

Suicide- or Homicide-Prone

A 1985 workshop and resulting report (*Surgeon General's Workshop on Violence and Public Health*) sponsored by the Surgeon General of the United States (Bureau of Maternal and Child Health and Resources Development, 1987), as well as a report titled *Injury Prevention: Meeting the Challenge*, by the National Committee for Injury Prevention and Control (1989), have served to heighten the salience of violence as a public health concern. They have also called attention to the importance of interdisciplinary cooperation in designing programs and research to address the interrelated problems of suicide, homicide, and family abuse.

In 1986 a National Research Council Panel published a two-volume report, *Criminal Careers and "Career Criminals"* (Blumstein, Cohen, Roth, & Visher, 1986a, 1986b), and in 1989 the Health and Human Services Secretary's Task Force on Youth Suicide issued a four-volume report (ADAMHA, 1989a, 1989b, 1989c, 1989d) detailing the risk factors, prevention interventions, and research needs in addressing the issues of youth suicide and lifelong patterns of violent or criminal behavior.

As discussed in Chapter Four, these studies emphasize that the root causes of violence often lie deep in the basic social or economic structure of human communities and families — areas that have traditionally been outside the domain of medical or public health practice. (See Table 5.6.)

Prevention-Oriented Care. Persistent poverty that results from lack of opportunities for entering the economic mainstream of society has historically been highly associated with rates of violence and homicide. Gurr (1989) pointed out that violent crime rates were high for many new groups of immigrants until opportunities opened for them to enter the industrial workforce. In the postindustrial U.S. society, the loss of relatively well-paying jobs for semiskilled laborers in manufacturing, the corollary movement of industry out of the heart of many U.S. cities, and the resultant disinvestments in inner-city schools and neighborhoods have exacerbated the problems of many minority youth in finding meaningful and well-paying employment. The poverty, sense of relative deprivation, and resentment resulting are cited as major contributors to the epidemic of violent behavior among these subgroups. Major interventions to prevent violence have, however, not tended to focus on these fundamental social and economic underpinnings and the structural and societal changes required to address them.

Table 5.6. Principal Programs and Services for Suicide- or Homicide-Prone.

Prevention-Oriented Care		Treatment-Oriented Care			Long-Term Care
	Ambulatory	Ambulatory	Institutional		
Public health system	Prevention-oriented	Treatment-oriented	Acute care	Long-term care	Home and community-based care
Legal deterrence	Case identification screening	Outpatient mental health services	Acute hospital care	Long-term inpatient mental health services	Child/adult protective services
Gun control	Psychological evaluation	Crisis intervention centers	Short-term inpatient mental health services	Residential treatment centers	Battered women's shelters
Capital punishment		Substance abuse cessation programs			Peer support self-help Save Our Sons and Daughters
Family planning					
Parenting skills education					
Substance abuse prevention					Correctional facilities
Stress reduction programs					Police and court systems
Violence prevention education					
Suicide prevention centers					

As in the area of substance abuse, philosophies regarding the prevention or reduction of homicides have tended to diverge in terms of means that emphasize more punitive, legal deterrence versus educational, skills building, or risk reduction strategies. Incarceration and capital punishment have, for example, been promulgated as means to either deter or incapacitate those who are likely to engage in violent interpersonal behavior.

Research investigating the impact of these methods has not demonstrated strong and consistent support for their success in reducing homicide rates (Blumstein, Cohen, Roth, & Visher, 1986a, 1986b; Kaplan, 1986; Layson, 1986; Lizotte, 1986; O'Carroll et al., 1991; Zimring, 1986). They are nonetheless the major devices available to the criminal justice system, which bears the major responsibility for addressing the consequences of individual and interpersonal violence.

Studies of the causes of suicide and homicide have identified a number of factors that have become the focus of public health–oriented prevention programs. Family planning and family life education programs have been encouraged to reduce unwanted pregnancies and teach parenting and problem resolution skills as alternatives to aggressive or injury-producing acts of physical violence. Alcohol and substance abuse prevention and stress reduction programs also have the secondary benefit of reducing or eliminating risk factors that are highly correlated with both individual and interpersonal acts of harm.

Curricula have been developed to teach junior and senior high school students how to alter their behaviors when cast in the role of aggressor, victim, or bystander in an effort to avert or diminish the lethality of incipient acts of interpersonal violence. Formal suicide prevention programs, available through a variety of public and private auspices (schools, community mental health centers, and private psychiatric hospitals, among others), are intended to assist in identifying individuals most at risk and to provide the individuals, families, and helping professionals information or resources to reduce the possibility of suicide (ADAMHA, 1989a, 1989b, 1989c, 1989d; Bureau of Maternal and Child Health and Resources Development, 1987; Center for Health Promotion and Education, 1990; Mercer, 1989; National Committee for Injury Prevention and Control, 1989; Osgood & McIntosh, 1986; Pfeffer, 1989).

The development of valid screening tools and training health care professionals, teachers, nursing home administrators, and protective service workers in how to use them can facilitate the design of early prevention-oriented interventions with those individuals most likely to inflict harm on themselves or others (Maltsberger, 1986, 1988; Orbach, 1988; Slap, Vorters, Chaudhuri, & Centor, 1989).

As with the legal-oriented approaches to deterring or averting violent behavior, more research is needed on what public health–oriented interventions are most likely to be successful in identifying and reducing the potential for violence.

Treatment-Oriented Care. Most treatment for suicide-related risks and behaviors has resided in the mental health services sector. "Treatment" for
violence-prone behavior leading to homicide has largely been provided
through the criminal justice system. Suicide crisis intervention programs
and hotlines, sponsored by a variety of public and private sources, provide
a resource for at-risk families or individuals. Mental illness and substance
abuse are important correlates of both suicidal and homicidal behavior. Programs and services to address these risk factors are also part of the continuum
of care for victims of intentional harm.

Long-Term Care. The principal philosophical focus of the criminal justice
system in dealing with individuals who have committed homicide or related
acts of intentional interpersonal injury is "incapacitation"—or imprisonment.
No particularly successful programs have been identified or implemented
to intercept or modify the "careers" of individuals who may be on their way
to a life of crime (Blumstein, Cohen, Roth, & Visher, 1986a, 1986b).
      Research and support for drug and vocational rehabilitation or other
programs that are likely to reduce rates of recidivism and/or postrelease criminal violence are very limited in poorly funded and overcrowded correctional
systems in many states. Residential treatment centers—many of which are
components of the criminal justice system—are an important source of treatment for emotionally disturbed, violent, and/or suicidal youths, though the
availability and nature of the treatment in these programs is quite varied
(Flanagan & Maguire, 1990; U.S. Department of Justice, 1988).
      Important components of community-based systems of support to avert
violent intentional injury include child, elder, spouse, or other family member
abuse services. Suicide, homicide, and family abuse and neglect appear to
be closely interrelated forms of individual and interpersonal violence. Volunteer groups, such as S.O.S.A.D. (Save Our Sons and Daughters) in Detroit,
provide social and emotional support for those whose family members have
been victims of violent death. Such support groups are also important components of the aftercare process, or "postvention," to assist family members
of suicide victims to deal with the socioemotional impact of the event (Osgood & McIntosh, 1986).

Abusing Families

The issue of child, spousal, elder, and other abuse among intimates has come
into political and social salience principally during the past twenty to thirty
years. The publication of findings in the medical literature during the 1960s
documenting the "battered child syndrome" led to the passage of child abuse
reporting laws in each of the fifty states between 1963 and 1967. In 1974,
Congress enacted the Child Abuse Prevention and Treatment Act, which
established the National Center on Child Abuse and Neglect within the Children's Bureau. The act also set out a budget for research and demonstration

projects and the development of a baseline national survey (Study of National Incidence and Prevalence of Child Abuse and Neglect), as well as a routine system of reporting for episodes of child abuse and neglect (National Study on Child Neglect Abuse and Reporting) (Gelles & Cornell, 1990).

In 1980, joint Congressional hearings called for the introduction of adult protective service laws and the establishment of a National Center of Adult Abuse. Following these hearings, the Administration on Aging identified elderly abuse as a priority research area (Filinson & Ingman, 1989). By 1990, a total of forty-five states or jurisdictions (including the District of Columbia, Guam, and the Virgin Islands) had laws requiring mandatory reporting of suspected elder abuse in domesting settings, while eight states had statutes governing the voluntary reporting of such incidents (Tatara, 1990).

The development of policies and legislation addressing the issue of wife abuse has lagged behind those in the areas of child and elderly abuse and neglect. The identification of wife abuse as a social problem began as a grass-roots effort on the part of women's groups first in England and then in the United States during the early 1970s. As early as 1972 in the United States, safe houses or battered women's shelters were established through the volunteer efforts of feminist-oriented organizations. In 1975, the National Organization for Women created a task force to examine wife battering. At the federal level, the Office of Domestic Violence, established in 1979, was closed in 1981. The National Domestic Violence Prevention Act was passed into law in the early 1980s, though funding has tended to be minimal. In 1984, the U.S. Attorney General established a Task Force on Family Violence, which published a major report dealing with this issue—*Attorney General's Task Force on Family Violence: Final Report* (U.S. Department of Justice, 1984a). Despite these grass-roots and federal programmatic efforts, and in contrast to the child and elder abuse areas, only a few states currently have mandatory reporting laws governing wife battering (Gelles & Cornell, 1990). (See Table 5.7.)

Prevention-Oriented Care. As indicated in Chapter Four, the propensity to abuse innocents and intimates lies deep in the structure of human society. Correspondingly, the interventions recommended to alter the likelihood of these behaviors occurring lie outside the domains traditionally encompassed by public health, and certainly medical care, practice.

Such proposals include, among others:

1. Altering the social and familial norms that legitimize and glorify violence (such as the acceptability of corporal punishment, media violence, and the ready availability of handguns)
2. Reducing violence and stress-provoking social and economic inequalities resulting from differential educational or employment opportunities
3. Mediating the sexist character of family and society, manifest in the

Table 5.7. Principal Programs and Services for Abusing Families.

	Prevention-Oriented Care		Treatment-Oriented Care		Long-Term Care	
	Ambulatory		Ambulatory	Institutional	Institutional	
Public health system	Prevention-oriented	Treatment-oriented	Acute care	Long-term care	Home and community-based care	
Legal deterrence	Screening and risk assessment	Emergency medical services	Acute hospital care	Long-term inpatient mental health services	Child/adult protective services	
Mandatory reporting			Short-term inpatient mental health services		Battered women's shelters	
Presumptive arrests	Counseling	Crisis response services				
Restraining orders	Individual				Peer support self-help	
Gun control	Family	Outpatient medical care services			Parents Anonymous	
Media campaigns	Group				Men's groups	
Family planning		Outpatient mental health services			Foster care	
Sex education	Substance abuse cessation programs				Home visiting	
Parenting skills education					Caregiver respite	
Substance abuse prevention					Day care	
Stress reduction programs					Child	
Violence prevention education					Adult	
					Housekeeping services	
					Transportation services	
					Housing alternatives	
					Legal assistance	
					Job placement	
					Police and court systems	
					Welfare services	
					Case management	

definition of rigid sex-role expectations and differential social status and rates of pay for "women's work" (such as child care, teaching, social work, or nursing) relative to "men's work" (administration, management, accounting, or medical practice)

4. Facilitating the linkage of isolated individuals and families (such as single-parent heads of households or the elderly living alone) with networks of community-based social support services (Gelles & Cornell, 1990)

The fundamental changes entailed in this series of recommendations require a social consciousness and political commitment not yet manifest in policy-making in this and related areas affecting the health and health care of vulnerable populations.

Nonetheless, programs have been developed or suggested to intervene categorically to prevent or treat the effects of intimate violence. Interventions that have emanated from the legal versus the public health or social service sectors tend to mirror conflicting philosophies, grounded in the contrasting values of "control" versus "compassion" toward abusers.

Methods of legal deterrence, such as mandatory reporting laws, presumptive (meaning mandatory) arrests when actual abuse is suspected, the imposition of civil protection (restraining) orders or peace bonds on those actually convicted, and the support of gun control legislation, represent efforts to forcibly (or legally) "control" or inhibit the likelihood of the (re)occurrence of violent behaviors.

Community media campaigns and associated hotlines have been used as means to enhance the public's knowledge and awareness of the family violence problem, as well as to encourage the reporting of suspected or actual incidents of abuse to the police or other proper authorities (Gelles & Cornell, 1990; Langan & Innes, 1986).

Public health and social service interventions, such as family planning, sex and sex abuse education, parenting skills education, substance abuse prevention, and stress reduction and violence prevention programs, attempt to reduce the risks associated with unwanted or unplanned pregnancies or other interpersonal or behavioral stressors within the family. Home visitation by nurses or other social service professionals has also been demonstrated to be an effective means for reducing the likelihood of child abuse and neglect in high-risk families. These and related service-oriented programs attend to the more "compassionate" orientation that abusers may themselves be victims of their environments, and that it is important to reduce the risks and increase the coping resources they need to avert the prospect of intentional or unintentional injury to an intimate in their care (Binder & McNiel, 1987; Cohn, 1982; Daro, 1988; Epstein, 1990; GAO, 1990d; Helfer, 1982, 1987; Neergaard, 1990; Olds, Henderson, Chamberlin, & Tatelbaum, 1986; Taylor & Beauchamp, 1988; Upsal, 1990; Wurtele, 1987).

The 1988 *Surgeon General's Letter on Child Sexual Abuse* (Koop, 1988), as well as the conference and resulting proceedings sponsored by the Bureau of Maternal and Child Health, *Family Violence: Public Health Social Work's Role in Prevention* (St. Denis & Jaros, 1988), encouraged a greater role on the part of public health and health care professionals in identifying and treating, or appropriately referring, cases of intrafamily violence and abuse. Family and individual counseling or substance abuse cessation programs are also often directly or indirectly intended to avert the risk of potential violence, in addition to addressing mental health or addiction problems within multiproblem families.

Such interventions may, for example, view the stress associated with social or economic factors (such as unemployment or cultural norms toward violence) as independent variables and personal and psychological variables (tendency to see violence as a problem-solving strategy, poor interpersonal or coping skills) as intervening variables that are most likely to predict which families or individuals will react to these stresses with acts of violence toward other family members (Justice & Justice, 1990; Straus, Gelles, & Steinmetz, 1981).

Treatment-Oriented Care. Cases of child, spousal, elder, or other intrafamilial abuse often land in outpatient medical care facilities—particularly big-city emergency rooms. For example, approximately 22 to 35 percent of women who visit emergency departments have been estimated to be there because of an injury from or manifestation of living in an abusive relationship (Randall, 1990). Especially severe cases may require inpatient admissions for the treatment of injuries incurred during the abusive incidents. Though poorly developed or nonexistent in most U.S. communities, hotlines or crisis response programs provide another avenue for dealing with the family or medical emergencies precipitated by incidents of abuse.

Approaches to treating child sexual and other types of abuse include the lay or paraprofessional approach utilizing peer counseling and support, the group approach emphasizing group therapy and education, and social work that relies on individual counseling. New emphases in trying to address the multicausal and multiproblem maltreatment in many families include multidisciplinary teams of medical care and social service professionals and interagency cooperation to develop networks of case identification, treatment, and referral for at-risk families and individuals (Asen, George, Piper, & Stevens, 1989; Carney, 1989; Justice & Justice, 1990; Keller, Cicchinelli, & Gardner, 1989; Taylor & Beauchamp, 1988).

Long-Term Care. Child and adult protective and welfare agencies are the major social service–oriented governmental institutions charged with identifying and intervening with abusing families and individuals. The level of funding and staffing for these agencies is uneven and generally inadequate across states, and the resultant caseloads often too large for agency case workers to attend closely to families most at risk.

Shelters or safe houses are one of the key sources of community-based, private sector support for battered women and their children. These agencies are largely supported by private donations and volunteer efforts and have slim operating budgets. Because of the need in many communities, the number of community-based alternatives for battered women has grown substantially over the past twenty years—from only five or six battered women's shelters in the early 1970s to, in 1987, 935 shelters, 550 safe houses, and 303 nonresidential treatment centers (Gelles & Cornell, 1990; PHS, 1990).

Protective service, welfare, and voluntary community groups concerned with abusing families attempt to identify and/or provide an array of support services. These may either mediate the stresses on families that appear to be productive of violence or permit the victims of abuse to gain sufficient independence to extricate themselves from the abusive environment. These services include foster care, caregiver respite, day care, housekeeping, alternative housing, transportation, legal, and job placement services, among others.

Peer support self-help groups, such as Parents Anonymous or men's groups formed to provide peer counseling for abusers, are also important components of the treatment and long-term service continuum for this population. Sometimes convicted offenders' participation in such groups is mandated by the courts. The dropout rates for both voluntary and nonvoluntary participants are nevertheless quite high in these groups.

The police and courts remain the front lines of intervention for many incidents of domestic violence—particularly spousal abuse. Domestic disturbances have come to be diagnosed as the "common cold" of police work. Mandatory (or presumptive) arrests for suspected intrafamilial abuse are permitted in some municipalities, though how local police departments choose to handle these cases remains quite variable. To attempt to deter convicted offenders from committing acts of violence once released from custody, the courts may issue restraining orders or peace bonds (in which the defendants are obligated to pay should they violate the court's ruling restricting their contact with the persons they abused previously) (Finn & Colson, 1990; Garner & Clemmer, 1986; Gelles & Cornell, 1990; Goolkasian, 1986; U.S. Department of Justice, 1984b; Whitcomb, 1985).

Homeless

The "new" homeless began to become more and more visible in U.S. cities during the early 1980s. In the absence of significant public and private initiatives in this area at the national level, the burden of caring for the homeless fell to local voluntary organizations (such as rescue missions or sectarian or nonsectarian charitable organizations) and municipalities. The major programs serving the homeless still rely to a large extent on these locally, largely privately funded, and in many cases, volunteer-based initiatives (IOM, 1988c; National Alliance to End Homelessness, 1990; U.S. Commission on Security and Cooperation in Europe, 1990).

Over time, however, private foundations as well as the federal government have assumed more of a role nationally in funding programs in general and for certain categories of the homeless (such as the chronically mentally ill). These include the Robert Wood Johnson Foundation Health Care for the Homeless Program (jointly funded by the Pew Foundation), the RWJF Project for the Chronically Mentally Ill (jointly funded by the U.S. Conference of Mayors and the Department of Housing and Urban Development, or HUD), and the RWJF Homeless Families Program (jointly funded by HUD) (Brickner, Scharer, Conanan, Savarese, & Scanlan, 1990; IOM, 1988c; Public Health Reports, 1990b).

The Stuart B. McKinney Homeless Assistance Act of 1987 provided support for the Health Care of the Homeless Program within the Bureau of Health Care Delivery Assistance, the Mental Health Services for the Homeless Block Grant Program, and the NIMH Community Mental Health Service Demonstration program, among others (DSPPD, 1990b, 1991; Sargent, 1989; Stephens, Dennis, Toomer, & Holloway, 1991). Public Law 100-6 authorized the creation and funding of the Veterans Administration Homeless Chronically Mentally Ill (HCMI) Veterans program, implemented in 1987 (Rosenheck, Gallup, Leda, Gorchov, & Errera, 1990). The Department of Health and Human Services has recently joined with HUD and NIMH in programs combining housing assistance with mental health services, and with NIAAA in supporting research and demonstration projects on alcohol and drug abuse treatment among the homeless (Public Health Reports, 1991).

These and other initiatives, as well as a 1988 IOM report on the homeless, *Homelessness, Health, and Human Needs* (IOM, 1988c), served to increase the visibility of this particularly vulnerable population nationally, and to present solutions for addressing their needs. As will be seen in Chapter Seven, the development of programs for the homeless falls far short of "curing" the problem of homelessness and of addressing the needs of those for whom it is already a fact of life. (See Table 5.8.)

Prevention-Oriented Care. As with other vulnerable populations, preventing homelessness requires societal and political investments that lie outside the domain of traditional public health and medical care practice.

The IOM (1988c) report on homelessness pointed out three major types of housing that could be effective in preventing homelessness: low-income, supportive, and emergency housing. Federal policy has manifested a decade-long retreat from ensuring decent housing for low-income Americans. There is also a paucity of specialized or supportive housing for vulnerable subgroups of the homeless that other systems of caring have failed — such as the physically disabled, mentally ill, abused women and children, and alcohol and drug users, among others. Emergency housing is particularly important for the new homeless (many of whom are mothers and children) who find themselves suddenly without a roof over their heads because of a family (domestic violence) or economic (job layoff) crisis.

Table 5.8. Principal Programs and Services for Homeless.

| | Prevention-Oriented Care | | Treatment-Oriented Care | | Long-Term Care | |
| | | Ambulatory | | Institutional | Long-Term Care | |
Public health system	Prevention-oriented	Treatment-oriented	Acute care	Long-term care	Home and community-based care
Housing	Prenatal care	High-risk mother and infant care services	Acute hospital care	Long-term inpatient mental health services	Homeless shelters
Low-income	Immunizations	Chronic disease management	Short-term inpatient mental health services	Convalescent care	Housing alternatives
Supportive	Health screening			Residential placement	Food assistance
Emergency	Infectious disease	AIDS treatment therapies			Education
Street and community outreach	Chronic disease				School-based programs
	Psychological evaluation	Outpatient mental health services			Vocational
Family planning					Battered women's shelters
Parenting skills education		Substance abuse cessation programs			Child/adult protective services
Nutritional services		Emergency medical services			Welfare services
AIDS education		Outpatient medical care services			Case management
Substance abuse prevention		Dental care services			

In addition, a variety of other outreach and prevention-oriented services are needed to prevent and/or ameliorate the complex, and often serious, health problems experienced by the homeless. Street and community outreach—particularly for mentally ill adults and runaway or homeless youth—are useful in identifying those individuals who may be most at risk of harm from living on the streets (victims of robbery, violence, or sexual exploitation, for example).

Homeless women and adolescent female runaways are much less likely to either be able to afford or to use birth control than are other women. They are also quite likely in many cases to be escaping abusive family environments. The provision of family planning and associated parenting skills education are then increasingly important for the growing number of women of childbearing ages among the homeless.

The homeless—particularly homeless youth—are more likely to be at risk of substance addiction and AIDS. Behaviorally oriented interventions, such as providing free condoms or sterile needles, may be more effective than traditional educational or attitude change approaches for altering high-risk behaviors among these subgroups. There is, however, a paucity of both demonstration projects and research exploring the utility of these or other approaches among the homeless.

Many of the homeless not only do not have a roof over their heads but also do not know the source of their next meal. Soup kitchens, pantries, and shelters have been mainstays in providing food for the homeless, as well as for other groups of the poor (Bowering, Clancy, & Poppendieck, 1991; Clancy, Bowering, & Poppendieck, 1991; Rauschenbach, Frongillo, Thompson, Anderson, & Spicer, 1990). Many of the health problems of the homeless, particularly among homeless children (under- or malnutrition, anemia, skin disorders, developmental delays), are associated with inadequate nutrition. Poor nutrition also puts pregnant homeless women at risk of having low-birthweight babies or other adverse birth outcomes. Expanding and targeting existing federal food programs for the poor, such as WIC or food stamps, are avenues for ameliorating the health effects of poor nutrition among the homeless (Alperstein & Arnstein, 1988; Alperstein, Rappaport, & Flanigan, 1988; American Academy of Pediatrics, Committee on Community Health Services, 1988; Bassuk & Rubin, 1987; CDF, 1991c; Hu, Covell, Morgan, & Arcia, 1989; Miller & Lin, 1988; Wood, Valdez, Hayashi, & Shen, 1990).

A related and important component of medical care for the vulnerable homeless is prenatal care and well-child care for homeless pregnant women and children. Homeless children are much less likely to have received routine immunizations. Respiratory ailments, tuberculosis, skin conditions, venereal, and other infectious diseases are more prevalent among homeless adults, relative to the general population, as are dental and mental health problems. Mobile vans and shelter-based and freestanding clinics have been used in a number of communities to provide screening and referral services for the homeless (Brickner et al., 1986; Brickner, Scharer, Conanan, Savarese, & Scanlan, 1990; Dennis, 1989).

Treatment-Oriented Care. The Institute of Medicine report on health care for the homeless points out a number of unique characteristics of homelessness that exacerbate the effective delivery of medical care and other services to this population (IOM, 1988c). These include the circumstances of living on the street, which make it difficult to implement a successful treatment plan (problems include trying to keep a supply of medication or dealing with the resulting side effects, such as drowsiness, that might make them more vulnerable to exposure or violence). The multiplicity and diversity of their health and social and economic needs (including mental, physical, and substance abuse problems, as well as inadequate incomes) also need to be taken into account. Other factors include their isolation resulting from the lack of supportive family or friends, and their distrust of traditional health and mental health care or other professionals because of bad experiences while under care previously.

The Robert Wood Johnson Foundation Health Care for the Homeless (RWJF-HCH) project attempted to incorporate principles in the design of health care programs for the homeless that would better match their serious and multifaceted needs. The nineteen projects differed considerably in design — evolving primarily according to the model deemed most appropriate by the local broad-based community coalitions responsible for the programs. The RWJF-HCH programs did tend to share the following elements in common, however: a holistic treatment approach that took into account the social and economic, as well as medical care, needs of the homeless (such as where they slept and got food and the benefits to which they were entitled); street and community outreach to establish a conduit for service or benefit provision; a well-trained and empathetic staff and continuity in the personnel seen; a multidisciplinary team approach and range of services to address their diverse medical, mental, social, and economic needs; and case management and coordination to facilitate continuity and follow-up.

Other major federally funded programs to serve the homeless, such as the Health Resources and Services Administration Health Care for the Homeless (HRSA-HCH) program (DSPPD, 1990b, 1991; Stephens, Dennis, Toomer, & Holloway, 1991), the NIMH Community Mental Health Services Demonstration Program (Sargent, 1989), and the Veterans Administration Homeless Chronically Mentally Ill (VA-HCMI) Program (Rosenheck, Gallup, Leda, Gorchov, & Errera, 1990), among others, have also incorporated many of the key components of the RWJF-HCH projects.

Hospital emergency rooms remain the major source of care for the homeless on an urgent or episodic basis in many U.S. cities or localities. Many homeless have not applied for, or have failed to retain eligibility for, benefits such as AFDC, SSDI, or SSI (because of the lack of a permanent address or the red tape required). This might entitle them to coverage for health care services through Medicaid or Medicare as well. Having such coverage may be particularly important when acute medical or mental health care is needed. Otherwise, the homeless are likely to be inadequately served or go unserved ("dumped") by institutions unwilling or unable to assume a larger financial burden for patients who cannot afford to pay for their care (IOM, 1988c; U.S. Commission on Security and Cooperation in Europe, 1990).

Long-Term Care. Particular problems experienced by the homeless with complex, chronic mental or physical problems are that they have neither a home nor supportive caregivers to provide them home care, and nursing homes may refuse to take them because they have no means of paying for their care and/or the institution is unwilling to take on caring for what they perceive to be problem patients. The homeless themselves are often unwilling to consider being cared for in traditional institutional settings because of prior negative experiences or a preference for a more independent life on the streets (even though viewed as an extremely tenuous or threatening way of life by middle-class health care providers).

Through volunteer or local municipal efforts, converted apartment buildings or shelters have been used to establish convalescent or respite units linked to, but separate from, health care institutions. These can provide a place for homeless seriously ill persons to go after discharge. A residential placement program of the Veterans Administration secures supervised housing alternatives in the community—either in private residences or personal board-and-care homes—for patients who are to be discharged from VA facilities. Creative and resourceful discharge planning is a particularly important need for the homeless (IOM, 1988c).

Shelters have provided the backbone of community-based service provision for the homeless in many U.S. cities. A 1988 National Survey of Shelters for the Homeless estimated that there were approximately 5,400 homeless shelters throughout the country. This represents a tripling in the number of shelters (from 1,900), and a corollary increase in bed capacity (from 100,000 to 275,000) since 1984. Around one-fourth (25 percent) of the shelters serve unaccompanied men, and the balance families with children (36 percent) or other (or more mixed) groups of the homeless (39 percent) (USDHUD, 1984, 1989c).

Soup kitchens, food pantries, and other emergency food assistance programs are important initiatives for addressing the paired problems of hunger and homelessness. The Stewart B. McKinney Homeless Assistance Act and associated Federal Emergency Management Agency funds were used by all of the twenty-eight cities surveyed in the 1991 U.S. Conference of Mayors' Task Force Survey of Hunger and Homelessness to support emergency food assistance activities. Locally generated revenues, state grants, and the Community Development and Community Services block grants were also important sources of support for these programs (U.S. Conference of Mayors, 1991).

Protective service agencies and battered women's shelters, as well as school-based programs and vocational educational or job placement programs, could be links in the chain of service provision for the homeless. This is particularly true with regard to homeless women and children, though in most cities, communication and coordination between agencies serving these populations is either poorly developed or nonexistent (Anderson, Boe, & Smith, 1988; Bachrach, 1987; Chenoweth & Free, 1990; Hagen & Ivanoff, 1988).

Outreach and case management are key components of the major public and private programs described earlier for serving the homeless (such as RWJF-HCH, HRSA-HCH, and VA-HCMI). Case management for the homeless has been viewed as a critical means to identify and coordinate a diverse and fragmented array of services on their behalf. It has also been judged a poor and unsatisfying substitute for the failure to undertake fundamental reforms of the systems (actually nonsystems) of care for the homeless as well as the array of other vulnerable populations numbered among them (the physically or mentally ill, persons with AIDS, alcohol and substance abusers, and victims of family abuse or neglect, among others) (IOM, 1988c).

Immigrants and Refugees

Most immigrants — legal or otherwise — confront many cultural, social, and economic barriers in adjusting to life in the United States. The programs and activities developed to serve immigrants depend, to a large extent, on the values and political objectives underlying U.S. foreign and immigration policies.

One set of opinions, for example, is guided by the strongly held values and attitudes of nativism, racism, protectionism, and xenophobia, which attempt to exclude or limit the influx of the foreign-born to the United States as well as the assumption of any collective or societal responsibility for their welfare.

An opposite perspective calls for a more open policy, principally due to the fact that many of those who were forced or sought to leave their homeland did so as a direct or indirect consequence of U.S. foreign political, military, or economic policy. This point of view argues that since those seeking refuge were made vulnerable by our collective (foreign) policies, there is a corollary collective (or societal) responsibility to attempt to address and provide for their needs.

Still another opinion is that certain categories of immigrants, such as foreign workers, should be encouraged to come to the United States because they bring a specialized set of skills or are willing to work for lower wages than U.S. citizens and thereby enhance the competitive position of U.S. industry and agriculture. In this case, they are assumed to be entitled to those benefits they earn through participation in the labor market and the corollary social class of which they become a member.

These and other values have variously guided the formulation of U.S. immigration policies at different times, as well as the programs and services to which immigrants and refugees are entitled (Bean, Vernez, & Keely, 1989; Guttmacher, 1984; Rumbaut, Chavez, Moser, Pickwell, & Wishik, 1988; Simon, 1991). (See Table 5.9.)

Table 5.9. Principal Programs and Services for Immigrants and Refugees.

Prevention-Oriented Care		Treatment-Oriented Care			Long-Term Care
	Ambulatory		Institutional		
Public health system	Prevention-oriented	Treatment-oriented	Acute care	Long-term care	Home and community-based care
Family planning	Prenatal care	Emergency medical services	Acute hospital care	Long-term inpatient mental health services	Education
Nutritional services	Immunizations	Outpatient medical care services	Short-term inpatient mental health services		Literacy/language training
Health education	Health screening	Outpatient mental health services			Housing alternatives
Infectious disease control	Infectious disease	Dental care services			Transportation services
Environmental risk abatement programs	Chronic disease				Legal assistance
Housing	Psychological evaluation				Job placement
Sanitation					Voluntary agency (Volag) refugee assistance
					Child/adult protective services
					Welfare services
					Case management

Prevention-Oriented Care. Many immigrant and refugee populations are exposed to substantial health risks as a function of inadequate public health or preventive-oriented care, as well as the hazardous, overcrowded, and unsanitary living and working conditions that characterized their lives prior and/or subsequent to arrival in the United States (Sandler & Jones, 1987; Toole & Waldman, 1990).

Those most socially and economically disadvantaged (legal or illegal) immigrants and refugees may in particular benefit from basic traditional public health services. This includes the maintenance of community standards and services regarding housing, sewage, and garbage pickup in those areas in which large immigrant or refugee populations reside. Though many cultural factors come into play in designing and delivering such services, basic health education and nutritional services may help to prevent the onset or spread of preventable diseases.

Refugees are required to undergo health screening, and to demonstrate a level of physical and mental health and/or associated support necessary to ensure their ultimate economic self-sufficiency once they are permanent residents of the United States. Undocumented (illegal) aliens are very unlikely to have any screening of this kind (such as for TB or hepatitis). Substantial proportions of subgroups of migrant and refugee children are also not likely to have had routine immunizations (for DPT, polio, or measles, for example), which greatly increases their risk of contracting these preventable childhood diseases.

The fertility rates of certain refugee and immigrant women are quite high. However, substantial educational and cultural barriers may exist to providing family planning and prenatal care services to such populations (Kulig, 1990; Rumbaut, Chavez, Moser, Pickwell, & Wishik, 1988).

Treatment-Oriented Care. Many (particularly illegal) immigrants often seek care only in emergencies that might be precipitated by accidents, injuries, or the complications of childbirth. The burden on the large public hospitals that tend to serve these populations is, as a result, substantial in many communities (FAIR, 1986).

Access to outpatient medical care services through private or institutional providers is limited by the same financial and organizational barriers that exist for other groups in the community with a similar profile of socioeconomic status and associated entitlements (such as Medicaid). In addition, however, cultural or language factors may also dictate where immigrants and refugees can or choose to go for care, such as community or neighborhood health centers, rather than hospital outpatient departments, or to private providers of the same race or cultural background, rather than to "foreign" (U.S.) physicians.

As mentioned earlier, both legal and illegal refugee groups have often experienced serious psychological, in addition to physical, trauma resulting from themselves or family members being tortured, or from witnessing loved ones killed. U.S. immigration policies have also contributed to the stresses experienced by refugees by scattering family members or providing very time-limited support for resettlement, for example. Policies and programs to treat as well as prevent posttraumatic stress syndrome and the associated psychological manifestations resulting from extremely stressful premigration or resettlement experiences are needed for many subgroups of refugees (Westermeyer, 1987; Westermeyer, Callies, & Neider, 1990).

The dental health needs of immigrants and refugees—particularly children—have been found to be substantial, due to inadequate nutrition or preventive or treatment-oriented dental care services (Chavez, Cornelius, & Jones, 1985; Pollick, Rice, & Echenberg, 1987).

Long-Term Care. One of the major problems many immigrants and refugees experience is the fact that they are unable to speak, read, or write English, or in some cases are illiterate even in the language spoken in their country of origin. English language and literacy classes are an important component of community support for these subgroups of new arrivals. Other important support services and resources for refugees and immigrants include job placement, housing, transportation, or welfare or in some cases legal assistance in these or related areas. Refugee status formally confers benefits such as Medicaid for the first eighteen to thirty-six months of residence, as well as English as a second language (ESL) courses and job training. In an effort in some communities to develop a comprehensive, family-oriented approach to these programs, efforts have been made to tie them to Head Start or other ongoing childhood education activities (Broughton, 1989; Rumbaut, Chavez, Moser, Pickwell, & Wishik, 1988).

Voluntary refugee assistance agencies (Volags), sponsored by religious, cultural, or human rights groups, among others, play a large role in obtaining the necessary sponsorship and support (for housing and employment, for example) needed by groups and individuals seeking admission to the United States under an official refugee status. Groups of volunteers also serve as a kind of underground railroad for "refugees" who are fleeing their homeland but who are not eligible for official refugee status under existing U.S. immigration policy.

Child or adult protective services agencies may be drawn into dealing with cases of apparent abuse or neglect on the part of immigrant or refugee families that are reported by health care or other professionals. These cases may, however, often be surrounded with ambiguity and misunderstanding due to language barriers, differing childrearing norms, or folk or indigenous medical care practices that may not be fully understood by the accusing professional. Formal or informal case management services are provided refugee populations through public (CPS, welfare) or voluntary (Volag) refugee assistance agencies.

The next chapter examines who pays for the current complex and diverse array of programs and services to care for the vulnerable.

6

Who Pays for Their Care?

Major legacies of the health and social legislation that proliferated in the mid to late 1960s are the Medicare and Medicaid programs. Medicare is a federal social insurance program that provides essentially universal entitlement to selected health care benefits for persons sixty-five and over through the social security system. Medicaid is a means-tested (or income eligibility–based) program for categories of individuals eligible for benefits through state public assistance programs. These programs include Aid to Families with Dependent Children (AFDC) and the federal Supplemental Security Income (SSI) program for the aged, blind, and disabled. Medicare provides uniform benefits across states, while Medicaid—a combined state-federal program—is characterized by wide variability in the services covered in different states.

Medicare and Medicaid are the principal payers for health care services for the vulnerable who happen to qualify for these programs. Private health insurance benefits are mainly available to people who are working full time and their dependents, though the majority of the uninsured are in households with either full- or part-time workers. The number of Americans with no private or public health insurance has increased dramatically in the past decade. The major cause has been cutbacks in health benefits in both the governmental and industrial sectors, which reflect an effort to contain the accelerating costs of medical care.

This chapter profiles the patchwork of public and private sources of payment for the care of the vulnerable and shows which groups are likely not to have any safety net of coverage.

Cross-Cutting Issues

The profile that emerges for many vulnerable Americans is that of a sieve, rather than a safety net, of coverage for care delivered through a financially constrained, publicly supported tier of institutions and providers.

Public Payers

Medicaid is a major source of coverage for many of the vulnerable—particularly high-risk mothers and infants, the chronically ill and disabled, persons with AIDS, and those with official refugee status. Recent legislation has, in particular, attempted to expand coverage to low-income women and children. The aged, blind, and disabled in financial need who qualify for SSI are automatically eligible for Medicaid. About half of those receiving SSI are eligible because of mental disorders or retardation. The actual benefits provided by Medicaid are, however, quite variable across states, and they have become more restrictive in some states during the past decade because of a diminished federal role in financing that program. In the mid 1970s, around six out of ten of the poor were covered by Medicaid. Now about six out of ten are not.

Medicare covers physician and hospital services for the elderly, but it provides limited support for long-term care services for this or other categories of eligibles. People who qualify for Social Security Disability Insurance (SSDI) are eligible for Part A of Medicare (which covers hospitalizations), but only after a two-year waiting period.

State governments assume a large role in financing mental health services and patient care services for persons with AIDS—particularly for those with no public or private insurance coverage.

Private Payers

Private insurance is primarily available to people who work and their dependents. Many of the vulnerable are not employed because physical, psychological, or social limitations in functioning preclude their doing so or they have lost their jobs as a result of associated illnesses or injuries. Certain groups who are working (such as illegal immigrants or refugees) are likely to be employed in jobs that do not offer health benefits. The private health insurance benefits for certain categories of problems (such as mental illness or substance abuse) have traditionally been more limited, and they have become even more so in recent years. Private insurers have also developed a variety of devices for ensuring that high-risk groups (such as persons who are HIV positive or technology-assisted children) are either excluded from coverage or have constrained benefit ceilings or high cost-sharing provisions.

The Uninsured

As many as thirty-seven million Americans have been estimated to be without public or private insurance of any kind. Certain categories of the vulnerable (such as the homeless, illegal aliens, and young minority victims of violence) are likely to be uninsured. Clearly distinct tiers of service are available for the poor or medically indigent who have mental health or substance abuse problems. This is also increasingly the case in the medical care system, as publicly supported hospitals and clinics face increased demands in providing care for the array of vulnerable groups studied here, who have neither the financial resources nor coverage to pay for it.

The final chapter presents recommendations for knitting together a more effective safety net of coverage out of the current patchwork of public and private financing. (See Table 6.1.)

Population-Specific Overview

The insurance coverage status of the array of vulnerable populations examined here will be reviewed in the discussion that follows.

High-Risk Mothers and Infants

Medicaid is the primary source of payment for pregnant poor women. Nonetheless, over one out of four women in the reproductive ages has no coverage for maternity-related care.

Public/Private Payers. The Omnibus Budget Reconciliation Act (OBRA) of 1981 eliminated many of the working poor and their dependents from eligibility. The act limited deductions for work-related expenses, child care, and earned income and tightened the AFDC resource requirements. Since that time, in the context of worsening trends in child and infant health indicators, a series of expansions have been directed at increasing the proportion of low-income women and children eligible under Medicaid.

The Deficit Reduction Act of 1984 mandated state Medicaid coverage for all children under five, including those in two-parent families, whose family incomes met the state's AFDC financial eligibility test; it also mandated this coverage for all pregnant women who qualified for AFDC. OBRA 1986 gave states the option to raise income eligibility as high as the federal poverty level for pregnant women, for infants, and optionally for children up to five years of age. OBRA 1987 expanded optional authority to raise the threshold to 185 percent for pregnant women and infants and include children up to eight years of age who were within 100 percent of the federal poverty level. Under provisions retained in the Medicare Catastrophic Coverage Act of 1988, the states were mandated to cover all pregnant women and infants within 100 percent of the poverty level. OBRA 1989 mandated extension of Medicaid coverage for children under six at or below 133 percent of the federal poverty level and gave states the option of extending coverage to children born after September 30, 1983. OBRA 1990 expanded coverage to all children age eighteen and under in families with incomes below the poverty level.

By and large, these laws expanded program eligibility but did not directly address issues related to the accessibility and quality of care provided

Table 6.1. Principal Payers for Vulnerable Populations.

Vulnerable Populations	Payers		
	Public payers	Private payers	The Uninsured
High-risk mothers and infants	Medicaid is primary payer for low-income pregnant women.	Private insurers provide limited coverage for maternity care.	26% of women in the childbearing years did not have maternity benefits (1985): 17% = no insurance 9% = private insurance without the benefit
Chronically ill and disabled	Medicare is primary payer for 65+ and for disabled under 65 through SSDI. Medicaid is primary payer for nursing homes for 65+ and disabled poor through SSI, medical indigence.	Private insurers provide very limited or no coverage for long-term care.	17% of disabled children and 19% of disabled working age adults were uninsured (1984).
Persons with AIDS	Medicaid is primary payer for PWAs through AFDC or SSI.	Private insurers largely refuse to insure PWAs and those who are HIV positive.	Around 23% of PWAs may be uninsured (1987).
Mentally ill and disabled	State governments are primary payers for specialty mental health services.	Private insurers tend to provide more limited coverage for mental than for physical health care benefits.	Vast majority of clients in public tier are uninsured. Around 10% in private tier may be uninsured.
Alcohol or substance abusers	Federal, state, and local governments are primary payers for public tier of services.	Private insurers are primary payers for private tier of services.	Vast majority of clients in public tier are uninsured. Around 11-13% in private tier may be uninsured.
Suicide- or homicide-prone	Criminal justice system is primary payer for costs of homicide-related deaths. Medicare may be payer for most elderly suicides.	Private insurers are payers for subset of suicide-related deaths.	Majority of homicide victims are likely to be uninsured.
Abusing families	Criminal justice and social service systems are primary payers for costs of family abuse. Medicaid may be major payer for abused children and Medicare for the elderly.	Private insurers are payers for subset of abuse victims.	Many of the victims of abuse in two-parent families with an unemployed wage earner may be uninsured.
Homeless	Public entitlement and insurance programs cover very small number of the homeless.	Private insurers have little or no role in providing coverage for the homeless.	Vast majority of homeless have no insurance.
Immigrants and refugees	Medicaid provides time-limited coverage for those with official refugee status.	Private insurers cover only immigrants and refugees in jobs with benefits.	Vast majority of illegal immigrants and many employed legal immigrants are uninsured.

to Medicaid-eligible women. The types of benefits covered vary greatly by state, eligibility determination and application procedures are generally complex and cumbersome, the rate of reimbursement to providers is lower than their average fees, and an estimated 27 percent of doctors providing obstetric services refuse to accept Medicaid patients. Many poor women do not have Medicaid coverage because of program access barriers or the fact that their income falls above restrictive state income eligibility guidelines (Barber-Madden & Kotch, 1990; Cunningham & Monheit, 1991; Hill, 1990; Mitchell, 1991; Sardell, 1990; Schlesinger & Kronebusch, 1990).

Using data from the 1977 National Medical Care Expenditure Survey and 1987 National Medical Expenditure Survey, Cunningham and Monheit (1991) estimated changes in insurance coverage for children between 1977 and 1987 based on their income and family composition. Children in poor and low-income two-parent families with only one parent working experienced the greatest estimated decline in private coverage—from 71 percent in 1977 to 47.3 percent in 1987. The diminished coverage for these children was attributed to the decline in real earnings for full-time male workers and the loss of jobs in the industrial sector to the services sector, where employers were less likely to offer health insurance.

For poor and low-income children in single-parent families, the decline in coverage resulted principally from a loss in public coverage—from 67.7 percent in 1977 to 51.4 percent in 1987. This decline was even more dramatic for working single parents. The diminished coverage for these children was attributed to the more stringent Medicaid eligibility requirements enacted earlier in the decade and the failure of subsequent expansions to keep pace with the growing number of poor and near-poor children—particularly in single-parent families.

The Uninsured. Thirty-six percent of poor children (those with incomes below federal poverty level guidelines) had neither public nor private coverage in 1987, compared to 21.8 percent in 1977. Most of the increase in the proportion uninsured was attributed to a substantial loss of Medicaid coverage. Around half (50.3 percent) of poor children were covered by public insurance (primarily Medicaid) in 1977, compared to 37.6 percent in 1987. The percentage of low-income children (those with incomes from 100 to 199 percent of the federal poverty level) with no insurance also increased from 20.9 percent in 1977 to 27 percent in 1987. This increase was due principally to their loss of private insurance. Sixty-two percent had private insurance in 1977, compared to 49.3 percent in 1987 (Cunningham & Monheit, 1991).

A study conducted by the Alan Guttmacher Institute estimated that in 1985, 26 percent of women (or 14.6 million) in the reproductive ages had no insurance to cover maternity care. Seventeen percent had no insurance of any kind, and 9 percent had private insurance that did not cover maternity services. Those without coverage were disproportionately young, unmarried, minority, and poor. An estimated 3.2 million women with incomes below the poverty level and another 2.8 million with near-poverty incomes had neither public nor private coverage for maternity care. By the time they gave birth, the percentage of women who were uninsured was reduced from 26 to 15 percent, because they became eligible for Medicaid once the pregnancy was recognized. The Medicaid eligibility determination process generally resulted in their seeking care later in their pregnancy, however (Alan Guttmacher Institute, 1987; Gold & Kenney, 1985; Gold, Kenney, and Singh, 1987).

Chronically Ill and Disabled

Three principal types of programs provide direct or indirect financial support for the chronically ill and disabled. These include the following: (1) income assistance programs, such as SSDI, SSI, and Veterans Administration (VA), Civil Service, and black lung disability programs; (2) health insurance programs, including Medicare and Medicaid as well as VA and CHAMPUS (coverage for dependents of U.S. military personnel); and (3) supportive service programs, funded through Social Services and Maternal and Child Health block grants, the Administration on Developmental Disabilities, the Department of Education, and Child Welfare (Office of Assistant Secretary for Planning and Evaluation, 1990).

Public/Private Payers. SSDI benefits are available to disabled persons under sixty-five who have previously been employed and their dependents. The definition of disability for SSDI eligibility is "the inability to engage in any substantial gainful activity by reason of any medically determinable physical or mental impairment which can be expected to result in death or has lasted or can be expected to last for a continuous period of not less than 12 months" (Office of Assistant Secretary for Planning and Evaluation, 1990, p. 5).

Only persons who are totally disabled and whose disability is expected to be long term can qualify. The major disabling conditions for new SSDI awards in 1988 included mental, psychoneurotic, and personality disorders (22 percent); neoplasms (16 percent); disease of the circulatory system (18 percent); and skeletal-muscular conditions (14 percent).

SSDI beneficiaries are eligible for coverage under Medicare, Part A. However, there is a twenty-four-month waiting period after qualifying for SSDI to become eligible for this benefit.

The SSI program provides monthly cash benefits to aged, blind, and disabled workers who are in financial need. Unlike SSDI beneficiaries, SSI recipients do not have to have worked. As a result, the SSI program covers a beneficiary population that SSDI does not tend to cover—disabled children. The SSDI definition of disability (cited earlier) also applies in determining SSI eligibility. Financial need is based on countable income (including both income and assets). States, at their option, can provide supplementary payments to federal SSI. The amount of these subsidies varies considerably from state to state.

About two-thirds of the SSI population were eligible on the basis of the disability (rather than age or blindness) criterion. Based on 1987 data on about three-fourths of the disabled SSI beneficiaries under sixty-five, about half had a primary disabling condition related to their mental, rather than physical, functioning: 27 percent had mental retardation (42.5 percent for SSI disabled children) and 24 percent had mental disorders.

Most SSI recipients are automatically eligible for Medicaid on receipt of SSI benefits. Unlike Medicare, with Medicaid there is no waiting period to establish eligibility.

Medicaid is the largest third-party payer for institutionalized long- term care, accounting for 43.1 percent of the expenditures for nursing home care (Lazenby & Letsch, 1990). Of the approximately 24.7 million persons who received services funded by Medicaid in 1989, 15 percent (3.6 million) were eligible because of their disability (3.5 million) or blindness (95,000) (Office of Assistant Secretary for Planning and Evaluation, 1990). The role of Medicaid in financing nursing home care came about largely due to the failure of Medicare or private insurance to cover these services for the chronically ill and disabled. But substantial gaps and variability in eligibility continue to exist in the coverage provided for individuals in nursing homes and other long-term care institutions (Carpenter, 1988).

The Medicaid Home and Community-Based (Section 2176) Waiver Program (enacted in 1981) and the TEFRA Section 134 Option for Disabled Children ("Katie Beckett" waiver enacted in 1982) provide more flexibility for providing long-term care services at home, rather than in institutional settings. The 2176 waiver permits certain home care services to be covered if they are budget neutral (do not cost more than institutional care). The Katie Beckett waiver permits family income-eligibility criteria to be waived in covering home care services for categories of individuals, such as ventilator-dependent children. In fiscal year 1985, forty-two states were covering a broad array of health and social services under the 2176 waiver: thirty-four served aged and physically disabled populations, thirty-five served the developmentally disabled or chronically mentally ill, six served other populations (Laudicina & Burwell, 1988). The Omnibus Budget Reconciliation Act of 1990 provided an alternative to the 2176 waiver in financing home and community-based care under Medicaid—through incorporating them as optional services for individuals with severe physical or cognitive impairments who were eligible for Medicaid (Lipson & Laudicina, 1991).

Medicare is a major payer for hospital and physician services but has a more limited role in financing long-term care for the chronically ill and disabled. Medicare's share of national spending for nursing home care grew from 2.3 percent in 1988 to 7.5 percent in 1989—principally due to provisions under the Medicare Catastrophic Coverage Act of 1988, which were subsequently repealed (Lazenby & Letsch, 1990). Of the 33.6 million people covered under Medicare in 1989, around 10 percent (3.2 million) were disabled people under sixty-five. The vast majority (around 93 percent) were also covered for physician's services under Part B.

The expansion of home health care benefits under Medicare since 1974 in particular has resulted in substantial increases in expenditures for that benefit under Medicare as well. Approximately 1.6 million persons were served by home health agencies under Medicare in 1988 — up from 0.3 million in 1974 (Silverman, 1990).

Approximately 25 to 30 percent of all disabled Medicare enrollees under age sixty-five are covered by Medicaid based on a variety of benefit and/or income criteria. Disabled Medicare enrollees with incomes below the poverty level are also entitled to have Medicare Part B premiums, coinsurance, and deductibles covered through Medicaid in many states (Ellwood & Burwell, 1990; McMillan & Gornick, 1984; Office of Assistant Secretary for Planning and Evaluation, 1990).

Programs funded under Maternal and Child Health block grants, particularly Programs for Children with Special Health Care Needs, play a significant role in the care of chronically ill children. Services vary across states, but most fund screening and treatment of handicapping conditions, case management, and counseling. Compared to funding for health and health-related services, financial support for community-based support services for families of children with impaired mobility (such as respite care, after-school care, homemaker services, and summer camp) is largely lacking, however (Walker, Palfrey, Butler, & Singer, 1988).

A 1987 national survey of firms offering health insurance to employees and their dependents found that though the range of covered services for chronically ill children had expanded in recent years, many benefits were limited and the deductible and coinsurance rates were high. This has forced families to bear an increasing share of the costs of their child's care. Over two-thirds of the firms covered comprehensive home health services, while only one-third covered long-term care services, such as skilled nursing homes (Fox & Newacheck, 1990).

The Uninsured. Children and working-age adults with substantial limitations in functioning are much less likely than their nondisabled counterparts to be covered under private insurance. According to the 1984 Survey of Income and Program Participation (SIPP), 16.6 percent of children with disabilities — including 21.4 percent of children with mental or emotional limitations and 12.1 percent with physical limitations — lacked health insurance coverage either through private plans or Medicaid. Almost one in five (18.6 percent) of working age adults with serious functional limitations lacked either public or private coverage (Office of Assistant Secretary for Planning and Evaluation, 1990).

A study conducted by ICF, Inc. and the Brookings Institution on alternatives for financing long-term care endorsed the growth of both public and private risk-sharing options. That study called for a universal social insurance–based long-term care program to be added to Medicare, rather than one linked to the more categoric, welfare-based Medicaid program, which is de facto currently the system of financing long-term care (Rivlin, Wiener, Hanley, & Spence, 1988; Wiener & Rubin, 1989). Though the Medicare Catastrophic Coverage Act of 1988, which attempted to operationalize aspects of such a scheme, was subsequently repealed, the issue of long-term care insurance continues to be a salient one in universal health care debates. These debates have included the 1990 Pepper Commission deliberations on national health insurance, among others (AARP, 1989; Burke, 1988; Jazwiecki, 1986; McCall, Knickman, & Bauer, 1991; Meiners, 1984; Pepper Commission, 1990; Rice, 1987; Somers, 1987; Somers & Merrill, 1991; Wallack, 1988; Wiener & Hanley, 1990; Wilson & Weissert, 1989).

Persons with AIDS

Medicaid is the largest payer for persons with AIDS. HIV-infected women and children may be eligible for Medicaid through the AFDC program. Nonelderly adult males and others have to meet the financial eligibility requirements for SSI to obtain Medicaid benefits.

Public/Private Payers. The proportion of persons with AIDS with Medicaid varies considerably by state because of differing eligibility requirements and covered benefits. Estimates of the percentage of patients dying of AIDS covered by Medicaid have ranged from 20 to 60 percent, and Medicaid's share of the total expenditures for AIDS has been estimated to range from 10 to 30 percent (Pascal, Cvitanic, Bennett, Gorman, & Serrato, 1989). The Health Care Financing Administration (HCFA) estimated that in fiscal year 1988, overall, Medicaid covered about 40 percent of AIDS patients and paid about 23 percent of their total expenditures for care (Baily, Bilheimer, Wooldridge, Langwell, & Greenberg, 1990).

Based on a 1987 nationwide survey of public and private teaching hospitals, Medicaid was the primary payer for 44 percent of all AIDS admissions. The percentage for other payers was as follows: private insurance (29 percent), self-pay (23 percent), Medicare (2 percent), prisoners (2 percent). The proportion covered by Medicaid was even higher among patients in public hospitals (52 percent) than in private facilities (34 percent) (Andrulis, Weslowski, & Gage, 1989). In 1985, the 1981 Omnibus Reconciliation Act was amended to permit states to apply for home and community-based (Section 2176) waivers for persons with AIDS. Only a few states have applied for these waivers, however (Lindsey, Jacobson, & Pascal, 1990).

In 1988, HCFA estimated that Medicare covered about 2 percent of persons with AIDS and paid about 1 percent of their estimated expenditures. To become eligible for Medicare, persons with AIDS or AIDS-related complexes must meet the requirements for "insured status" and "disability" under SSDI. As with the general disabled population, they must wait twenty-four months after qualifying for SSDI before they can receive this benefit. However, many persons with AIDS do not live long enough to qualify (Baily, Bilheimer, Wooldridge, Langwell, & Greenberg, 1990).

Practically all private insurance companies refuse to insure individual health insurance applicants with AIDS, and over 90 percent refuse to insure those with HIV antibodies. According to a 1988 OTA survey of a sample of commercial insurers, Blue Cross/Blue Shield plans, and HMOs, 86 percent either screened or planned to screen individual applicants for AIDS. Methods to further reduce their exposure to the financial risk of AIDS included tighter underwriting guidelines, expanding the use of AIDS testing, adding questions about AIDS to enrollment applications, and refusing to insure individuals with a history of sexually transmitted diseases (OTA, 1988a). In 1987, around three out of ten AIDS admissions (29 percent) were covered by private insurance. The proportion of privately insured AIDS admissions was much higher in private (48 percent) than in public hospitals (13 percent) (Andrulis, Weslowski, & Gage, 1989).

State budgets are also a substantial source of funds for AIDS-related programs. In 1989, state governments contributed $252 million, or just over half of the $495 million spent at the state level, for AIDS—excluding Medicaid. States were most likely to use the remaining (federal) share of these expenditures ($233 million) for surveillance and testing and counseling programs, which were heavily supported through cooperative agreements with the Centers for Disease Control. States were more likely to use their own non-Medicaid funds for patient care, support services, and administrative activities. Support for AIDS education and information programs was relatively evenly divided between federal and state sources of funding (Rowe & Keintz, 1989).

The Uninsured. Though no direct national estimates are available, the proportion of persons with AIDS who have no insurance, because of the restrictive eligibility criteria imposed by both public and private insurers, is likely to be quite high. Based on a 1987 national survey of teaching hospitals, patients directly responsible for the costs of the hospitalization (who largely represent people who are indigent or uninsured) accounted for more than one out of five admissions (23 percent). The proportion of other nonhospital costs (physician visits, pharmaceuticals, home health care) that people with AIDS have to pay themselves is likely to be even higher.

In 1989, HCFA published an eight-volume report examining the economic consequences of HIV infection for the Medicaid and Medicare programs, based on alternative scenarios of the development of AIDS cases, treatment methods, and the distribution of sources of payment (HCFA, 1989). This and other studies, focusing on the state and private sector role in financing, are needed to determine equitable and affordable ways of paying for the array of services needed by persons with AIDS.

Mentally Ill and Disabled

State budgets are the largest sources of funding for mental health care services. The types of coverage provided by these and other sources have, however, tended to encourage the use of institutional care rather than outpatient or community-based care.

Public/Private Payers. The principal payers for specialty mental health services in 1986 were as follows: state mental health agencies (42.5 percent) or other state (5.6 percent) or local government sources (7.8 percent); Medicaid (9.0 percent), Medicare (3.0 percent), or other federal sources, such as CHAMPUS or the VA (10.3 percent); client fees (16.7 percent); and miscellaneous other sources (5.0 percent) (Scallet, 1990, p. 119).

The benefit design of Medicaid and Medicare and the deficit financing role of state mental health authorities (meaning they are the payer of last resort for patients not covered from other sources) have resulted in the respective payers mainly covering certain types of services. State psychiatric hospitals are principally funded by state mental health authorities. Those funded by a mix of state mental health authorities and local governments primarily include psychiatric outpatient clinics, psychiatric day/night facilities, multiservice mental health organizations, state- and local government–operated general hospital psychiatric units, and other residential treatment centers. Residential treatment centers for emotionally disturbed children tend to be supported by state and local sources of funds for education or criminal justice, rather than mental health per se. Private psychiatric hospitals and general hospital psychiatric units are mainly supported through private insurance and patient fees (Taube, 1990).

Federal income support programs, such as SSDI, SSI, AFDC, and food stamps, assist mentally ill individuals in obtaining nonmedical support services. SSI and SSDI in particular help to defray the living expenses of residents in facilities not covered by Medicaid. The largest federal block grant funding sources for services and resources for the mentally ill and disabled are Alcohol, Drug Abuse, and Mental Health; Community Development; and Social Services block grants (Craig, 1988b).

Most mentally ill Medicaid beneficiaries qualify through being eligible for SSI benefits. Mandatory services provided under Medicaid cover the basic mental health care needs of acutely ill patients in hospitals and nursing homes. Considerable variability exists across states in the optional services covered to facilitate the care of the mentally ill in the community (such as reimbursement for freestanding outpatient clinic services, prescription drugs, case management, rehabilitation, and home health care). Small residential facilities, such as halfway houses, adult foster homes, and crisis centers cannot qualify for Medicaid. The Medicaid program also specifically excludes payments to persons ages twenty-two to sixty-four in an institution for mental disease — those facilities in which more than half of the residents of a facility with sixteen or more beds are mentally ill (GAO, 1990e; Taube, Goldman, & Salkever, 1990).

Medicare coverage for mental health services is limited. Mentally disabled individuals become eligible for Medicare principally through their enrollment in the SSDI program. As mentioned earlier, mental illness is the reason reported most often by (22 percent of) SSDI-eligible individuals. It does not cover many of the social support and other long-term care services needed by the chronically ill in general, nor mentally ill individuals in particular.

Part A of Medicare imposes a lifetime limit of 190 days of care in freestanding psychiatric hospitals and 90 days in a general hospital within a benefit period. Medicare Part B coverage for physician services in inpatient settings is the same for mental and physical treatment. Coverage in outpatient settings differs, however. Part B pays 80 percent of approved charges after a deductible is met for treatment of physical disorders, but only 50 percent of treatment for mental disorders (with the exception of Alzheimer's disease, to which the 80 percent coverage rule applies).

In 1987, 2.7 percent ($2.2 billion) of total Medicare payments ($79.8 billion) went for identifiable mental, alcohol, and drug services. Approximately 88 percent of the mental health service expenditures were under Part A, compared to 63 percent of overall Medicare expenditures — reflecting the more generous coverage for inpatient than for outpatient psychiatric care services (Lave & Goldman, 1990). Currently, psychiatric facilities are excluded from the Medicare prospective payment system, though consideration is being given to how such a system could be applied in those settings (Jencks, Horgan, Goldman, & Taube, 1987).

Bureau of Labor Statistics Surveys of the availability of private coverage for mental health services for the period from 1979 to 1984 showed that 99 percent of medium and large firms in the private sector offered coverage for inpatient psychiatric care. However, in 1984 fewer than half (48 percent) of the employees had coverage that was equal to (had parity with) their coverage that provided for other illnesses — down from 58 percent in 1979. The percentage with outpatient coverage increased from 87 percent in 1979 to 96 percent in 1984. This coverage was quite limited, however. Only 7 percent had coverage comparable to that for other illnesses in 1984 — down from 10 percent in 1981. In 1984, the vast majority (89 percent) had coverage that was subject to severe limitations (on the numbers of visits or dollars covered, or high coinsurance rates, for example) — an increase from 82 percent with such restrictions in 1981 (Brady, Sharfstein, & Muszynski, 1986; Ridgely & Goldman, 1989).

Capitated systems of financing (based on payments per enrollee) are increasingly being considered as a mode of financing services for groups of employees or program-eligibles through both the public and private systems of financing care (Mechanic & Aiken, 1989b). A 1986 national survey of health maintenance organizations (HMOs) showed that 97 percent offered mental health service coverage and two-thirds offered substance abuse coverage to their enrollees. Slightly more than half (58 percent) covered at least thirty days of inpatient mental health care services per member per year. Four out of five (79 percent) provided for twenty ambulatory mental health visits. Most (85 percent) of the HMOs provided inpatient coverage without deductible or copayment requirements, while outpatient mental health coverage required an additional average copayment of $15 per visit (Levin, Glasser, & Jaffee, 1988).

The Uninsured. Data from the National Center for Health Statistics and National Institute of Mental Health showed that a larger proportion of psychiatric patients than of medical-surgical patients are uninsured. Based on the 1986 National Hospital Discharge Survey, 9.5 percent had no insurance, compared to 7.6 percent of all patients. According to 1981 NIMH data on the mental health services sector, 10.4 percent of discharges from general psychiatric units, 5 percent from psychiatric hospitals, and 62 percent from public mental hospitals were not insured (Frank, 1989). Problems of the absence or inadequacy of coverage are greatest for the long-term chronically mentally ill, who require a comprehensive array of inpatient and outpatient mental health as well as related social services (Frank, 1989; Frisman & McGuire, 1989; Grazier, 1989; Robinson, Meisel, & Guthierrez, 1990).

Alcohol or Substance Abusers

Although the proportion of alcohol and substance abuse services covered by private third-party insurance has increased substantially in recent years, the largest overall source of support continues to be federal, state, or local funds. However, distinct types and tiers of services have emerged in response to the evolution of private versus public sources of funding.

Public/Private Payers. Federal funding for drug abuse grew substantially from 1969 to 1974, stabilized, and then declined before beginning to grow again in 1986. From 1969 to 1975, the federal government put the majority of its anti–drug abuse resources into treatment and prevention rather than criminal justice. In the mid 1970s, the trend was reversed, and in 1989 the lion's share (69 percent) of federal anti–drug abuse expenditures was in the criminal justice area.

In 1976, the federal government paid for 42.5 percent of drug treatment and state and local governments paid for 48.2 percent. The balance came from private sources (5.0 percent) or other donations (4.3 percent). In 1989, the federal share was down to 17.4 percent—which included Medicaid, Medicare, or other public insurance (10.6 percent), welfare and social service payments (3.7 percent), and federal categoric grants (3.1 percent). The state and local share declined to 34.8 percent, while the percentage covered by private sources increased considerably, to 42.4 percent. This included 29.3 percent by private third-party payers, 11.2 percent by client out-of-pocket payments, and 1.9 percent private donations. The balance (largely donations) not paid by governmental or private sources was 5.4 percent (Gerstein & Harwood, 1990, pp. 210–217; NIDA, 1990b, p. 65).

Two distinct tiers of drug abuse treatment have emerged, which are linked directly to the means of paying for care. The public-tier programs are either publicly owned or private not-for-profit programs that obtain their revenues mainly from local, state, or federal agencies. This public tier of some 3,846 facilities is comprised mainly of large, multisite residential and methadone programs and outpatient clinics. They principally serve clients who are indigent or uninsured, and are largely an adjunct to the criminal justice system.

The private tier of 1,275 facilities primarily contains private providers who serve patients with private insurance or sufficient resources to pay for treatment themselves. This tier evolved primarily from hospital inpatient units that focused on alcohol treatment but now include a substantial outpatient and aftercare focus. The private tier treated 22 percent of all reported admissions and received 41 percent of system revenues. It averaged $2,450 in revenues per admission, compared to public system revenues of $1,240 per admission (Gerstein & Harwood, 1990, pp. 201–206).

The funding of alcohol treatment has followed trends similar to that of drug abuse treatment in terms of diminished federal support relative to increased private support over time. In 1982, the percentage distribution of funding sources compared to 1989 was as follows: federal programs (16.8 percent versus 4.8 percent), state or local (34.7 percent versus 35.3 percent), public welfare (1.6 percent versus 1.5 percent), public insurance (6.9 percent versus 8.5 percent), private insurance (26.4 percent versus 31.9 percent), client fees (9.8 percent versus 13.2 percent), and other (3.7 percent versus 4.7 percent) (IOM, 1990, p. 188; NIDA, 1990b, p. 65).

Separate public and private service systems also exist for the treatment of alcohol problems. A 1987 State Alcohol and Drug Abuse Profile (SADAP) survey of programs receiving government funding from state alcoholism agencies showed that 79 percent of the funds for treatment came from state, local, or federal sources, with the balance (21 percent) from private health insurance, client fees, or other sources. In contrast, according to a 1986 survey of private sector specialty programs conducted by the National Association of Alcoholism Treatment Programs (NAATP), the vast majority of the admissions were covered by private insurance (67 percent) or patient fees (11 percent), while the balance (22 percent) came from public sources (IOM, 1990, pp. 197–201).

Medicare and Medicaid pay a relatively small (around 10) percent of alcohol and drug abuse treatment costs overall. Neither Medicare nor Medicaid has specific benefits for the treatment of alcohol or drug abuse. Both programs tend to categorize treatment of these problems under mental disorders, with attendant limitations in coverage and benefits under Medicare and wide variability in optional services covered under Medicaid. Neither provides coverage for the educational, vocational, and psychosocial services that are generally considered to be an important component of rehabilitation and maintenance for substance abuse (relapse prevention) (IOM, 1990).

A 1988 survey of medium- and large-sized companies showed that 74 percent of employees with insurance through work had drug treatment coverage. Of the 20.6 million employees with benefits, the proportions having coverage for the major types of treatment modalities were as follows: detoxification (96 percent), outpatient rehabilitation (81 percent), and inpatient rehabilitation (77 percent). Most plans imposed substantial limitations on benefits. The most frequently imposed inpatient limit was thirty days per year; the most frequent outpatient limit was twenty to thirty visits per year (Gerstein & Harwood, 1990, pp. 278–280).

The Uninsured. The vast majority of clients seen in the public drug and alcohol abuse treatment sectors have no insurance. Around 11 to 13 percent of the treatment costs for those seen in the private sector were paid directly by the clients themselves.

Suicide- or Homicide-Prone

The agencies and institutions that bear the costs associated with attempted or completed suicides and homicides reside in a variety of sectors. A number of the correlates and predictors of violent deaths, such as depression, suicidal ideation or attempts, aggressive behavior, and family discord or abuse, among others, tend to be treated within the mental health care sector. Alcohol and substance abuse is treated within both the general mental health and alcohol and drug abuse treatment sectors. The extent of coverage for mental health and substance abuse services, like the direct medical care costs for individual victims of suicide and homicide, is a function of the type of plan and benefits for which they might be insured.

Public/Private Payers. Those individuals most likely to be suicide victims (white males) usually have private insurance coverage or Medicare.

Other sectors, such as the criminal justice and social service systems, absorb a great deal of the costs of dealing with the consequences of violent death due to homicide and suicide. Total public expenditures for the criminal justice system increased 147.6 percent (approximately 18.4 percent per year on average) between 1971 ($10.5 billion) and 1979 ($26.0 billion) and 134.6 percent (approximately 14.9 percent per year on average) between 1979 and 1988 ($61.0 billion) (Flanagan & Maguire, 1990; U.S. Bureau of the Census, 1991c). These expenditures encompass a variety of criminal justice activities other than those related directly to homicide and suicide. However, violent (and particularly drug-related) crime is an important component of expenditures within the criminal justice system.

Major social services activities administered by the Department of Health and Human Services that also provide direct or indirect support for programs to prevent suicide and related violent or abusive behaviors include the Social Services, Community Services, and ADAMH block grants; Head Start; Child Welfare Services; Foster Care; the Child Abuse and Neglect Program; the Older Americans Act; the Runaway Youth Act; and the Adolescent Family Life Program (Silverman, 1989).

The Uninsured. Those most likely to be both the perpetrators and victims of homicide (black and Hispanic males) are least likely to have insurance. In some cases, they may qualify for publicly subsidized coverage (through the VA or possibly Medicaid, for example). A 1989 GAO study of eight urban trauma centers found that 52 percent of patients who were victims of gunshot or stabbing wounds had no insurance and 26 percent were eligible for medical care assistance under government programs that did not fully reimburse trauma costs (GAO, 1991b). As indicated in the discussion of coverage for mental health and substance abuse services earlier in this chapter, the coverage provided for these services under both public and private plans remains limited as well.

Abusing Families

The principal payers for the costs associated with maltreatment are the agencies and institutions that address the short-term and long-term needs of abusing families. These include the child protective services and welfare systems, foster care programs, regular and special education programs, police departments, juvenile and adult court and detention facilities, substance abuse treatment programs, and public health departments, in addition to medical care and rehabilitation services providers (Daro, 1988).

Public/Private Payers. The medical care costs of the injuries resulting from abuse—many of which are treated in hospital emergency rooms—are covered by the family's or the individual's insurance. Daro (1988, p. 155) projected the hospitalization costs for all those children reported to have suffered serious physical injury from maltreatment during 1983 ($N = 23,648$). The resulting impairments included brain damage, skull fractures, bone fractures, internal injuries, poisoning, and burns. Assuming that only half of the children required hospitalization for an estimated 5.2 days (the average length of stay for children with bone fractures), Daro estimated that the inpatient costs of treatment would exceed $20 million. The vast majority would be paid by Medicaid, since many of the children on which the estimates were based received public assistance.

Medicare is the principal payer for the medical care costs associated with injuries or illness experienced by noninstitutionalized abused dependent elderly (Filinson & Ingman, 1989; Quinn & Tomita, 1986; Steinmetz, 1988).

The Uninsured. Estimates of the number of uninsured among victims of intimate abuse are not available. Unemployment, underemployment, and associated economic stresses often characterize such families. The rates of uninsurance are likely to be highest among those families (such as those with two parents) that do not qualify for benefits through AFDC, but in which the main wage earner is either out of work or employed in a low-paying or part-time job with no benefits.

Homeless

The vast majority of homeless have no means of paying for care. Most are uninsured. A very small number have some form of public or private insurance coverage.

Public/Private Payers. Data on the homeless seen at the 109 Health Resources and Services Administration Health Care for the Homeless (HRSA-HCH) projects during calendar year 1989 showed that only 13 percent of those served received or were eligible to receive Medicaid, 1 percent had Medicare coverage, and 1 percent had private insurance. The percentage receiving other types of benefits was also minuscule: AFDC (4 percent), SSI (3 percent), WIC (1 percent) (DSPPD, 1991).

The Homeless Eligibility Clarification Act, which was part of the Anti–Drug Abuse Act of 1986, provided that people without fixed home or mailing addresses could not be denied eligibility for Medicaid, food stamps, AFDC, SSI, veterans' benefits, job training, or other programs (U.S. Commission on Security and Cooperation in Europe, 1990). A focus of the HRSA-HCH, as well as other programs serving the homeless, is to assist those who are eligible in obtaining benefits.

The Uninsured. The vast majority of homeless continue to slip through the cracks of the fragmented and inadequate safety net of support of health and social services that do exist for the poorest of the poor in our society—among whom the homeless are clearly numbered.

Immigrants and Refugees

"Overdocumented" immigrants (those with official refugee status) have the most formalized guarantees of support and coverage (for a period at least), and the "undocumented" (illegal aliens) the least.

Public/Private Payers. Public policy regarding the health care of refugees was detailed in the Refugee Act of 1980 (Public Law 96-212). Title III of the act authorized the Office of Refugee Resettlement (ORR) within the Department of Health and Human Services to (1) monitor health screening and immunization activities in overseas centers before refugees enter the United States, (2) inspect the health documents of refugees at the port of entry, (3) notify local health departments of refugees resettling in their communities, (4) provide health assessments after relocation, and (5) facilitate refugees' access to timely treatment through appropriate health and mental health services.

Federal support for the medical treatment of refugees is based on either Title XIX of the Social Security Act (Medicaid) or the Refugee Medical Assistance (RMA) program. The 1980 Refugee Act guaranteed 100 percent federal reimbursement to states for the costs of those refugees who qualify for Medicaid, usually up to a thirty-six-month period. Medically indigent refugees who do not qualify for Medicaid (such as those who do not meet the family composition requirements for AFDC or have disabilities that entitle them to SSI) may be covered under the RMA program directly. The Office of Refugee Resettlement pays all the costs for those refugees during the first eighteen months in the United States. After that period, ORR will reimburse states for another eighteen months only if there is a state or local General Assistance program available for this purpose.

Needy refugee families with children may qualify for AFDC benefits, and aged or disabled refugees may be eligible for the SSI program on the same means-tested basis as citizens. Such assistance is usually conditioned on the refugee's willingness to accept appropriate employment and to attend English-as-a-second language (ESL) or job training classes (Rumbaut, Chavez, Moser, Pickwell, & Wishik, 1988).

Considerable controversy exists regarding whether undocumented aliens should have any guaranteed access to medical care. The 1966 statute authorizing Medicaid, unlike the Medicare statute, contained no express restrictions on eligibility based on citizenship. An amendment to the Medicaid statute (H.R. 5300, Section 4607), passed in 1985 in the closing days of the 99th Congress, however, expressly made undocumented aliens ineligible for benefits under that program. Subsequent changes have allowed more discretion to the states, but in 1992 New York was the only state in which undocumented alien women were eligible for Medicaid except in the case of life-threatening medical emergencies (APHA, 1992; Nickel, 1986).

The cost of providing uncompensated care to undocumented aliens has fallen most heavily on cities and counties. Communities and health care providers along the U.S.-Mexico border have complained bitterly that the federal government has done little to stop the flow of illegal aliens, and yet has withdrawn from any fiscal responsibility for the costs incurred in dealing with the serious health care needs they present. For example, in 1986, El Paso County, Texas, Commissioners sent President Reagan a bill for $10 million — the estimated costs of treating illegal aliens at the R.E. Thomason General Hospital in El Paso, where 20 percent of the patients were estimated to be illegal (FAIR, 1986; Nickel, 1986).

A great deal of variation exists across other federal and local programs with respect to their position on providing services to illegal aliens. Federally funded community and migrant health centers provide care irrespective of immigration status. On the other hand, pregnant women without social security numbers are not eligible for the federally supported WIC supplementary feeding program, even though undocumented immigrant and refugee women may be most in need of this service. The citizenship requirements for eligibility for public health department and indigent care services in different states and localities vary considerably. Like legal immigrants and refugees, those who are in the country illegally may sometimes travel to states with more general eligibility requirements or benefits to obtain needed care for themselves or other family members (Guttmacher, 1984; Nickel, 1986; Rumbaut, Chavez, Moser, Pickwell, & Wishik, 1988).

Many immigrants, as well as refugees and illegal aliens, are working. Those who are paid through regular payrolls have social security and state and local income taxes withheld. Working or not, they pay sales taxes on their regular purchases; excise taxes on gas, cigarettes, or liquor; and property taxes on property they rent or own. Overall, legal and illegal immigrants and refugees may well contribute more to the public coffers through these means than they take through various entitlement or income transfer programs (Nickel, 1986).

The Uninsured. Legal immigrants are generally entitled to the same benefits as U.S. citizens. But like illegal aliens and refugees, they are nonetheless often employed in jobs or industries that pay low wages and have few or no health and other benefits. Substantial proportions have no private insurance through their places of employment and do not qualify for coverage for Medicaid or other welfare benefits because what they do earn is too high and/or they do not fit the specific (AFDC, SSI) criteria for eligibility (Chavez, Cornelius, & Jones, 1985; Rumbaut, Chavez, Moser, Pickwell, & Wishik, 1988). This dilemma is reflected particularly in the high rates of Hispanics nationally (41 percent) with no form of public or private insurance coverage (Short, 1990).

The next chapter examines the impact of organizational and financial barriers on access to needed services for this and other categories of vulnerable populations.

7

How Good Is
Their Access to Care?

Access implies that people have a place to go and the financial and other means of obtaining care. The way services are organized and the methods that exist to pay for them may not always facilitate either entry or continuity, however.

Chapters Five and Six described the programs and payers that exist to provide a continuum of care for the vulnerable. This chapter reviews the evidence of organizational and financial barriers to access in the context of evaluating how well they have succeeded.

Cross-Cutting Issues

In general, the following picture emerges: (1) institutional doors are closed to many of the vulnerable; (2) for those who do gain entry, people with few resources are likely to enter through one door and those with more resources through another; and (3) the process of providing and paying for services itself does not always recognize the nonclinical causes or consequences of the problems that prompted them to seek care initially.

Organizational Barriers

Many doors are closed to the vulnerable because of fear. Such fears include providers' fears of medical malpractice lawsuits from high-risk mothers or of contracting HIV infection or losing patients due to treating persons with AIDS. Other examples of the barriers that inhibit access for the most vulnerable include a community's fears of having a halfway house for the mentally ill or a shelter for battered women or the homeless in its neighborhood, Mexican illegals' fears of being detected, or Southeast Asian refugees' fear of being referred to protective service authorities because of folk remedies used to treat a sick child.

Higher-income people and those with private insurance and their families are likely to be seen in private psychiatric hospitals or residential substance abuse treatment centers if they have mental health or substance abuse problems. The poor and uninsured, on the other hand, are more apt to receive care in overcrowded and underfunded state-supported facilities, to be reinstitutionalized in local jails or prisons, or to join the ranks of the homeless.

Systems of caring for the vulnerable are more aptly described as nonsystems, primarily because there is little integration or coordination of services across the variety of health and social service sectors required to address their needs. This is true for essentially all the categories of the vulnerable examined here.

As mentioned earlier, case managers are being utilized to create systems of care for individuals where none exist in the community. Consortia of institutions and agencies represent alternatives at the community level to build comprehensive, coordinated systems of care for vulnerable populations (such as those supported by the Ryan White legislation to improve services to persons with AIDS, the RWJF and HRSA Health Care Programs for the Homeless, and proposals for implementing the Year 2000 Objectives for the nation, among others). Categorically oriented state and federal funding have historically provided incentives favoring fragmented, rather than integrated, program development. The persistence of these fiscal disincentives, as well as traditional interagency rivalries and competition, makes building such consortia problematic, if not impossible, in many localities.

Financial Barriers

Some providers' doors are closed to people who cannot afford to pay the usual and customary fee for services. Almost three out of ten obstetrics providers refuse to see women on Medicaid. Diagnosis related group (DRG)–based reimbursement under Medicare has encouraged some providers to discharge chronically ill elderly patients in less stable condition. Private insurers have increasingly sought to exclude certain high-risk groups, such as persons with AIDS, from coverage, or to limit the benefits of others (those with mental health or substance abuse problems, for example).

The system of financing services can be characterized as having neither parity nor equity. Parity means that levels of third-party coverage and benefits are comparable for different types of services (such as acute medical care, mental health, substance abuse, or long-term care), and equity means they are comparable for different groups of people (based on race, employment status, or public versus private sources of coverage, for instance).

The physically disabled and other categories of the vulnerable who qualify for Medicare through SSDI, such as persons with AIDS, could go without having any coverage for needed care or fail to survive the two-year waiting period. People covered by Medicaid, which provides very low rates of reimbursement in many states, or those who work in jobs that provide

no coverage (as do many illegal aliens) are much more likely to confront substantial financial barriers to access than those with generous job-related
benefits.

The incentives provided by both public and private insurers have dis-
couraged, rather than encouraged, the growth of integrated systems of caring for the vulnerable. Most plans cover medically related hospital and physician expenses. Only limited benefits are provided either for prevention-
related services or for long-term home and community-based care.

Overall, a number of significant barriers currently exist to providing
and paying for care for vulnerable populations. (See Table 7.1.)

Population-Specific Overview

The major organizational and financial barriers to access for vulnerable populations are examined in the discussion that follows.

High-Risk Mothers and Infants

High-risk mothers face a number of barriers to obtaining adequate and appropriate care, including the lack of financial resources; an inadequate number and distribution of providers; a fragmented, uncoordinated, and incon-
venient delivery system; and cultural and personal factors that inhibit their
seeking formal medical care services (IOM 1985, 1988d; National Commission to Prevent Infant Mortality, 1988a; PHS, 1989).

Organizational Barriers. The Institute of Medicine report *Prenatal Care: Reaching Mothers, Reaching Infants* concludes that reducing financial access barriers
through expanded public or private coverage or even increasing the numbers of providers willing to offer maternal and child health care services still
does not address the fact that the U.S. maternity care system ("the complicated network of publicly and privately financed services through which
women obtain prenatal, labor and delivery, and postpartum care") is "fundamentally flawed, fragmented, and overly complex" (IOM, 1988d, p. 12).
This system is characterized by poor service coordination. A major problem is the absence of a systematic system of referrals between maternal and
child health or health department clinics and inpatient delivery sites, as well
as relevant human service systems such as welfare, housing, or schools. Other
problems include a lack of information about where to go for care, service
hours that do not accommodate women's work schedules, long waits for ap-
pointments or to be seen once at the site, language and cultural barriers,
lack of alternatives for child care, and transportation difficulties.

The IOM report, as well as other studies, documents that many women
who delay seeking prenatal care have unplanned or unwanted pregnancies.
They may also not think care is important or that it is needed only if a woman
becomes ill. Many poor, inner-city women, including the growing number

Table 7.1. Principal Access Barriers for Vulnerable Populations.

Vulnerable Populations	Barriers	
	Organizational	Financial
High-risk mothers and infants	The U.S. maternity care system is "fundamentally flawed, fragmented, and overly complex" (IOM, 1988d, p. 12).	Women who have no insurance or are on Medicaid face substantial financial and institutional barriers to access to maternal and child health services.
Chronically ill and disabled	The array of programs and services needed for caring for the chronically ill or disabled are either not available or not well coordinated in most communities.	Restrictive eligibility and coverage provisions on the part of both public and private payers limit financial access for the chronically ill and disabled.
Persons with AIDS	The main organizational barriers to care for PWAs in many cities include substantial service gaps, strained capacity, providers' fears of treating PWAs, and at-risk groups' lack of information.	Private insurers overtly exclude PWAs and HIV-positive individuals from coverage, and public insurers severely restrict eligibility or covered services for PWAs.
Mentally ill and disabled	The deinstitutionalization of the mentally ill without adequate community-based support services has resulted in a high risk of "reinstitutionalization" and homelessness.	The current system of financing mental health services lacks both *parity and equity*—that is, coverage *comparable to medical care services* and *across groups*, respectively.
Alcohol or substance abusers	Alcohol and substance abuse services are often poorly matched to needs due to the chronic relapsing nature of the problem, the lack of or fragmentation of services, or the unavailability of culturally sensitive treatment.	The private system sees fewer clients but receives more revenues, while the public system sees more, and more serious, cases of alcohol or substance abuse but receives fewer revenues.
Suicide- or homicide-prone	Both suicidal and homicidal behavior are dealt with in a fragmented and uncoordinated fashion across an array of discrete service delivery sectors in most communities.	Primary prevention programs for suicide and homicide are generally nonexistent, and the burden of caring for victims of violence tends to fall disproportionately on the public sector in most communities.
Abusing families	Programs for different categories of victims of intimate violence are poorly developed, fragmented, and uncoordinated.	Both public and private programs in family abuse tend to have limited funding, inadequate staffing, and poorly developed or supported systems of referral or placement.
Homeless	The organizational barriers to care for the homeless are exacerbated by their extreme poverty, unstable and unhealthy living conditions, and multidimensional health care needs.	Public support of programs and services for the homeless is limited and has failed to focus on the larger socioeconomic origins of the problem.
Immigrants and refugees	The main organizational barrier to care for immigrant and refugee populations is the unavailability of accessible and culturally sensitive providers and services.	Many immigrants and refugees experience substantial financial barriers to care due to low incomes or the time-limited availability of public coverage (refugees) or the unavailability of private coverage through their jobs.

of homeless women, are socially isolated and do not have a network of family or friends to support them emotionally or materially during their pregnancy. Women who abuse alcohol and drugs, or illegal immigrants and refugees, may also fear exposure to social or legal sanctions as a result of going for care.

The number of physicians willing to provide obstetrician-gynecologist services — particularly to low-income, uninsured, or Medicaid-eligible women — has decreased substantially in recent years. The number of such physicians in inner-city or rural areas has also declined. These trends are attributed to the low rates of reimbursement and the cumbersomeness of the payment process for Medicaid-eligible women, as well as the greatly increased risk and premiums associated with malpractice suits (Fossett, Perloff, Peterson, & Kletke, 1990; National Commission to Prevent Infant Mortality, 1988b).

A two-volume IOM report, *Medical Professional Liability and the Delivery of Obstetrical Care,* documented that there is a malpractice crisis nationally in the delivery of obstetrical care to high-risk women. It recommended a number of long-term reforms (such as developing alternatives to the existing tort system for resolving malpractice claims), as well as short-term solutions (directed toward those groups most at risk of inadequate maternity care) for addressing this problem (IOM, 1989a, 1989b).

Financial Barriers. Women with private insurance are much more likely to seek prenatal care than are women who have no insurance or are on Medicaid (Braveman, Oliva, Miller, Reiter, & Egerter, 1989; Fingerhut, Makuc, & Kleinman, 1987; IOM, 1988d; Oberg, Lia-Hoagberg, Hodkinson, Skovholt, & Vanman, 1990). A 1987 General Accounting Office (GAO) study of prenatal care access in thirty-two U.S. communities found that 81 percent of privately insured women began care in the first three months of their pregnancy and made nine or more visits, compared to 36 percent of the women with Medicaid coverage and 32 percent with no health insurance (GAO, 1987b). As pointed out in Chapter Six, the Medicaid enrollment process in many states is complex and cumbersome, and many low-income women may be well into their pregnancy before they can establish eligibility. Less than half of the women and children in families with incomes below the poverty level are covered by Medicaid. The proportions of uninsured women and children in general, and among the poor and low-income in particular, have increased over the past decade.

The availability of a full range of maternal and child health and family planning services has also been limited by restrictions and cutbacks in Title V and Title X funding (Fossett, Perloff, Peterson, & Kletke, 1990; Joyce, 1987; Rosenbaum, Hughes, & Johnson, 1988).

Since 1986, many states have attempted to reduce the administrative barriers to obtaining Medicaid by streamlining eligibility determination procedures. They have also initiated programs to enhance outreach to Medicaid-eligible women and to recruit obstetrical providers into participating in the program and have added enriched nonmedical prenatal benefits (Hill, 1990). The direction of these reforms acknowledges that simply establishing high-risk women's and children's eligibility for Medicaid will not be sufficient for enhancing their access to adequate perinatal care services. The availability, accessibility, and acceptability of these services must also be substantially improved (Caro et al., 1988; Cooney, 1985; IOM, 1988d; Lia-Hoagberg et al., 1990; Piper, Ray, & Griffin, 1990; Poland, Ager, & Olson, 1987; Sable, Stockbauer, Schramm, & Land, 1990; St. Clair, Smeriglio, Alexander, Connell, & Niebyl, 1990).

Chronically Ill and Disabled

The chronically ill and disabled face a number of barriers in obtaining needed medical and social support services — particularly for long-term or community-based care. These barriers are both organizational and financial.

Organizational Barriers. The array of programs and services for the chronically ill and disabled, which are listed in Table 5.2, are either not available in many communities or serve only limited subsets of those eligible for these services. This is particularly the case for the community-based primary and tertiary prevention-oriented programs, such as risk reduction education or intervention programs, day care, home delivered meals, home visiting, transportation services, and caregiver respite services, among others. Even when available, there is often poor communication about or inadequate coordination among services (such as transportation and day care) to ensure that those in need are aware of and are able to obtain access to them (Densen, 1991; Ireys, Hauck, & Perrin, 1985; Jones, Densen, & Brown, 1989; Krout, 1983a, 1983b; Nyman, Cyphert, Russell, & Wallace, 1989; Scanlon, 1988; Singer, Butler, & Palfrey, 1986; Wallace, 1990). Case management services are often devices for insurers to contain the costs of care — rather than for clients to have expanded access to needed services (Capitman, 1988). The Americans with Disabilities Act (ADA) enacted in 1990 is intended to reduce overt discrimination against the disabled primarily in the areas of employment, housing, and public accommodations (West, 1991).

The shorter lengths of stay and earlier condition-specific rates of discharge subsequent to the introduction of DRGs have highlighted the inadequate institutional and human services system capacity in many communities in providing adequate nursing home, as well as community-based, care (GAO, 1987a; Ho, 1987; Scanlon, 1988). Surveys of the elderly and disabled children have documented that large proportions (half to two-thirds) have substantial unmet needs for both medical and related social support services (GAO, 1988b, 1989e; Short & Leon, 1990). A particularly pressing need for many chronically ill and disabled and their families involves caregiver respite, housekeeping, or home visiting services to relieve the stress of caregiving for the large number of family members who care for their functionally restricted parent or child at home (Kosberg, Cairl, & Keller, 1990; McCann, 1988; Oktay & Volland, 1990; Romeis, 1989; Stone & Kemper, 1989; Stone & Short, 1990).

Financial Barriers. As mentioned in Chapter Six, almost one in five adults and children with serious functional limitations has no form of public or private insurance coverage. Both public and private insurers limit financial access for this population through either restrictive eligibility criteria, limitations of benefits, or the cost-sharing provisions and/or level of reimbursement provided for covered services (Doty, Liu, & Wiener, 1985; Feder, 1990; Griss, 1988, 1989; Newacheck & McManus, 1988; U.S. Congress, House Select Committee on Aging, 1985).

The two-year waiting period for Medicare eligibility for the SSDI population represents a significant barrier during a period in which their expenses are likely to be the greatest. About one-third of SSDI beneficiaries are estimated to be uninsured at some point during this period. Medicare is oriented toward paying for acute medical care—particularly physician and hospital services. Therefore, it does not cover many of the services required to prevent the onset of primary or secondary disabilities, such as preventive or wellness care (though pap smears were recently added as a covered service) or custodial or personal assistance services. It also provides very limited coverage for other services more likely to be needed by this population, such as outpatient mental health services, prescription drugs, and disposable and durable medical equipment.

Medicare pays for home health care and rehabilitation services, if these services are deemed "medically necessary" or permit "restoration of function," respectively. Neither of these criteria might, however, be met by individuals who have long-term, irreversible loss in physical and social functioning. Further, the prospective payment provisions enacted under Medicare have resulted in many elderly and disabled individuals being discharged into the community in less stable condition, without adequate posthospitalization care provisions.

More stringent cost-sharing provisions associated with Medicare through coinsurance, deductibles, and the Part B premium have increased the financial burden on many elderly and disabled beneficiaries as well. It is estimated that Medicaid covers these costs for only about one-third of the poor elderly, and that out-of-pocket expenses as a percentage of income are no less now for the elderly than they were prior to the enactment of Medicare (Ellwood & Burwell, 1990; Feder, 1990; Lubitz & Pine, 1986; Smeeding & Straub, 1987; U.S. Congress, House Select Committee on Aging, 1985, 1989).

Medicaid, not Medicare, provides coverage for one of the largest components of care for the elderly and disabled—long-term nursing home care. However, Medicaid's means-tested provisions have often increased, rather than diminished, the financial or cost-sharing burden on families. Families must "spend down" to poverty level to qualify for Medicaid coverage for nursing home care. But the Medicare Catastrophic Coverage Act of 1988 did increase the allowed amount of the nondisabled spouse's monthly income (to $786 per month) and the couple's assets (up to $60,000) that could be retained. The Katie Beckett waiver allowed states the option of not counting the parents' income in determining Medicaid's eligibility for services to be provided at home that were formerly covered only if the child was institutionalized. Only a few states have elected to implement this option, however.

One of the most significant equity issues with respect to the Medicaid program is the wide variability across states in optional benefits, such as physical therapy, occupational therapy, personal care, and rehabilitative services, among others, which may not be "optional" for the long-term chronically ill or disabled (Carpenter, 1988; Ellwood & Burwell, 1990; Griss, 1988, 1989; McMillan & Gornick, 1984).

The restrictive eligibility criteria for SSI and SSDI, and associated Medicare and Medicaid benefits, also do not fully take into account the probable inability of those deemed ineligible under those public programs to obtain or afford private insurance. Private insurers are increasingly using preexisting condition exclusion criteria, medical testing, and restrictive underwriting policies to exclude or drop categories of the disabled or seriously ill. As with the public insurers, most private policies also fail to cover the major services required to prevent primary or secondary disability, such as wellness and preventive care and long-term health and social support services (Griss, 1988, 1989).

Persons with AIDS

Persons with AIDS face an array of overt and purposeful organizational and financial barriers to needed services.

Organizational Barriers. A 1989 GAO study in five communities (New Haven, Philadelphia, Baltimore, New Orleans, and Seattle–King County) documented considerable variability in the resources available to care for AIDS patients. In all the communities, substantial service gaps or strained capacity existed. Unlike New York, the other cities did not experience an overall shortage of hospital beds for AIDS patients. However, hospitals that served as the principal providers of services for persons with AIDS in the communities did sometimes confront situations in which their AIDS caseloads exceeded their inpatient unit capacity. Many outpatient clinics had long waiting lists for services. In most of the communities, nursing homes did not admit people with AIDS because of limited bed capacity, the lack of facilities or staff to care for infectious patients, and low levels of Medicaid reimbursement. Long-term home and community-based care for persons with AIDS, including home nursing, attendant care, case management, mental

health services, substance abuse treatment, and dental care, were either extremely limited or nonexistent in most communities. The lack of housing
for people with AIDS was a serious problem in all of the cities studied (GAO,
1989a).

In 1990, the Ryan White Comprehensive AIDS Resource Emergency
and AIDS Prevention Acts were passed to help cities, states, and facilities that
were particularly burdened by the epidemic, through building community
consortia of providers to help address the problem (APHA, 1990a, 1991c).

A particularly important barrier to medical care for persons with AIDS
is the fear that health care providers themselves have of contracting the disease (Aoun, 1989; Daniels, 1991; Emanuel, 1988). According to a 1988 AMA
survey, though most physicians felt a responsibility to care for persons with
AIDS, some (such as surgical and obstetrician-gynecologist specialists and
older, married physicians) were less likely to feel a strong obligation to do
so (Rizzo, Marder, & Willke, 1990). A 1988 national survey of patients
documented a reticence on the part of providers to discuss AIDS with their
patients. Only 15 percent of the patients indicated that they had discussed
AIDS with their physician, and in the vast majority of these cases (72 percent), the patient, not the physician, introduced the topic (Gerbert, Maguire,
& Coates, 1990). Fear of AIDS has also had an impact on the willingness
of medical students and residents to treat AIDS patients, or to enter specialties
or establish practices with high concentrations of persons with AIDS (Cooke
& Sande, 1989; Link, Feingold, Charap, Freeman, & Shelov, 1988).

Data from a survey of clients of the RWJF AIDS Health Services Program in nine cities showed that whites, men, and non–IV drug users with
AIDS were more likely to obtain care through private physicians or outpatient clinics, while nonwhites, women, and IV drug users were more likely
to use hospital emergency rooms (Mor, Fleishman, Dresser, & Piette, 1992).

A number of studies have documented that those who may be most
at risk of AIDS also know the least about it (CDC, 1988a, 1990e; Hardy,
1990; NCHS, 1990c; Valdiserri, Arena, Proctor, & Bonati, 1989). The level
of knowledge on the part of subgroups of adolescents who are likely to be
most at risk (such as minorities or those who are in adolescent detention
facilities) has been found to be less than those at lower risk (DiClemente,
Boyer, & Morales, 1988; DiClemente, Lanier, Horan, & Lodico, 1991;
Goodman & Cohall, 1989). These studies highlight the need for targeted
and culturally sensitive educational and behavioral-risk interventions to those
who may be most at risk, but least informed, about modes of HIV transmission (Aruffo, Coverdale, Vallbona, 1991; Eskander, Jahan, & Carter,
1990; Kappel, Vogt, Brozicevic, & Kutzko, 1989).

Financial Barriers. A great deal of political controversy has surrounded defining the appropriate federal role in addressing the needs of persons with AIDS.
The Reagan administration and the public health and health care infrastructure were slow to react to the onset of the epidemic (Bayer, 1989, 1991;

Iglehart, 1987; Panem, 1988; Presidential Commission on the Human Immunodeficiency Virus Epidemic, 1988; Winkenwerder, Kessler, & Stolec, 1989). In recent years, there has been a backlash in response to increased levels of AIDS funding by opponents, who argue that "too much" is being spent on that illness since the death rate for other diseases, such as heart disease and cancer, is even higher (Murphy, 1991). In 1989, 45 percent of the Public Health Service AIDS budget was allocated for biomedical research, 49 percent for epidemiology and public health control measures, and only about 5 percent for patient care services (GAO, 1989a). A much larger share of state expenditures for AIDS programs (26 percent) is devoted to patient care services (Rowe & Keintz, 1989).

As mentioned in Chapter Six, substantial financial barriers exist for those who require care for AIDS. According to a 1987 survey of the fifty states and the District of Columbia, in many states there were no explicit constraints imposed by insurance commissions prohibiting private insurers from discriminating based on sexual orientation, asking about or performing HIV antibody testing, or excluding AIDS as a covered condition (Faden & Kass, 1988).

Daniels (1990) and others, such as Oppenheimer and Padgug (1986), point out that the concept of "actuarial fairness" that underlies the justification for these practices directly conflicts with the requirements of "social fairness" (or justice). Considerations of "fairness" from an actuarial point of view argue for the *exclusion* of those most at risk from a common insurance pool. But considerations of "fairness" from a social justice standpoint argue for the inclusion of this group. Medicaid benefits in general and for AIDS patients in particular are limited in many states. According to a 1988 national survey, forty-four states covered AZT—a drug that appears to have been successful in prolonging the survival of persons with AIDS. Most states placed some limit on coverage or reimbursement and did not have special Medicaid coverage for AIDS care (Buchanan, 1988).

Mentally Ill and Disabled

Major access and service availability problems for the mentally ill and disabled have resulted from shifting philosophical, political, and programmatic priorities regarding the types of facilities and services most appropriate for meeting their needs.

Organizational Barriers. The deinstitutionalization of mentally ill individuals without sufficient development of alternative community-based systems of care led early on to a revolving door of readmissions. More recently, concerns have arisen about the "transinstitutionalization" or "reinstitutionalization" of the mentally ill to an array of institutions, such as board-and-care homes, nursing homes, residential treatment centers, or jail, among others. This population is also at a higher risk of having no home at all.

The 1978 President's Commission on Mental Health *Task Panel Report on Access and Barriers to Care* pointed out that one of the fundamental barriers to adequate service provision for this population was the victim-blaming stigma associated with being mentally ill and its resultant impact on public and political support for programs and services to address their needs (President's Commission on Mental Health, 1978b).

The elimination of categoric support for CMHCs with their inclusion in block grants to states in the early part of the 1980s resulted in a number of centers closing or greatly reducing the scope of services they provided (Dowell and Ciarlo, 1989). A shortage of community-based services, as well as case management and coordination across service systems, exists. This is particularly true for children and the seriously mentally ill or retarded (Crocker, 1990; Knitzer & Olson, 1982; OTA, 1986).

A pressing need for the chronically mentally ill is community-based housing. Obstacles to developing an adequate continuum of alternatives include the absence of legislation to facilitate access to such housing, poor interagency cooperation, inadequate funding, a diminished supply of public and private low-income housing stock, and community resistance to having mentally ill individuals living in the neighborhood (Boyer, 1987; Levine & Haggard, 1989).

The rates and location of mental health services used vary substantially for different age, sex, race, and income groups, as seen for the treated rates reported in Table 3.6 (discussed in Chapter Three). The precise pattern of differences varies to some extent by the type of service and group of individuals being considered. In general, however, there is an inverted U-shaped use curve by age, with younger people (particularly children) and the elderly using fewer outpatient mental health services than middle-aged individuals. Women are also more likely to use outpatient mental health services (in both the general medical care and specialty mental health care sector) than are men. Blacks and Hispanics are less likely to have been seen on an outpatient basis than are whites, but blacks in particular may be more likely to be hospitalized, once in the system. Children and the elderly appear to use very different sources for inpatient psychiatric care, as do men and women (see Table 3.5) (Diehr, Williams, Martin, & Price, 1984; Ford, Kamerow, & Thompson, 1988; Hough et al., 1987; Mechanic, Angel, & Davies, 1991; Scheffler & Miller, 1989; Shapiro et al., 1984; Thompson et al., 1988; Wells, Hough, Golding, Burnam, & Karno, 1987; Wells, Manning, Duan, Newhouse, & Ware, 1986).

The magnitude of unmet need for mental health services is estimated to be high in many committees. Based on the Epidemiological Catchment Area study, around 30 percent of individuals with a diagnosable mental disorder go untreated, while 56 to 59 percent receive care in the general medical care sector and only 8 to 12 percent in the specialty mental health sector (Hough et al, 1987, p. 709). Rates of untreated disorders have been estimated to be higher for children, the elderly, blacks, and Hispanics (particularly among Hispanics who are migrant agricultural workers, those who are less acculturated, or those who lack insurance coverage) — compared to working-age adults and whites (Shapiro, Skinner, Kramer, Steinwachs, & Regier, 1985; Vega, Scutchfield, Karno, & Meinhardt, 1985; Wells, Golding, Hough, Burnam, & Karno, 1988; Wells, Hough, Golding, Burnam, & Karno, 1987). Based on 1980 data, the Office of Technology Assessment estimated that 70 to 80 percent of children in need were not receiving appropriate mental health services (OTA, 1986, p. 5).

Financial Barriers. During the 1965–1975 decade, there was considerable support for the development of mental health programs. Spending for mental health facilities grew at an average annual rate of 12 percent. However, from 1977, as the percent of the GNP spent for general medical care continued to grow, the share of the GNP devoted to mental health fell 28 percent (Marmor & Gill, 1989).

The current system of financing mental health services lacks both parity and equity. Parity means that mental health services are as accessible and available as are general health care services to those who need them. Equity refers to coverage being equally available to all groups, based on need, rather than factors such as their income, occupational status, race, or where they live (Ridgely & Goldman, 1989).

The extent of coverage and rates of reimbursement for providers under both public and private systems of financing programs are less for mental health than for general medical care services. For example, in Medicaid, the rate paid for specialty psychiatric services, when provided by physicians, is lower than that paid for general medical services delivered by the same providers (Taube, Goldman, & Salkever, 1990). For Medicare patients seen on an outpatient basis, those being treated for physical illnesses have to pay 20 percent of the charges for the visits themselves. Beneficiaries being treated for mental illness have to pay half (with the exception of recent exemptions for the medical management of prescription drugs and for treatment for Alzheimer's patients) (Lave & Goldman, 1990). Data from a Bureau of Labor Statistics Survey in 1984 documented that fewer than half (48 percent) of the employees in medium and large firms had coverage for psychiatric inpatient care equivalent to that for other illnesses, and even fewer (7 percent) had equivalent coverage for outpatient psychiatric care (Brady, Sharfstein, & Muszynski, 1986).

People's willingness to purchase mental health care is even more sensitive to how much it costs them out of pocket than is the case for general medical care services — regardless of the nature of the problem. The more they have to pay themselves, the less likely people who need mental health care services are to obtain them (Frank & McGuire, 1986).

Substantial differences exist across groups in how mental health care is financed. Per capita expenditures under the direct control of state mental health agencies (the major source of revenues for mental health services) ranged from a low of $10.51 in Iowa to almost nine times that amount

($90.12) in New York, based on 1985 data (Lutterman, Mazade, Wurster, & Glover, 1988). In 1986, state mental health agencies were the largest source of revenues for state psychiatric hospitals (73.4 percent), while patient fees and private insurance were the primary sources of funds for private psychiatric hospitals (67.3 percent) (Taube, 1990, p. 226).

The public and private third-party coverage has tended to provide disincentives for services other than inpatient services and inadequate or nonexistent attention to the comprehensive, longer-term social and health care service needs of the mentally ill and disabled (Elpers, 1987; Morrissey, 1989; Scallet, 1990).

Both deinstitutionalization and public financing through Medicaid have encouraged the use of nursing homes as a long-term institutional alternative for the seriously mentally ill. The Omnibus Budget Reconciliation Act of 1987 required preadmission screening, as well as an annual review of nursing home residents, for mental illness and mental retardation. New applicants or residents who had been in the home fewer than thirty months who were not deemed to need active mental health treatment would not be covered by Medicaid and would be considered for placement in other "less restrictive settings." Freiman, Arons, Goldman, & Burns (1990) have estimated that this could lead to a displacement of 37,890 to 65,600 nursing home patients—many of whom would not have adequate provisions for their housing or personal care needs in the community.

Alcohol or Substance Abusers

The delivery system for alcohol and substance abuse services is fragmented, poorly integrated, and variably funded and developed across states. Further, the unique characteristics of substance abuse addiction compound the problems in adequately addressing the needs of people with these disorders.

Organizational Barriers. Substance abuse has been characterized as a "chronic relapsing disorder," with identifiable stages of development (use, abuse, dependence, recovery, and relapse), that has an array of physical, psychological, and social correlates and consequences. Further, treatment itself may be mandated, rather than voluntary, for those affected. As a result, a variety of interventions and treatment modalities with different objectives, and focusing on different stages of the problem, have emerged to address the needs of individuals who use or abuse alcohol and drugs.

Methodologies and data sources for directly assessing the match of service availability with the actual need for alcohol and substance abuse services are not well developed. Correlational analyses examining the association between indicators of alcohol problems and treatment capacity (age-adjusted cirrhosis death rates and alcohol and chemical dependency beds per 1,000 persons) have, however, shown little or no relationship (IOM, 1990, pp. 163–182). A National Association of Addiction Treatment Providers (NAATP) study concluded there was evidence of underutilization of substance abuse services in the private sector: only 0.3 percent of eligible individuals received treatment for substance abuse during a two-year period, though estimates of the percentage of the national population in need ranged upward of 5.0 percent (MEDSTAT, 1991).

Jails, prisons, and the criminal justice system in general are also important sources of referral and treatment for the drug abusing population. There are no uniform standards or well-proven models in successfully treating drug abuse as a deterrence to recidivism. Further, the overcrowding in many state prison systems, often due to an increase in convictions for drug-related or drug-involved crimes, has created additional strains on an already overburdened system of corrections (Gerstein & Harwood, 1990).

In addition to wide variations in the availability and adequacy of treatment for substance abuse disorders, a further challenge is providing "culturally sensitive treatment" to groups most at risk, such as racial and ethnic minorities. Programs may fail to incorporate adaptations to those groups' culture or values that could facilitate the treatment process. Desirable measures include hiring bilingual staff, grounding the treatment in the client's own spiritual belief system, and/or locating or designing the facility itself in a manner compatible with cultural tastes and preferences (Knox, 1985; OSAP, 1990b; Vanderwagen, Mason, & Owan, 1986; Ziter, 1987).

Financial Barriers. The resources, services, and clients in the two (public versus private) tiers of care in the drug abuse treatment system differ significantly. The private system sees 22 percent of the clients in treatment but receives 41 percent of the revenues. In contrast, the public system sees 78 percent of the clients but receives only 59 percent of the revenues. The revenues for inpatient and residential treatment per client in the private system are approximately three to four times those in the public system, though average outpatient revenues are similar. Compared to the private sector, public sector clients are much more likely to be long-term, serious, multiproblem cases. They often have a recurrent history of drug abuse or dependence, tend to be unemployed, poorly educated, and in poor health, are likely to be from broken or disorganized families, and frequently have criminal records. Counselors in the public sector generally see more clients on an inpatient basis on average (9.7) than do those in the private system (7.2), even though inpatient treatment is more of a focus in the private sector.

The private sector has a much higher rate of unused (or excess) capacity (34 percent) than does the public sector (16 percent). However, the excess capacity in public methadone maintenance programs is, on average, much smaller (5 percent), and the capacity across states and localities varies substantially. In some states, the waiting times to obtain access to public drug treatment services are substantial (Gerstein & Harwood, 1990).

The NDATUS and SADAP surveys have documented wide variability across states in the availability and funding of alcohol treatment services that is not necessarily correlated with variations in the need for these services. The number of beds per 1,000 persons for inpatient/residential rehabilitation and recovery services (considered the standard treatment for alcohol problems) ranges from 0.49 beds per 1,000 in the District of Columbia to 0.09 in West Virginia. Per capita expenditures for treatments for all types of care vary from $23.54 in Rhode Island to $1.33 in Oklahoma. Programs serving clients with alcohol problems are also segmented according to a "continuum of [client] social competence" — paralleling the public and private tiers of drug abuse treatment. For example, clients seen in hospital-based aversion conditioning treatment programs are likely to have much higher levels of social functioning (have jobs, are in intact families, and do not have criminal records) than those served in county police–sponsored rehabilitation centers (IOM, 1990, pp. 163–182).

Both public and private insurance provides limited coverage of alcohol and drug abuse treatment services. Anywhere from thirty-one million to ninety-two million Americans have been estimated to have no or inadequate drug abuse treatment coverage. This assumes that thirty-one million people have no health insurance at all, and around forty-eight million people with private insurance and thirteen million people on Medicaid have no or very limited benefits (Gerstein & Harwood, 1990, pp. 225–226). Health insurance is also oriented toward covering medically oriented (particularly inpatient) services, which are only one part of the complex array of social and community-based services needed by substance abuse clients. Substantial variability also exists in the types of substance abuse providers and services that are eligible for reimbursement by private and public insurers (particularly Medicaid), which results in a crazy quilt of coverage across states and subgroups.

Suicide- or Homicide-Prone

Major impediments to the development of accessible and effective programs to reduce the likelihood of suicide or homicide include the lack of a clear consensus on how best to address what are purported to be multifactorial biological, psychological, and social origins of violent behavior. This consensus should be based on well-developed theories, empirical research, demonstrations, and program evaluations.

Organizational Barriers. At present, the problems of suicidal and homicidal behavior are dealt with in a fragmented and uncoordinated fashion across an array of discrete service delivery sectors. These include the public health, medical care, mental health care, substance abuse treatment, criminal justice, social service, and educational systems. The Public Health Objectives for the nation call for better coordination and integration of services across these sectors to effectively address the Year 2000 goals to reduce violent and abusive behavior (PHS, 1990). It is possible that more "indirect" interventions (such as economic development programs in inner-city neighborhoods or mental health or substance abuse services) may be even more effective than "direct" interventions (such as suicide prevention or crisis intervention centers) in affecting such behaviors (Rosenberg, Gelles, et al., 1987).

Nonetheless, direct suicide and homicide prevention programs are not well developed in many states. In 1987, only two (0.6 percent) of 325 injury-prevention programs based in state health departments focused on homicide. From 1986 to 1990, only one (0.2 percent) of 552 award-winning community-based health promotion projects included homicide (CDC, 1990f).

Prison overcrowding has become a major problem in many states and localities due to an increased focus on "incapacitation" as a means of dealing with offenders. The average square feet per inmate in local jails, for example, decreased from 54.3 in 1983 to 50.9 in 1988, and the average number of inmates per unit increased from 2.4 to 2.5 (Flanagan & Maguire, 1990, p. 79).

A 1988 nationwide survey of state units on aging, mental health commissioners, legislative reference bureaus, and crisis intervention centers conducted by the American Association of Retired Persons (AARP) showed that very few agencies focused suicide prevention programs on the elderly. The elderly continue to have the highest overall rates of suicide (Mercer, 1989).

Professionals such as physicians, teachers, social workers, pastors, and mental health and substance abuse counselors need to be better trained to identify those who may be most at risk of violent behavior. Such individuals could serve as "gatekeepers" to identify and channel high-risk individuals and their families to appropriate prevention- or treatment-oriented services (Maltsberger, 1986, 1988; PHS, 1990). Suicidal youth and victims of aggravated assault and family abuse are, for example, much more likely to be seen in hospital emergency rooms. Emergency room personnel could be trained in the use of protocols for identifying high-risk cases and given information regarding available channels and sources of referrals to assist them (ADAMHA, 1989b; Slap, Vorters, Chaudhuri, & Centor, 1989).

Financial Barriers. Socioeconomically disadvantaged subgroups have access to different types of prevention- and treatment-oriented services than do more advantaged subgroups. As mentioned earlier in this chapter, the public and private treatment tiers in the mental health and substance abuse treatment sectors clearly serve different socioeconomic classes. The population housed in correctional facilities is increasingly minority. The black population increased from 21 percent of admissions to state and federal prisons in 1926 to 44 percent in 1986 (Langan, 1991, p. 5).

Targeted primary prevention and broader social, economic, and educational programs—which could perhaps serve as a deterrent or alternative to criminal or violent behavior leading to incarceration—are either nonexistent or poorly developed in most high-risk minority and disadvantaged neighborhoods. Further, many interventions may not be sensitive to the cultural differences and norms that affect who is most vulnerable to different forms of violence within a community (ADAMHA, 1989c; Gurr, 1989; Kraus, Sorenson, & Juarez, 1988).

Over sixty trauma centers have closed in the past five years — many as a result of the financial burden of the costs of uncompensated care for individuals with violence-related trauma. These closings have placed additional burdens on other public and private community providers for the delivery of trauma care (GAO, 1991b).

Abusing Families

The major issues in caring for victims of intimate violence are inadequate services and programs and the fragmentation and lack of integration resulting from the fact that different programs focus on discrete categories of victims of violence (children, wives, the elderly, and so on). A further problem is the poor coordination across the array of sectors (medical care, public health, welfare, protective services, mental health, and criminal justice, among others) involved in service provision in general and for each group.

Organizational Barriers. Different paradigmatic approaches exist in the medical care, human services, and legal systems regarding how best to handle cases of intimate abuse. This greatly inhibits the prospect for communication and coordination of a multifaceted interagency approach to addressing the needs of both victims and perpetrators (Knudsen, 1988; Saunders, 1988).

Within child and adult protective services agencies, the values of "compassion" and "control" are often in tension or conflict. Program administrators have to weigh their agency's legalistic mandates to detect and investigate incidents of abuse against certain humanistic considerations. Safety concerns dictate the forcible removal of the victim or restraint of the offender, but this has to be balanced against the wishes of many "victims" to remain in situations that by agency or professional standards are abusive (Carney, 1989; Fritz, 1989; Knudsen, 1988; Solnit, 1987).

Similar tensions exist in considering the design of community prevention and treatment initiatives in this area. In most states and localities, the agencies and constituencies concerned with different victims of intimate abuse may rarely coordinate service and programs. For example, one agency (a battered women's shelter) may deal principally with addressing the needs of one affected family member (the mother), while another (the child protective services agency) deals principally with others (the children), and still another (the police) with the perpetrator of the violence (the father). Such a system further exacerbates the fragmentation, confusion, and lack of integration that already plagues many abusing families (Cohn, 1982).

Virtually no laws exist to explicitly protect certain categories of victims of "hidden violence," such as siblings, adolescents, or nonelderly parents. Local police are frequently reluctant to intervene in domestic disturbances because of the issue of family privacy and the fact that many victims often drop charges against the perpetrator prior to prosecution. Adult protective services are more likely to focus on the elderly, rather than on cases of spousal or nonelderly adult abuse.

Further, the laws governing elder abuse are variably implemented and understood by agency officials in many states. A 1989 survey of state health departments regarding awareness of state laws on procedures for elder abuse demonstrated that though 94 percent of respondents were aware of the laws, only 20 to 28 percent reported the use of written procedures or training materials specifically designed for health personnel. Part of the reason that state public health departments reported little activity in this area was the fact that elder abuse reporting laws tend to place implementing authority in human services, aging, or law enforcement agencies, rather than health departments (Ehrlich & Anetzberger, 1991).

Though physicians may be the front-line sentinels for identifying at-risk or actual victims of abuse, many are not adequately trained to appropriately diagnose them or refer them to suitable nonmedical networks of treatment or support (Jellinek, Murphy, Bishop, Poitrast, & Quinn, 1990; Randall, 1990).

School-based sex abuse education and related prevention-oriented efforts are variably available in most communities (Wurtele, 1987). The Year 2000 Objectives call for at least 50 percent of elementary and secondary schools to teach nonviolent conflict resolution skills and to extend coordinated, comprehensive violence prevention programs to at least 80 percent of the local jurisdictions with populations over 100,000 (PHS, 1990).

Financial Barriers. Both governmental and private volunteer efforts in this area tend to have limited funding, inadequate staffing, and poorly developed systems of referral, placement, or social and human services resources to provide for victims of intimate violence. In some states, shelters have to turn away two battered women for every woman who receives services, and in 1987, nearly 40 percent of battered women and children needing emergency housing were turned away because of lack of space (PHS, 1990).

Homeless

Access problems previously detailed for other vulnerable groups are multiplied for the homeless. Obvious problems include extreme poverty; inadequate, unstable, or unhealthy living conditions; poor nutrition; and the greater prevalence of mental illness, substance abuse, and sexual or physical exploitation and injury. All of these factors contribute to the poorer health of the homeless than of the U.S. population in general; the homeless are also in worse health than the housed poor in many cities.

Organizational Barriers. The homeless are much less likely to have a regular source of care or transportation and much more likely to have long waits, experience hostile attitudes, and/or to be told to go elsewhere when they do seek care. The lack of integration of the public health, medical care, mental health care, substance abuse treatment, social service, and other sectors caring for discrete categories of vulnerable populations makes designing an effective system of care for the multiproblem homeless even more difficult (IOM, 1988c; Miller & Lin, 1988; Padgett, Struening, & Andrews, 1990; Robertson & Cousineau, 1986; Roth & Fox, 1990; U.S. Commission on Security and Cooperation in Europe, 1990).

The publicly and privately funded Health Care for the Homeless projects described earlier (Chapter Five) attempted to design systems of care for the homeless that would eliminate or ameliorate many of these traditional access barriers to needed services. Early evidence suggests they have met with some success. Outreach and case management services have, for example, been particularly effective in getting eligible homeless in for care and encouraging return visits when needed (Brickner, Scharer, Conanan, Savarese, & Scanlan, 1990; Center for Health Policy Studies, 1989; DSSPD, 1991; Stephens, Dennis, Toomer, & Holloway, 1991; United Hospital Fund, 1990). The lack of a place to go postdischarge is a major problem for many chronically mentally or physically ill homeless. The VA-HCMI has facilitated the development of residential treatment alternatives for homeless veterans to address the needs of this subgroup of the homeless (Rosenheck, Gallup, Leda, Gorchov, & Errera, 1990).

The demand on major sources of support for the homeless in many cities—such as emergency food and shelter programs—is growing, and in many cases it exceeds the capacity of the system to meet it. The 1991 U.S. Conference of Mayors' *Status Report on Hunger and Homelessness in America's Cities* found that the demand for food assistance had increased 26 percent on average over the previous year in all but two of the twenty-eight cities surveyed. In 79 percent of the cities, emergency food assistance facilities turned away people in need because of lack of resources. On average across the cities, 17 percent of the requests for emergency food assistance went unmet. The requests for emergency shelter (or housing) by homeless families increased an average of 17 percent over the same period. Shelters turned away homeless families or individuals in 75 percent of the cities because of lack of resources. An average of 15 percent of the requests for emergency shelter were estimated to have gone unmet (U.S. Conference of Mayors, 1991).

In the 1988 HUD National Survey of Shelters for the Homeless, shelter managers reported that their facilities were at full capacity more than half (or an average of 192) of the nights during the year. The average number of nights the shelters were full was even greater for those serving families with children (259 nights), and somewhat lower for those serving unaccompanied men (131 nights) or other (or more mixed) groups (169 nights) (USDHUD, 1989c).

Financial Barriers. Private advocacy groups for the homeless and others have sharply criticized the federal government for its slowness in developing program and policy initiatives for the homeless (GAO, 1985; National Alliance to End Homelessness, 1988; Partnership for the Homeless, 1987, 1989). The agencies charged with the implementation and oversight of the McKinney Act have also been subject to severe criticism in Congressional hearings and reports. They have been chastised for the restrictions (relating to the complex application process, matching funds requirements, and funding stream, among others) that made it difficult for grantees to get programs in place in a timely fashion and for the lack of responsiveness of the programs to local needs and priorities. Other criticism has been aimed at the footdragging and delays on the part of agencies charged with both the expenditure and oversight of program funds (GAO, 1990c; U.S. Commission on Security and Cooperation in Europe, 1990; U.S. Congress, House Committee on Government Operations, 1988; U.S. Congress, House of Representatives, Government Activities and Transportation Subcommittee and the Employment and Housing Subcommittee, 1989). A 1990 GAO report on the programs supported under this act documented that though a number of barriers had been removed, some agencies were still slow in utilizing the funds that had been allocated and/or had not adequately monitored funded programs to see if the legislative intent of the act was being satisfactorily met (GAO, 1990c).

As with other vulnerable populations, the root causes of homelessness lie deep in the social, economic, and political structure. The question of "access" for the homeless then poses the corollary question of what it is most appropriate for at-risk groups and individuals to have "access" to in order to prevent or eliminate the problem of homelessness. A report titled *Homelessness in the United States* by the U.S. Commission on Security and Cooperation in Europe (1990, p. 68) concluded that "the Executive Branch and Congress should act to address growing poverty and larger socio-economic issues such as unemployment, an insufficient minimum wage, the lack of affordable housing and health care, and education deficiencies. The federal government should provide, in addition to funding, moral leadership and a comprehensive strategy designed to address larger socio-economic problems, of which homelessness is just a symptom."

Immigrants and Refugees

The type and magnitude of access problems differ for documented legal immigrants, overdocumented refugee populations, and undocumented illegal aliens. However, the common factors affecting access for all of these groups are the availability and affordability of services and their acceptability and adequacy for those in need of care (Rumbaut, Chavez, Moser, Pickwell, & Wishik, 1988).

Organizational Barriers. Availability refers principally to the types of providers that are present in areas where immigrants and refugees tend to live and to the question of whether the providers' doors are open to them. As indicated in the previous chapter, some providers require that patients present proof of citizenship or permanent residence status to be eligible for services. Undocumented aliens will be reluctant to seek care as a result, because of fears of detection and subsequent deportation. Further, some facilities make little or no accommodation to serving immigrant and refugee populations by failing to have bilingual providers or translators to facilitate patient-provider communication.

Community outreach as well as follow-up are important components in enhancing service availability, through identifying people at risk and facilitating their access to needed medical care. Mobile vans and storefront clinics have been used to provide health screening, immunizations, and referrals of at-risk immigrant and refugee populations in urban neighborhoods, as well as isolated rural communities along the U.S.-Mexico border.

As Rumbaut, Chavez, Moser, Pickwell, and Wishik (1988, p. 177) point out, "the delivery of health care to immigrants and refugees is, of course, not merely a technical-medical orientation or a bureaucratic-financial transaction, but also a social relation in a culturally defined situation." The acceptability and adequacy of services being offered to these populations is substantially affected by "social and cultural problems of miscommunication, misinformation, misunderstanding, and mistrust in the relationship between provider and patient" (Rumbaut, Chavez, Moser, Pickwell, & Wishik, 1988, p. 170). The principal factors that generate and/or exacerbate these problems include language barriers and cultural beliefs and practices that differ between the providers and the populations being served. These difficulties can give rise to a reluctance to seek care initially, a failure to follow prescribed medical regimens, a fear and distrust that inhibit the pursuit of subsequent follow-up care, and poor treatment outcomes (Ernst, Philip, Viken, & Blaisdell, 1988; Rumbaut, Chavez, Moser, Pickwell, & Wishik, 1988; Siddharthan, 1990).

Financial Barriers. The affordability of services is principally a function of whether people have insurance or other personal resources to pay for care. The federally supported guarantees of Medicaid coverage for medically indigent refugees do not extend beyond the first thirty-six months of residence, and in some cases only to a maximum of eighteen months in states that do not have General Assistance programs for the poor. The periods of adjustment to a new culture, the development of English-language proficiency, and the treatment of serious medical or psychological problems may, however, extend well beyond these fixed eligibility periods. Further, those who work may be in a "Catch-22" situation, in that they do not have insurance coverage provided through their place of employment and yet are earning too much to qualify for Medicaid. Many legal and illegal immigrants find themselves among the working poor, who are employed in low-paying jobs but have no health insurance for themselves or their families.

Uninsured illegal aliens in particular tend to seek care at free neighborhood clinics, staffed by volunteer providers, or on a cash-only basis from private or clinic providers who are willing to deliver services on this basis. Both uninsured legal and illegal immigrants make greater use of hospital outpatient departments and emergency rooms than people with private insurance. Some studies have suggested, however, that illegals are more likely to use emergency rooms than outpatient departments, mainly because they seek care either principally or solely in emergencies (Chavez, Cornelius, & Jones, 1985; Rumbaut, Chavez, Moser, Pickwell, & Wishik, 1988).

The availability and affordability of services — particularly the ability to pay for them — greatly affect whether or not immigrants and refugees seek care at all. The quality of the care provided is affected by its adequacy, as well as its acceptability, to those who are eventually served.

Chapter Eight reviews the evidence regarding the costs and Chapter Nine the quality of the care currently being provided to the vulnerable, to further explore the appropriateness and affordability of existing organizational and financial arrangements to serve this population.

8

How Much Does
Their Care Cost?

Little uniformity exists in how the costs of caring for the vulnerable are defined, or in the types of data available, across studies or groups.

In some studies, *costs* refer to the direct dollar expenditures by an agency or program. In others, *true economic costs* are estimated, based on assigning values to the amount of resources used or lost in a defined population as a result of illness. *Direct costs* in this case refer to those resources used in providing services (such as hospital, physician, or other treatment services), and *indirect costs* refer to those lost (due to absenteeism, death, or imprisonment, for example). In some cases, the out-of-pocket costs (or cash outlays) of the affected individuals or their families are an important component of the financial burden of care.

Cost-benefit (CB) and cost-effectiveness (CE) analyses are used to evaluate which programs yield the best outcomes relative to what they cost. In *cost-benefit analyses,* both costs and benefits are expressed in dollar terms, while in *cost-effectiveness analyses,* benefits are expressed in nonmonetary units (such as days of hospitalization, numbers of physician visits, level of functioning, or quality-adjusted life years).

This chapter reviews the evidence that is available regarding the costs of care (however defined) for each group, as well as cost-benefit and cost-effectiveness studies that attempt to determine which programs yield the best outcomes relative to their cost.

Cross-Cutting Issues

For some groups and/or programs, clear conclusions can be drawn. For others, the evidence is mixed, and for still others, it is nonexistent.

Overall Costs

Sophisticated efforts to estimate the economic costs of mental illness and alcohol and drug abuse have yielded relatively clear-cut generalizations regarding the major resources used or lost due to these problems. The bulk of the economic costs resulting from mental illness and alcohol abuse are the indirect costs of lost productivity, as well as the direct institutional, provider, and other treatment expenses, while the social costs associated with crime-related expenditures and losses comprise the bulk of the economic costs of drug abuse.

Estimates of the true economic costs of other problems are not readily available. However, the evidence that does exist suggests that the economic and social consequences of infant deaths and those resulting from suicides and homicides, reflected in years of productive life lost, are substantial, as are the medical care and related expenses of caring for persons with AIDS and victims of family abuse and neglect.

The financial burden on many of the vulnerable, as well as the institutions that care for them, is clearly reflected in the substantial out-of-pocket outlays assumed by the chronically ill and disabled and their families, as well as the disproportionate share of uncompensated expenditures borne by public hospitals in caring for persons with AIDS.

Little evidence of the costs of care for homeless and immigrant and refugee populations exists beyond reports of the expenditures and budgets of programs and agencies most directly involved with these populations.

Cost-Benefit/Cost-Effectiveness

Even less data are available regarding the cost-benefit or cost-effectiveness of alternative programs for caring for the vulnerable.

The clearest evidence of cost-beneficial effects are for selected prevention-oriented services. The cost-benefit and cost-effectiveness of prenatal care and other primary prevention-oriented services for high-risk mothers and infants have been clearly demonstrated. Studies of child abuse and neglect services also confirm that early interventions, such as parenting skills education and peer support, among others, are much more cost-effective than programs that attempt to deal with treating these problems once they occur.

Cost-benefit and cost-effectiveness analyses of case management or noninstitutional alternatives for the chronically physically or mentally ill have yielded mixed results. In a number of cases, the costs of these alternatives were higher than those for institutional care, and the outcomes were better according to some indicators and unchanged according to others.

Research on the costs of alternative programs relative to outcomes is either quite limited for certain groups, such as persons with AIDS or alcohol or substance abusers, or virtually nonexistent for others, including suicide or homicide victims, the homeless, and immigrant and refugee populations. In many cases, the objectives of the programs serving these populations are mixed or ill-defined, as are the political or theoretical perspectives on the origins (or causes) of the problems underlying the design of these programs. (See Table 8.1.)

Table 8.1. Principal Costs of Care for Vulnerable Populations.

	Costs	
Vulnerable Populations	*Overall costs*	*Cost-benefit/cost-effectiveness (CB/CE)*
High-risk mothers and infants	The costs for low-birthweight and high-risk infants are substantially higher than for normal deliveries.	Every dollar spent on prenatal care could save as much as $3.38 in the medical care costs of low-birthweight infants (IOM, 1985).
Chronically ill and disabled	The out-of-pocket cost burden is high for many of the chronically ill and disabled due to the lack of coverage for long-term care services.	CB/CE studies of home- and community-based alternatives to institutionalized care have yielded mixed results regarding program costs and outcomes.
Persons with AIDS	The lifetime costs of medical care for PWAs are estimated to be around $85,000 (Hellinger, 1991), with public hospitals assuming a disproportionate burden of the costs of their care.	Little data exist on the CB/CE of alternatives for organizing and delivering care to PWAs.
Mentally ill and disabled	About half of the economic costs of mental illness are due to the indirect costs resulting from lost productivity.	CB/CE studies of case management and other community-based alternatives for long-term care for the mentally ill and disabled do not clearly confirm that costs are less (offset) under these arrangements.
Alcohol or substance abusers	The vast majority of the economic costs for drug abuse are the social costs associated with crime-related expenditures; for alcohol abuse, they are the direct costs of treatment and the indirect costs of death and disability.	Both the availability and findings of CB/CE studies of substance abuse treatment alternatives vary across types of programs and public versus private tiers of service.
Suicide- or homicide-prone	In addition to direct expenditures by the criminal justice, social service, and other sectors, the major personal and societal costs of homicides and suicides are the years of potential life lost (YPLL).	CB/CE studies of alternatives for either preventing suicide or homicide or treating the perpetrators or victims of intentional violence are a largely neglected area of research.
Abusing families	Though a paucity of data are available on the costs of the array of categories of family abuse, the available evidence suggests that both the personal and social costs are high.	CB/CE studies of child abuse and neglect in particular suggest that primary prevention-oriented services provide a much greater prospect for savings and success than do programs to treat families in which abuse has already occurred.
Homeless	The direct and indirect costs of homelessness have not been estimated directly, though the burden of caring for them has fallen disproportionately on local and state governments and voluntary, nonprofit providers.	The precise goals of programs to serve the homeless must be better defined before meaningful CB/CE analyses can be conducted.
Immigrants and refugees	The costs of caring for immigrants and refugees are borne principally by federal agencies charged with their entry, resettlement, and support; programs to which they seek entitlement; state and local agencies that assume responsibility for their care; as well as families.	As with the homeless, the goals of programs to address the complex health and social service needs of immigrants and refugees must be better defined before meaningful CB/CE analyses can be conducted.

Population-Specific Overview

The overall costs and cost-benefit and cost-effectiveness of programs to serve the vulnerable will be reviewed.

High-Risk Mothers and Infants

Prenatal care and related primary prevention-oriented services are much more cost-effective investments than hospitalized neonatal intensive care for low-birthweight or high-risk births that could have been prevented.

Overall Costs. The overall expenditures for maternity care and delivery have increased in recent years. This trend has resulted from the overall rise in health care costs, increased use of neonatal intensive care units, rising malpractice fees and claims, and the growing burden of uncompensated care—an estimated 40 percent of which is due to uncompensated maternity care costs.

 A 1989 survey of 173 community hospitals, 70 childbirth centers, and 153 licensed midwives conducted by the Health Insurance Association of America (HIAA) found that the average cost of maternity care for a normal delivery was $4,334. This figure included $2,842 for hospital charges and $1,492 for the physician's fee. These amounts were higher for cesarean delivery: total = $7,186; hospital = $5,133; physician's fee = $2,053. The charges for both freestanding ($2,111) and hospital-based birthing centers ($3,233)— including practitioners' fees—as well as midwives' fees for normal delivery ($994), were substantially lower than those for physician deliveries (HIAA, 1989b).

 The costs for low-birthweight and other high-risk infants are substantially higher than for normal deliveries. An Office of Technology Assessment study estimated that in 1984, the average hospital costs ranged from $11,666 to $39,421 for low-birthweight infants in neonatal intensive care units and from $26,737 to $60,015 for very-low-birthweight newborns. The cost on average for newborns requiring assisted ventilation for more than seventy-two hours was around four times that for all low-birthweight infants cared for in neonatal intensive care units (OTA, 1987b).

Cost-Benefit/Cost-Effectiveness. A number of studies have documented the cost-benefit and cost-effectiveness of programs to reduce teenage pregnancy, low-birthweight births, and infant mortality. Burt (1986) calculated that in 1985, the American public paid an average of $13,902 per family over a twenty-year period for each first birth to a teenager—principally through Aid to Families with Dependent Children, food stamp, and Medicaid program support for these mothers, many of whom drop out of school and are unemployed. If all teenage births were delayed until the mother was twenty or older, the cost would be $8,342—a net savings of $5,560 per birth.

 A 1988 Office of Technology Assessment report, *Healthy Children: Investing in the Future,* estimated that for each low-birthweight birth that was prevented from $14,000 to $30,000 could be saved in the costs of newborn hospitalization, rehospitalizations in the first years, and the long-term costs of institutional care, foster care, early intervention, special education, and services for individuals one to thirty-five years of age (OTA, 1988b).

A 1985 Institute of Medicine study documented that for mothers on public assistance from high-risk socioeconomic groups, every additional dollar spent on prenatal care would result in savings of $3.38 in the medical care costs of low-birthweight infants (IOM, 1985). The Institute of Medicine study was based on achieving the 1990 objective of 9 percent low-birthweight births. A study in New Hampshire projected a savings of $2.26 for every dollar spent on prenatal care for mothers with less than a high school education. Target rates in that study were the actual low-birthweight rates for New Hampshire women who received adequate prenatal care (Gorsky & Colby, 1989).

Joyce, Corman, and Grossman (1988) estimated an infant health production function across large counties in the United States in 1977, to compare the cost-effectiveness of various health programs (including prenatal care, neonatal intensive care units, WIC [women, infants, and children] supplemental food programs, and others) in reducing race-specific neonatal mortality rates. Early initiation of prenatal care was found to be the most cost-effective means of reducing neonatal mortality rates. Neonatal intensive care saved more newborn lives but cost substantially more than the other programs and hence was found to be the least cost-effective. With few exceptions, WIC was the second most cost-effective program, followed by abortion, family planning, community health center programs, and finally neonatal intensive care. In general, the most successful programs were even more cost-effective for African-Americans than for whites.

Chronically Ill and Disabled

The out-of-pocket burden of care is substantial for many of the chronically ill and disabled—principally because of the limited coverage available for long-term care services. Cost-benefit and cost-effectiveness studies of home- and community-based alternatives to long-term institutionalized care have yielded mixed results regarding program costs and outcomes.

Overall Costs. Particularly significant components of the costs of long-term care for the chronically ill and disabled include nursing home, home health care, and associated community and supportive services. The nation spent $53.3 billion on nursing home and home health care in 1989. Of the $47.9 billion spent on nursing home care, residents and their families paid the largest share (44.4 percent, or $21.3 billion)—only $8.7 billion of which represented monthly social security payments paid directly to nursing homes or through the patients' families. Other payers included Medicaid ($20.6 billion), Medicare ($3.6 billion), private insurance ($0.5 billion), and other private and governmental sources ($1.9 billion). The average annual cost of a nursing home stay was about $30,000, and the average daily rates were higher for private pay than for Medicaid patients (AARP, 1991a; Lazenby & Letsch, 1990).

Of the $5.4 billion spent for home health care, Medicare paid the most ($2.1 billion), followed by Medicaid ($1.0 billion), private health insurance and out-of-pocket payments ($1.3 billion), and state and local sources ($0.9 billion) (AARP, 1991a; Lazenby & Letsch, 1990).

A particular concern in evaluating the costs of care for the chronically ill and disabled is the direct and indirect economic burden on the individuals themselves and their families. Out-of-pocket health care costs for the elderly in 1988 were estimated to average $2,934 per person, which represented 18.1 percent of their income. This reflects an increase from the 12 to 13 percent of their income spent in the 1977–1980 period (U.S. Congress, House Select Committee on Aging, 1989). Analyses of the 1985 National Nursing Home Survey data showed that among the elderly who incurred $3,000 or more in out-of-pocket expenses, 82.5 percent was due to uncovered outlays for nursing home expenses and the balance for acute care expenses (hospital, physician, dental, prescription drugs) (Rice, 1989).

Out-of-pocket expenditures for the community-dwelling elderly are less than for the institutionalized population. However, those in poor health and who have more limited activity, are poor, and live in two-person families where only one is elderly are at a greater risk of paying a higher percentage of their income out-of-pocket for care. Hospitalization and related expenses are a significant component of out-of-pocket costs for the community-dwelling elderly (Kovar, 1986; Liu, Manton, & Liu, 1985). The out-of-pocket costs of care for chronically ill children—particularly those who are technology dependent—have been cited as one of the major stressors on families in caring for these children at home (Aday, Aitken, & Wegener, 1988; Jacobs & McDermott, 1989).

Cost-Benefit/Cost-Effectiveness. Providing less restrictive alternatives to long-term stays in acute care hospitals or nursing homes has been hypothesized to reduce costs and enhance the well-being of the chronically ill elderly or disabled. The experience with Medicaid Section 2176 home and community-based waivers, which were designed to be budget neutral, has failed to show that they result in no additional Medicaid spending for services (Vertrees, Manton, & Adler, 1989).

Hedrick and Inui (1986), in an information synthesis of experimental or quasi-experimental studies of the cost and effectiveness of home care, pointed out that home care appears to have had no impact on mortality, patient functioning, or nursing home placement. Further, the costs of care were not reduced and may have in fact been greater by as much as 15 percent when home care services were utilized. They also pointed out that limitations of the research designs, sample sizes, and resultant rival hypotheses (sample subject attrition and selection, for example) created serious problems with interpreting and generalizing the results of these studies.

Kemper, Applebaum, and Harrigan (1987) reviewed the results of sixteen major community care demonstration projects, all of which, though varied in design, shared the common objective of substituting community care (adult day care, homemaker services, home health care, and so on) for nursing home care. Case management and an expanded package of community services were the key program elements in each of the demonstrations. Overall, there were small reductions in nursing home costs for some people. But these were more than offset by the increased costs of providing expanded community services to those who were likely to have remained at home anyway in the absence of these services. These expanded community services did, however, result in some improvements in participants' levels of satisfaction with care, social interaction, and quality of life as a whole.

Weissert and Cready (1989a) subjected over two dozen controlled experiments of home and community-based long-term care services conducted over the past thirty years to a break-even analysis. They concluded that improved targeting of high-risk elderly patients (particularly to avert hospitalization) and better controls on utilization could lead to more efficient service provision.

Persons with AIDS

Public hospitals bear a disproportionate share of the burden of uncompensated care resulting from constrained public and private third-party coverage of persons with AIDS. Varying estimates of the overall costs of care exist, and little research is available on the cost-effectiveness or benefits of alternative models for organizing and delivering services for persons with AIDS.

Overall Costs. Estimates of the average lifetime medical care costs of AIDS have varied widely—from, for example, a high of $147,000 for the United States as a whole for the period from 1981 to 1985 to a low of $27,000 based on a 1984 study done in San Francisco. A range of factors has contributed to variations in these estimates across studies, including differences in the time period on which the analyses are based, the case mix and components of services included, the use of costs in some studies versus charges in others, and changes in the methods of treatment over time—particularly the greater use of AZT and a shift to outpatient or community-based services (Fox & Thomas, 1989; Hellinger, 1988a, 1988b, 1990; Scitovsky & Rice, 1987; Scitovsky, 1988, 1989a, 1989b). Estimates in 1991 of the lifetime costs of medical care for AIDS were around $85,000 (Hellinger, 1991).

Projections of the total direct national costs of AIDS also vary—both as a function of variability in the estimates of the average lifetime costs and as a function of the projected total numbers of AIDS cases (Fox & Thomas, 1989; GAO, 1989b). Hellinger (1991) estimated that the cumulative lifetime medical care costs of treating all people diagnosed with AIDS in 1991 was $5.8 billion. Approximately $1.4 billion was estimated to be spent on people who were HIV positive but did not have AIDS, and the balance of $4.4 billion on persons with AIDS.

Hospital inpatient costs are the major component of expenditures for persons with AIDS. Public hospitals bear a disproportionate share of the uncompensated costs of care for PWAs. According to the 1987 U.S. Hospital AIDS Survey, the average cost per inpatient day was $681. The cost per patient per year was $17,190, and the total estimated cost of AIDS inpatient care during 1987 was $486 million. Revenues averaged 80 percent of costs ($545 per day). The average losses per day were significantly higher for public ($218 per day) than for private ($92) hospitals (Andrulis, Westlowski, & Gage, 1989).

Little data are available on the costs of AIDS by risk groups, geographical location, or type of provider, or for HIV-infected persons other than persons with AIDS. There is some evidence, however, that IV drug users are more likely to present with pneumocystis carinii pneumonia (PCP), while homosexual and bisexual males are more likely to have Kaposi's sarcoma (KS). Patients with PCP often require inpatient care, while KS can largely be treated on an outpatient basis, resulting in a lower level of expenditures for individuals with this diagnosis. The limited number of studies on children with AIDS estimate that the lifetime cost of their care is likely to be higher, compared to adults, due to the absence of noninstitutional alternatives (such as foster care) to their remaining in the hospital (Scitovsky, 1988, 1989a, 1989b).

Other important components of the costs of care for persons with AIDS include direct nonpersonal costs (for instance, research, screening, health education, and support services) and indirect costs, such as lost output due to illness and premature death. The magnitude of nonpersonal direct cost outlays is largely dependent on future policies to support these services. Most of the indirect costs result from lost earnings due to premature death. This may differ, however, for different risk groups (homosexual white males versus minority IV drug users, for example) (Scitovsky, 1988, 1989a, 1989b).

Cost-Benefit/Cost-Effectiveness. An important research question related to the care provided people with AIDS is the cost-effectiveness of alternative models for organizing and delivering services—such as comparisons of hospital-based, community-based, and/or managed care case management models (Knickman, Benjamin, & Duhman, 1988). Cost-benefit analyses of premarital and blood donor screening programs for HIV antibodies have shown that the latter, but not the former, is worth doing—given the cost of screening relative to the numbers of cases likely to be detected (Eisenstaedt & Getzen, 1988; Petersen, White, & Premarital Screening Study Group, 1990).

Mentally Ill and Disabled

Almost half of the economic costs of mental illness have been estimated to be due to the indirect costs resulting from lost productivity, with most of the rest being due to direct institutional, provider, and related treatment expenses. The results of studies of the cost-benefit and cost-effectiveness of case management and other alternatives for long-term care of the mentally ill and disabled do not clearly confirm that other costs are less (or offset) under these arrangements, which parallels the conclusions from cost-benefit and cost-effectiveness studies of related programs and services for the chronically physically ill and disabled.

Overall Costs. The magnitude of the costs of mental illness and the methods for estimating these costs have varied over time and across studies (Frank & Kamlet, 1985; Levine & Levine, 1975; Levine & Willner, 1976; President's Commission on Mental Health, 1978b; Rice, Kelman, Miller, & Dunmeyer, 1990). The estimates discussed here are principally based on a 1990 report supported by the Alcohol, Drug Abuse, and Mental Health Administration, *The Economic Costs of Alcohol and Drug Abuse and Mental Illness: 1985* (Rice, MacKenzie, & Associates, 1990).

Mental illness was estimated to have resulted in $103.7 billion in economic costs to the U.S. economy in 1985. For 1988, the total cost was estimated to have been $129.3 billion. Direct costs—which included the personal health care costs for institutional and provider services and prescription drugs, as well as costs for support services such as research and training for providers and administration—comprised 41.0 percent (or $42.5 billion) of 1985 costs. Over 75 percent of the direct costs was for services provided by mental health care institutions: mental health specialty and federal institutions (30.2 percent), short-stay hospitals (20.7 percent), nursing homes (24.9 percent), professional services (13.2 percent), prescription drugs (3.4 percent), and other support costs (7.6 percent).

Indirect costs include the illness (morbidity) and death (mortality) resulting from mental illness. Indirect costs due to morbidity, measured by the value of reduced or lost productivity, accounted for almost half—45.7 percent (or $47.4 billion)—of the $103.7 billion in total economic costs. A total of 39,707 deaths were estimated to have been due to mental disorders, representing more than one million person-years lost (26.4 years of life per person) and a loss of $9.3 billion to the economy (8.9 percent of total costs). The balance of the total economic costs (4.3 percent or $4.5 billion) was for other related costs—particularly the amounts spent by caregivers in providing care to mentally ill family members ($2.5 billion), as well as criminal justice–related expenses ($1.3 billion).

Total economic costs for men ($57.1 billion) are more than one-third higher than for women ($42.1 billion), and the largest share (50.2 percent) was spent on individuals fifteen to forty-four years of age, compared to other age groups: under fifteen (2.1 percent), forty-five to sixty-four (30.3 percent), and sixty-five and over (17.4 percent). These relative distributions of costs reflect the greater prevalence of more serious disorders requiring institutional care among men, as well as larger estimates of lost productivity among men and working-age adults (Rice, MacKenzie, & Associates, 1990).

As mentioned in both Chapters Six and Seven, for those covered by either public or private plans, the out-of-pocket share of the cost for mental health care is higher than for general medical care, and publicly supported institutions are particularly likely to bear a disproportionate burden of caring for those who have no resources to pay for it themselves.

Cost-Benefit/Cost-Effectiveness. The cost of mental health services varies across delivery settings. The cost of outpatient psychiatric services delivered in organized settings (such as hospital outpatient departments) has been found to be higher than those delivered in private physicians' offices (Rupp, Taube, Bodison, & Barrett, 1987). The median costs of most services in community mental health centers (with the exception of psychiatric evaluations and medication reviews) were also higher than in hospitals or freestanding clinics providing comparable services (Dowell & Ciarlo, 1989).

Treatment cost variations across delivery settings are not necessarily a function of differences in the health and mental health of the types of patients seen in the respective settings. An unanswered question with respect to these variations, then, is whether more effective or more cost-effective care is being delivered in certain settings than in others (Frank & Kamlet, 1990).

An argument for providing third-party coverage for mental health services is the hypothesized "medical offset effect"—that is, the use of specialty mental health care services could result in a corresponding reduction in the use of and expenditures for physical health care services. There is, however, no strong empirical support for this hypothesis (Fiedler & Wight, 1989). Further, as with case management–based systems of care for the chronically ill and disabled, evaluations of case management programs for the mentally ill have documented increased costs without substantially measurable improvements in functional outcomes (Franklin, Solovitz, Mason, Clemons, & Miller, 1987; Jerrell & Hu, 1989). Much more research is needed on both the efficiency and effectiveness of general and specialty mental health services, and on how both costs and outcomes should be measured (Dickey et al., 1989; Fiedler & Wight, 1989; Frank & Kamlet, 1990).

Alcohol or Substance Abusers

The social costs associated with crime-related expenditures comprise the lion's share of the costs of drug abuse, whereas the direct costs of treatment and the indirect costs of death and disability account for the bulk of outlays associated with alcohol abuse. Both the availability of cost-benefit and cost-effectiveness studies of substance abuse treatment alternatives, and the results of the research that has been conducted, are quite variable across types of programs and (public versus private) tiers of service provision.

Overall Costs. The total economic costs of drug abuse nationally were estimated to be $44.1 billion in 1985 and $58.3 billion in 1988. Social costs (other related costs) comprised most ($32.5 billion or 74 percent) of the economic burden of drug abuse in 1985. Direct crime-related expenditures for public police protection, private legal defense, and property destruction amounted to two-fifths ($13.2 billion) of these social costs. Other social costs included the productivity losses associated with engaging in a criminal career or being incarcerated rather than having legal employment. Other direct and indirect costs constituted a much smaller share of the overall price tag of drug abuse: indirect morbidity costs (14 percent), mortality costs (6 percent), direct treatment and support costs (5 percent), and the costs of AIDS (2 percent). The direct and indirect costs of AIDS associated with intravenous drug use were estimated to be almost $1 billion in 1985 — mainly due to the high death rates among persons with AIDS (Rice, MacKenzie, & Associates, 1990).

Alcohol abuse was estimated to have cost the nation $70.3 billion in 1985 and $85.8 billion in 1988. In contrast to the costs of drug abuse, in 1985, core costs (the direct costs of treatment and indirect costs of death or disability), rather than other related (social) costs, accounted for the largest proportion (83 percent) of the economic burden of alcohol abuse. Of these core costs ($58.2 billion), the bulk ($51.4 billion) was due to the indirect costs of illness ($27.4 billion) and loss of life ($24.0 billion) associated with alcohol use and abuse. Around 95,000 deaths due to alcohol were estimated to have occurred in 1985, representing 2.7 million person-years lost or 28.2 years per death.

The majority of the direct costs ($6.8 billion) associated with alcohol abuse represented expenditures for treatment ($6.3 billion) and the balance for the support costs associated with research, training, and program administration. Social costs amounted to $10.5 billion (15 percent) of the total economic costs, with the largest components being expenditures for alcohol-related crime and motor vehicle crashes. The balance of total costs (2 percent or $1.6 billion) was due to fetal alcohol syndrome, which results in serious physical and mental deficiencies that require costly rehabilitation and long-term care services for affected infants (Rice, MacKenzie, & Associates, 1990).

Smoking was estimated to have cost the nation $52.3 billion in 1985. The major components of these costs were direct morbidity ($23.7 billion), indirect morbidity ($10.2 billion), mortality ($17.8 billion), and pediatric mortality (0.6 billion). The annual per capita cost of smoking-related diseases was $221 nationally — ranging from $284 per person in Rhode Island to $56 per person in Utah (Public Health Reports, 1990c).

As indicated in Chapter Six, an increasing share of the costs of substance abuse treatment — particularly in the private service tier — is being borne by third-party payers as well as by the clients themselves, since the cost-sharing provisions, even for those with coverage, are higher for these services than for general medical care.

Cost-Benefit/Cost-Effectiveness. Limited data are available on the cost-benefit and cost-effectiveness of substance abuse prevention and treatment programs. Very few randomized clinical trials or even quasi-experiments have been conducted to examine the effectiveness of different treatment alternatives, much less their cost in relationship to benefits.

In the drug abuse area, the limited number of evaluations conducted have demonstrated that the benefits (in terms of clients' increased employment and lower involvement in crime) of methadone maintenance, residential therapeutic communities, and to some extent outpatient nonmethadone treatment programs equaled or exceeded the costs of these programs. Virtually no systematic cost or outcome data exist for chemical dependency programs. Results from the limited numbers of evaluations of treatment programs in correctional institutions (which are an increasingly important component of drug treatment as the proportion of individuals imprisoned for using drugs or committing drug-related crimes increases) have shown either no or equivocal evidence of "success" (Gerstein & Harwood, 1990).

The principal focus of research on the cost-benefit of alcohol treatment programs has been on "medical offset effects"—that is, whether the overall costs of medical care associated with alcohol problems are lessened when treatment for the underlying problem is provided. Reviews of the literature in this area have demonstrated that for groups of employed individuals and those enrolled in private insurance or prepaid health plans, savings in medical care costs do result and are sustained over the long term. The evidence is more ambiguous for publicly insured populations (those with Medicaid or VA coverage, for example). These groups are much more likely to be low income, to have deferred seeking treatment until the medical complications of alcohol abuse have become severe, and to bring fewer personal and social resources (in terms of self-esteem and social networks or family support) to the treatment and recovery process (Holder, 1987; IOM, 1990; Jones & Vischi, 1979; Luckey, 1987).

Even less research has been conducted on the cost and benefits of prevention-oriented interventions for alcohol and substance abuse. Some studies have demonstrated that advertising by the alcohol and tobacco industry increases and higher excise taxes and minimum-age provisions decrease adolescents' consumption of these substances. However, much more research is needed that examines the impact of prevention-oriented substance abuse programs (Casement, 1987; Coate & Grossman, 1987; Goplerud, 1990; IOM, 1989c; Lieberman & Orlandi, 1987; U.S. Department of Education and U.S. Department of Health and Human Services, 1987).

Suicide- or Homicide-Prone

In addition to expenditures by the criminal justice, social service, and other sectors that deal with the effects of suicide and homicide, other major personal and societal costs include the years of potential life lost (YPLL) due to early death, the direct costs of hospitalization and associated medical costs for severe injury, and the resulting impact on the quality of life of the family and community.

Overall Costs. In 1985, homicides accounted for 612,556 years of potential life lost before age sixty-five. Assault by firearms and explosives accounted for 61.4 percent of YPLL due to homicide. Seventy-six percent of the homicide-attributable YPLL occurred in males. The YPLL rate per 100,000 persons was highest for black males (1669.3) and lowest for white females (99.4). As a proportion of total YPLL, homicide-attributable YPLL increased 93 percent from 1968 through 1985—from 2.7 to 5.2 percent (CDC, 1988c).

In 1980, there were 26,689 reported suicides, or a rate of 11.9 per 100,000, corresponding to 619,533 years of potential life lost before age sixty-five (Rosenberg, Gelles, et al., 1987). The national costs of youth suicide (among those fifteen to twenty-four years of age) resulted in fifty-three years of life lost per suicide or forty-two years (217,000 YPLL) before age sixty-five. These figures were somewhat higher for females than males, whites than nonwhites, and fifteen- to nineteen- compared to twenty- to twenty-four-year-olds, due to the longer life spans of the former subgroups (Weinstein & Saturno, 1989).

In 1980, successful and unsuccessful suicide, homicide, and aggravated assault attempts accounted for 1.8 million hospital days and $754.4 million in health care costs. At least 355,500 victims were hospitalized in connection with homicides or aggravated assaults; the hospital costs for those who survived plus those who eventually died totaled approximately $606 million. The cost of physician visits raised the cost to $638 million. No data were available to estimate the costs of emergency room treatment, pharmaceuticals, extended care, or other treatment for offenders who were injured during the assault. The cost of health care for treating suicide attempts was estimated to be approximately $110.2 million in hospital costs and $6.2 million for physician visits (Rosenberg, Gelles, et al., 1987).

The indirect costs to families and society of violent deaths resulting from suicide and homicide are also substantial. Children who are victims of or witnesses to violence often suffer delays in physical, social, and emotional development and/or posttraumatic stress disorders. Battered women are at greatly elevated risk of alcoholism, drug abuse, attempted suicide, child abuse, rape, and mental health problems. The death of a wage-earning spouse can also result in serious economic deprivation for the surviving spouse and dependent children.

Surviving family members of suicide victims often experience shame and guilt, as well as fears regarding the prospect of other family members' making such attempts. Suicide can result in survivors' inability to collect life insurance benefits, or in the instance of suicide attempters, to increased financial burdens resulting from mental health or medical care treatment costs.

The "suicide contagion" that appears to be precipitated in some communities in response to a suicide and the movement of middle-class residents and businesses out of neighborhoods that have high rates of violent crime are examples of broader community or societal costs that result from suicide- and homicide-related violence (Rosenberg, Gelles, et al., 1987; Sampson, 1986).

Cost-Benefit/Cost-Effectiveness. Cost-benefit and cost-effectiveness analyses of alternatives for either preventing suicide and homicide or treating the perpetrators/victims of these intentional acts of harm represent a largely neglected area of research.

Abusing Families

Little systematic data are available on the direct, indirect, and related social costs of the array of categories of family abuse and neglect. The evidence that does exist, however, suggests that the human and personal costs of family abuse and neglect are substantial. Primary prevention-oriented services appear to provide a greater promise of savings and success than do programs to provide treatment in families in which abuse has already occurred.

Overall Costs. Based on the National Clinical Evaluation Study of nineteen clinical demonstration projects conducted between 1979 and 1981, the prevalence of specific health or emotional problems among abused children under thirteen years of age was as follows: chronic health problem (30 percent); cognitive or language disorder (30 percent); socioemotional problem, such as low self-esteem, lack of trust, and so on (50+ percent); self-mutilative or other self-destructive behaviors (14 percent); difficulty in school, including poor attendance or misconduct (50+ percent); and learning disorders requiring special education (22 percent). The prevalence of these disorders was even higher among adolescent victims (Daro, 1988, p. 154). The socioemotional and physical impact on adult victims of abuse and neglect has also been documented to be substantial (McLeer & Anwar, 1989).

Daro (1988) estimated both the immediate and longer-term financial costs of child maltreatment. Immediate costs included hospitalization for injuries associated with serious maltreatment, such as skull or bone fractures, internal injuries, and burns, among others ($20 million); rehabilitation and special education services ($7 million); foster care ($460 million); and other immediate costs of educational, juvenile court, and private therapeutic services. Longer-term costs included those associated with juvenile courts and detention ($14.8 million); long-term foster care ($646 million); loss of future earnings (from $658 million to $1.3 billion); and other costs associated with adult criminal courts and detention, drug or alcohol abuse–related treatment, and potential welfare dependency.

Analyses of the National Crime Survey yielded the following estimates of the annual morbidity associated with domestic violence: 21,000 hospitalizations, 99,800 days of hospitalization, 28,700 emergency room visits, and 39,900 visits to physicians. The total annual health care costs resulting were $44,393,700, with indirect costs of 175,500 lost days from paid work (Inter-University Consortium for Political and Social Research, 1981).

Cost-Benefit/Cost-Effectiveness. Studies examining the cost-benefit and cost-effectiveness of alternative prevention and treatment services for child maltreatment have concluded that prevention-oriented services provide greater promise of both success and savings than do those that are oriented toward treating individuals and families in which abuse has already occurred (Daro, 1988; Dubowitz, 1990).

Based on a review and synthesis of research in this area, Daro (1988) concluded that from a cost-effectiveness point of view, those programs that provide parenting education, educational and skills development, lay therapy, peer support groups, and group and family therapy yielded the greatest benefits relative to per-client costs. Group or family therapy appeared to be a much more cost-effective treatment alternative than individual therapy, particularly because of the much higher costs and generally poorer outcomes associated with the latter intervention. In a review of related research, Dubowitz (1990) concluded that home health visitors and medical foster care were more cost-effective alternatives to prolonged hospitalization in preventing abuse among chronically ill or handicapped children.

Prevention services that are linked to existing universal service systems, such as public schools, public health care providers, community-based family service agencies, or churches, are much more likely to be cost-effective than those requiring new categoric institutions for dealing with the problem.

Homeless

The burden of caring for the homeless has largely fallen on local and state governments and voluntary, nonprofit providers. The direct and indirect economic and social costs of homelessness have not been estimated directly. They are, however, likely to be substantial.

Overall Costs. A Federal Interagency Task Force on Food and Shelter, created in 1983, endorsed the policy that homelessness was essentially a local problem, and that federal agencies should principally work with the private sector and with local governments to inventory and coordinate potential resources to serve the needs of the homeless.

In 1983, one of the first major federal funding initiatives in this area, the Federal Emergency Management Agency (FEMA), provided $100 million to distribute to nonprofit groups and state governors, under the direction of a National Board of representatives from major charitable organizations (the United Way, the Salvation Army, the National Council of Churches, and others). This funding was significant in catalyzing the establishment of a network of emergency shelters that became the backbone of the service system for the homeless. Approximately 90 percent of the shelters are operated by private, nonprofit organizations, particularly religious groups, and about 80,000 volunteers served thirty million hours in such shelters in 1988 (USDHUD, 1989c).

Subsequent federal initiatives for the homeless have largely been encompassed within the provisions and amendments of the Stewart B. McKinney Homeless Act (P.L. 100-77) (DSPPD, 1990b, 1991; GAO, 1990c; USDHUD, 1988a, 1988b, 1989a, 1989b, 1990). Funding for the McKinney Act programs increased substantially, from $198.6 million in fiscal year 1989, to $599.1 million in 1990, and to $681.8 million in 1991. Total funding for all federal programs targeted at homelessness (including the McKinney Act) was $807.1 million in 1991. Other federal programs serving the homeless included nutritional programs within the Department of Agriculture, the Department of Defense surplus and food bank programs, and Department of Health and Human Services programs for the homeless mentally ill, substance abusers, and runaway youths, among others (USDHUD, 1991).

The McKinney Act also catalyzed a larger role on the part of both states and municipalities in caring for the homeless. Because of limited resources in most states, the Council of State Governments has stressed the importance of designing prevention-oriented programs that attempt to address the root causes of homelessness (U.S. Commission on Security and Cooperation in Europe, 1990; USDHUD, 1988a, 1989a).

Based on the twenty-eight cities surveyed in 1991 by the U.S. Conference of Mayors Task Force on Hunger and Homelessness, all the cities used funds available through the McKinney Act, 75 percent used locally generated funds (including ones based on funding devices, such as a one-cent tax on cigarettes), 68 percent used state grants, 68 percent used Community Development block grant funds, and 28 percent drew on Community Services block grant funds (U.S. Conference of Mayors, 1991).

The direct and indirect economic costs of homelessness have not been measured as such. These include the direct costs of medical care for the homeless for conditions that in many cases are preventable or that would be less likely to become serious with proper treatment. The burden of providing medical care for the homeless also falls most heavily on those institutions (such as county or inner-city teaching hospitals) that are already assuming a disproportionate burden of caring for those who cannot afford to pay for care. Growth in the direct and indirect costs of mental illness, substance abuse, AIDS, and family abuse described earlier is exacerbated by the increasing number of homeless with these problems. As the numbers of children and women of childbearing ages continue to grow among the homeless, the lost productivity and resulting burden of caring for vulnerable, multiproblem homeless infants and children loom as a substantial, long-term societal, economic, and human cost.

Cost-Benefit/Cost-Effectiveness. Programs to serve the homeless have a range of goals and objectives, including providing permanent housing, providing emergency shelter or food relief, reducing the prevalence of physical health problems, treating associated risks such as mental illness or substance abuse, or providing social support, among others. Conducting cost-benefit or cost-effectiveness analyses of programs to serve the homeless requires a clear delineation of their major intended benefits.

Immigrants and Refugees

The costs of caring for immigrants and refugees are borne by the federal agencies charged most directly with their entry, resettlement, and support (such as the Immigration and Naturalization Service in the Department of Justice and the Office of Refugee Resettlement in the Department of Health and Human Services). The costs are also borne by the programs to which they seek entitlement (such as Medicaid, Medicare, AFDC, or SSI), the state and local institutions and providers that assume a large burden of their (often uncompensated) care, and the families and individuals themselves who seek to pay for care out of their own (often limited) resources.

Overall Costs. To implement enforcement of the Immigration Reform and Control (IRCA) Act of 1986, the Immigration and Naturalization Service substantially increased its total direct program budget and full-time equivalent personnel — from $594 million and 11,656 staff in 1986 to an estimated $1.0+ billion and 16,000+ staff in 1990. The State Legalization Impact Assistance Grants (SLIAG) program under the IRCA authorized $1 billion per year for four years (beginning in fiscal year 1988) to reimburse state governments for the costs of public assistance, health, and educational services to newly legalized citizens. A related IRCA program — Systematic Alien Verification and Entitlements (SAVE) — requires that states verify the immigration status of all aliens applying for selected federally funded public assistance benefits (Bean, Vernez, & Keely, 1989).

    A major concern on the part of many refugees is the possibility of losing insurance coverage, after a designated period of Medicaid eligibility, or of being dropped once they start working, in jobs that nonetheless provide no health insurance benefits. Legal or illegal immigrants and refugees who do not have insurance coverage are much less apt to seek medical care. The mortality and morbidity associated with the resultant failure to treat what are often preventable or curable diseases among foreign-born men, women, and children is substantial (Ahearn and Athey, 1991; Chavez, Cornelius, & Jones, 1985; Gibney, 1987; Kulig, 1990; Rumbaut, Chavez, Moser, Pickwell, & Wishik, 1988; Sandler & Jones, 1987; Toole & Waldman, 1990; Westermeyer, 1987; Wilk, 1986).

Cost-Benefit/Cost-Effectiveness. As with the homeless, studies examining the cost-benefit and cost-effectiveness of programs to serve immigrants and refugees must take into account their complex health and social service needs. Such studies must also recognize that individually oriented service programs to address these needs are essentially treating the symptoms of problems that have roots deep in other social or political domains.

    Chapter Nine reviews the evidence regarding the quality of the care delivered by programs and services directed toward the vulnerable.

9

What Is the Quality
of Their Care?

Considerations of the quality of medical care have traditionally focused on the structure, process, and outcomes of the care provided. Structure refers to the characteristics of the institution or providers delivering services. Process criteria relate to the treatment protocols or standards recommended or used by providers. Outcomes refer to the actual health consequences of the care delivery process for patients (Donabedian, 1980).

The measurement of outcomes is an increasingly salient consideration in evaluating the quality of medical care as well as related programs and services. The relationship of the structure and process of care to outcomes is an especially important issue. As with research on the costs and cost-benefits and effectiveness of care for the vulnerable, the evidence regarding structure, process, and outcome evaluations of quality is generally scanty.

This chapter reviews what is known and what still needs to be learned about the quality of care provided to the vulnerable in the context of structure and process, as well as outcome, criteria of quality.

Cross-Cutting Issues

The results suggest that structure and process criteria have tended to dominate evaluations of the quality of care being delivered for certain groups and/or in certain settings. The development of indicators of the outcomes of care and the linkage of structure and process criteria to outcomes is the emerging frontier of quality-of-care assessment in general, as well as in programs and services to care for the vulnerable in particular.

Structure/Process

For some groups, structure and process criteria have been utilized to a considerable extent in assessing quality. Such criteria have, for example, tended to predominate in assessments of the quality of care being provided the chronically ill and disabled in nursing homes. This has primarily been in response to licensure, reimbursement, or other external requirements. Evaluations of the quality of care in the mental health, alcohol and substance abuse, and family abuse fields have often focused on the training and qualifications of providers.

Mental health professionals have attempted to promulgate treatment protocols and standards, through the auspices of local provider groups or national agencies or associations. These standards have been accepted and implemented in various ways, however. Studies have clearly demonstrated a relationship between the receipt of prenatal care and good birth outcomes. But only recently have there been attempts to clearly specify the content of prenatal care (procedures or protocols) likely to be most effective for women with different profiles of risk.

Structure, and particularly process, criteria are poorly developed for certain populations (persons with AIDS, the homeless, immigrants and refugees). These criteria have a mixed record of success in improving outcomes for others (alcohol or substance abusers and perpetrators and victims of suicide, homicide, and family abuse, for example). Cultural barriers and prejudices or misunderstandings on the part of providers may play an important role in the care received by many of these groups. Further, new standards and protocols are needed as new services and treatment modalities (such as home care or case management) come to be utilized.

Outcomes

Considerable ambiguity surrounds the specification of outcome criteria of quality. One particularly problematic aspect for essentially all of the groups examined here is the specification of the desired program or treatment outcomes (or objectives). These are relatively clear for high-risk mothers and infants (to reduce the incidence of low-birthweight infants or the number who die) and the chronically physically or mentally ill (to maximize physical or cognitive functioning), for example. But they are extremely ill-defined or ambiguous for others (persons with AIDS, victims of abuse or violence, or the homeless).

In addition, the theoretical and associated empirical underpinnings to guide the design of interventions in these areas are also weak, due to limited research or ambiguous or conflicting theories and findings regarding the origins (or causes) of the underlying problem being addressed.

Further research that clarifies what outcomes are desired, how the outcomes should be measured, and which interventions are most likely to be successful in effecting these outcomes is needed in evaluating the quality of care being provided the vulnerable. (See Table 9.1.)

Population-Specific Overview

The structure, processes, and outcome indicators of the quality of care for vulnerable populations are discussed in the following paragraphs.

Table 9.1. Principal Quality-of-Care Issues for Vulnerable Populations.

Vulnerable Populations	Quality	
	Structure/process	*Outcomes*
High-risk mothers and infants	Two major issues regarding the structure and process of care for high-risk mothers and infants are (1) what should the content of prenatal care be, and (2) what and how much technology should be used at birth?	Though the magnitude of the relationship varies, prenatal care is generally associated with better birth outcomes. High-technology delivery and neonatal intensive care can further harm as well as help high-risk infants.
Chronically ill and disabled	Protocols and criteria for evaluating long-term care tend to focus on what regulating or accrediting bodies require.	Though not well developed, outcomes-oriented research focuses on the impact of long-term care arrangements on patient functioning and quality of life.
Persons with AIDS	"Caring," not "curing," is the major focus of much AIDS-related care.	The desired *clinical* outcomes of care for persons with AIDS are ill-defined.
Mentally ill and disabled	Because of the array of providers and facilities involved in providing mental health care, there is considerable variability in the standards and norms of practice in this area.	Standards and guidelines development in the mental health area has not adequately related program or therapeutic practices to hypothesized or desired outcomes.
Alcohol or substance abusers	Quality assurance and assessment procedures in the alcohol and substance abuse area are either nonexistent, implicit, or limited in application.	As with the mental health care area, the nature of the alcohol and substance abuse treatment system exacerbates problems in clearly defining desired outcomes and how best to achieve them.
Suicide- or homicide-prone	There is no widely shared consensus regarding how best to prevent or treat intentional violence, primarily because of the lack of an integrated theoretical base regarding its causes.	Individually oriented interventions may have little overall effect on community suicide or homicide rates.
Abusing families	Medical, social service, and related personnel may be inadequately trained to detect and/or intervene in cases of family abuse.	A multitude of outcomes may be the focus of interventions in the area of family abuse: increased knowledge of situations that might prompt it, behavioral evidence of change, reduction in reported prevalence, or increase in underreports of abuse.
Homeless	The problem of establishing quality-of-care norms for the homeless is exacerbated by their overall lack of basic support, as well as medical care, services.	The precise outcome objectives for programs to serve the homeless must be specified in evaluating the extent to which they effectively deal with the origins and/or consequences of the problem.
Immigrants and refugees	The quality of care obtained by immigrants and refugees is greatly affected by its accessibility, adequacy, and acceptability to these populations.	Knowledge of social and cultural factors in caring for foreign-born populations will enhance the prospect of better patient compliance and outcomes.

High-Risk Mothers and Infants

Structural considerations of the quality of maternal and child health emphasize comparisons of perinatal outcomes across different types of prenatal care and birthing delivery sites. Process evaluations examine the relationship of prenatal care and the technologies and procedures associated with delivery and high-risk newborn care to perinatal outcomes. Evaluations of the effectiveness of interventions to improve birth outcomes have focused on overall infant mortality and low-birthweight indicators. They have also focused on more refined rates of birthweight-specific mortality and congenital or birth-related morbidity and/or disability. Two major questions with respect to relating the structure and process of care to perinatal outcomes include (1) what exactly should the content of prenatal care be, and (2) what types of and how much technology should be used at birth and particularly in trying to sustain extremely low-birthweight infants?

Structure/Process. The recommendations of the Public Health Service Expert Panel on the Content of Prenatal Care extended beyond traditional measures of the number and timing of prenatal visits to the utility of preconception and postpartum visits, psychosocial assessment and follow-up, early and continuing risk assessment, and health promotion interventions (to quit smoking, for example). The panel also recommended varying the number, timing, and content of visits based on the assessed risk of the mother and fetus (PHS, 1989).

The wider availability of neonatal intensive care units is credited with the decline in birthweight-specific neonatal mortality rates over the past twenty-five years (OTA, 1987b). Further, there is evidence that low-birthweight infants born in hospitals with neonatal intensive care units experience substantially lower mortality than those born in hospitals that do not have these facilities (Mayfield, Rosenblatt, Baldwin, Chu, & Logerfo, 1990; Paneth, 1990).

The research on deliveries in maternity or birthing centers, compared to those in hospitals, suggests that these centers offer a safe alternative for many women and may in fact be less likely to result in cesarean deliveries for women with comparable risk profiles (Baruffi, Strobino, & Paine, 1990; Rooks et al., 1989).

Outcomes. Research on the effectiveness of prenatal care includes (1) observational studies based on birth and death records, either from vital statistics or clinical data bases, and (2) evaluations of programs offering enriched or augmented prenatal care services (OTA, 1988b).

The observational studies have, as a whole, found a positive relationship between the use of prenatal care and birth outcomes. The magnitude of the association varies, however, due to differences in the care and outcome variables used in each study.

Specific programs that have been evaluated with respect to their impact on birth outcomes include federally sponsored initiatives, such as Maternity and Infant Care Projects, the Improved Pregnancy Outcome Projects, and WIC. Private foundation–supported efforts, such as the Robert Wood Johnson Foundation Perinatal and Rural Infant Care Programs, among others, have also been studied. The findings from evaluations of specific programs are less consistent — one reason undoubtedly being that the programs themselves represent varying types of prenatal and associated perinatal interventions.

The implicit assumption that more technology at birth necessarily means better care is being challenged. Shy, Luthy, Bennett, & Whitfield (1990) found that the use of electronic fetal monitoring (EFM) was associated with a threefold greater risk of cerebral palsy compared to the conventional practice of a nurse using a stethoscope to check the unborn infant's heart rate during delivery.

Sophisticated neonatal intensive care unit technology can also precipitate iatrogenic (care-induced) conditions. Examples include bronchopulmonary dysplasia resulting from prolonged exposure to mechanical ventilation and retinopathy of prematurity associated with administering high concentrations of oxygen to premature newborns. The tiniest newborns (those less than 750 grams) are least likely to survive neonatal intensive care and most likely to have long-term disabilities and handicaps when they do (OTA, 1987c).

Rosenblatt (1989) has pointed out the perinatal paradox in the United States of ensuring de facto entitlement of high-risk infants and their mothers to high-cost neonatal intensive care, but not to guaranteeing access to lower-cost and more effective prenatal care services.

Chronically Ill and Disabled

Kane and Kane (1988) have argued that the nature of long-term care (LTC) differs from acute care along a number of dimensions that create special difficulties in developing criteria of quality. For example, LTC has a longer time horizon and represents a series of interrelated rather than discrete events of care, and the goals of care (maintenance versus enhanced functioning versus rehabilitation) are not well defined. Also, LTC is largely comprised of low-technology services provided by lay caregivers or paraprofessionals, rather than highly technical care provided by skilled professionals. Finally, because of the likely transitions among a variety of providers, the quality of care for LTC consumers lies outside the control of any one provider.

Structure/Process. Protocols and criteria for evaluating the quality of long-term care for the chronically ill and disabled are not well articulated. Efforts to assess the quality of LTC have focused most often on nursing homes, and in more recent years, on home health care providers and board-and-care homes. As with quality assessment activities in the acute care area, most efforts have focused on structure and process measures of quality.

The principal quality assurance activities for nursing homes include regulation-oriented approaches, such as licensure by the states, focusing principally on safety and fire codes, and certification as skilled nursing or intermediate care facilities to meet Medicare and/or Medicaid program standards. These activities also include annual inspections to ensure that all care reimbursed by Medicaid and Medicare is medically necessary and of acceptable quality; Ombudsman Programs, required by the Older Americans Act, which serve as nursing home patient advocates; and the training, licensure, and regulation of personnel, such as nursing home administrators (AARP, 1991b; Kane & Kane, 1988).

In his book *Unloving Care: The Nursing Home Tragedy* (1980), Bruce Vladeck pointed out that standards of quality for nursing homes were almost exclusively concerned with inputs (such as staffing and physical facilities) and process (such as paperwork), rather than outcomes. He quoted a former state official as saying, "'there is nothing in our regulations that says a nursing home may not permit a patient to starve to death'; they only require three meals a day meeting minimal standards" (Vladeck, 1980, p. 156).

Standards for evaluating the structure and process indicators of quality for other major categories of long-term care, such as home care, case management, and board-and-care homes, are even less well developed than those for nursing homes.

GAO studies have documented considerable variability in the training and experience of employees of home health agencies providing high-risk infusion therapies, for example (APHA, 1990b), and a range of quality problems in board-and-care homes, including physical abuse, unsanitary conditions, and the lack of medical attention to meet residents' needs (GAO, 1989c).

The National Maternal and Child Health Clearinghouse (NMCHC) has developed a workbook to summarize standards of quality across the array of providers and agencies potentially involved in the care of children with special needs. Items covered include individualized services, health professional and team characteristics, health care facility responsibilities, state health department responsibilities, and community and societal supports (NMCHC, 1990).

Outcomes. There is an increasing interest in specifying and measuring outcome indicators of quality for LTC. An outcomes approach to assessing nursing home quality would focus on actual, relative to possible, improvements in the patients' status, given their level of functioning—such as enhanced personal satisfaction, participation in enjoyable activities, and improved mobility and rates of discharge home. In this context, structure and process measures of quality become relevant as points of intervention to produce improvements in patient outcomes. Examples of these measures include inadequate medical supervision of patients' health status; low levels of training and high turnover among the principal immediate caregivers—nurses' aides; the overutilization of medications, especially psychoactive drugs; and lack of stimulating social or recreational activities (Kane, 1990; Kane & Kane, 1988; Libow & Starer, 1989).

As indicated in Chapter Eight, outcomes research on the quality of home care and other community-based services has principally been undertaken in the context of evaluating the cost-effectiveness of these programs. A meta-analysis of studies focusing explicitly on the outcomes of home care showed a small beneficial but nonsignificant effect on mortality rates, and somewhat stronger evidence of a reduction in nursing home placement (Hedrick, Koepsell, & Inui, 1989). However, there is a need to develop more formal, conceptual frameworks for understanding the correlates and outcomes of home care, as well as more explicit outcome and process measures of the quality of care being provided to people at home (Kramer, Shaughnessy, Bauman, & Crisler, 1990).

Persons with AIDS

The continuum of caring needed by persons with AIDS resembles that of the chronically ill and disabled. People with AIDS require long-term care entailing a complex array of social and medical services, and "caring"—not "curing"—is the major focus of the caregiving process itself (Benjamin, 1989). As indicated in Chapter Seven, however, a comprehensive, coordinated continuum of care is available only in fragments for the elderly and is practically nonexistent for persons with AIDS in most U.S. communities. The traditional problems of measuring structure, process, and outcome indicators of quality are then made worse when the structures are ad hoc, the norms for the process of care are evolving, and the desired outcomes of the caregiving process are ill-defined.

Structure/Process. In surveying AIDS case managers in forty-two cities, Piette, Fleishman, Mor, and Dill (1990) found that case managers in community-based organizations were more likely to focus on expanding the range of services available to persons with AIDS and monitoring the provision of services that had been promised than their hospital-based counterparts. The latter more frequently emphasized working with medical personnel and providing psychological counseling.

A small number of studies examining the success of various public health interventions in increasing levels of knowledge and reducing the behavioral risks associated with AIDS have provided preliminary evidence of success (Gerbert & Maguire, 1989; Hardy, 1990; Montgomery, Freeman, & Lewis, 1989; Moran, Janes, Peterman, & Stone, 1990; NCHS, 1990c). Preliminary evidence from evaluations of interventions to reduce high-risk behaviors among groups most at risk (such as homosexual/bisexual men and IV drug users) have demonstrated increased awareness of risks and/or reductions or modifications of high-risk behaviors. This has been true in general,

[handwritten margin note: In general ↑ of awareness but not in subgroups?]

though not necessarily for particularly at-risk demographic subgroups (such as adolescents, young heterosexual adults, those with less education, and minorities) (Becker & Joseph, 1988; Dengelegi, Weber, & Torquato, 1990; Solomon & DeJong, 1989; Stephens, Feucht, & Roman, 1991). The National Research Council Panel on the Evaluation of AIDS Interventions has pointed out the absence of strong experimental and quasi-experimental designs of the studies to date in this area, however. The panel has urged the formulation of a rigorous research agenda focusing on the structure, process, and outcome of major public health interventions to prevent the spread of AIDS (Coyle, Boruch, & Turner, 1991).

Outcomes. What little clinical research that has been done to date on the quality of AIDS patient care has focused on the efficacy and effectiveness of particular therapies, such as AZT or routine immunizations of persons with AIDS (AHCPR, 1990c).

[handwritten margin note: location]

Studies in a limited number of sites have pointed to the impact of the location of services on the outcome of care provided. A study in a small sample of California hospitals found that the odds of dying in a hospital that had less experience in caring for AIDS patients were greater than in a hospital with more experience. The authors also pointed out, however, that there were significant limitations with the data, including the absence of information on the quality of care as well as on the severity of the patient's condition prior to admission (Bennett, 1990; Kanouse, Mathews, & Bennett, 1989).

Kanouse, Mathews, and Bennett (1989) outlined the major clinical issues to be considered in developing a research agenda to evaluate the quality of care of people with AIDS: (1) focus the research on major groups based on the stage and/or diagnoses associated with the condition, such as those with early HIV disease, opportunistic infections, AIDS-acquired dementia complex, and those in the terminal stages of the illness; (2) conduct research on a range of alternative therapies to establish their effectiveness; and (3) encompass both inpatient and outpatient components of care in the process.

The Agency for Health Care Policy and Research has encouraged investigators to address HIV/AIDS-related quality-of-care issues through its AIDS Medical Care Effectiveness Program (AMCEP) and associated clinical guidelines development activities. The results of initiatives funded through this program, as well as projects currently in progress under that agency's auspices, can begin to address many of the unanswered questions concerning the correlates and outcomes of care being provided persons with AIDS (AHCPR, 1990b).

Mentally Ill and Disabled

Quality assessment activities in the mental health care sector have, in particular, been fragmented and reactive. The development of standards or quality review procedures has often been in response to external demands for accountability from insurers, program funders, or institutional accrediting bodies, such as Professional Standards Review Organizations, the Joint Commission on the Accreditation of Health Care Organizations, or state funding agencies. Further, there is a paucity of both strong experimental, as well as quasi-experimental, evaluations of the efficacy and effectiveness studies of mental health treatments and programs (Cohen & Stricker, 1983; Hamilton, 1985; Mattson, 1984; Wells & Brook, 1989).

Structure/Process. Quality-of-care issues relating to the structure of mental health services focus on the characteristics of the providers and facilities from which services are received. An array of providers with widely varying educational and licensure credentials deliver mental health care services. These providers include M.D.-trained psychiatrists, master's and Ph.D. psychologists, M.S.W.-level social workers, psychiatric nurses, bachelor's-level counselors and therapists, and associate-degree-level certified alcohol and drug abuse counselors (CADAC), among others.

As mentioned in previous chapters, a great deal of mental health care is rendered by primary care physicians in general medical care settings. Considerable controversy exists regarding the adequacy of training and the quality of care delivered by this array of mental health care providers. Further, no well-developed uniform standards exist for what types of services should be in place within particular mental health care delivery sites (psychiatric hospitals, residential treatment centers, outpatient treatment settings, and so on) to ensure high-quality care in those discrete facilities, much less in relationship to a comprehensive, integrated continuum of care for the mentally ill (Gottlieb, 1989).

Two major types of studies on assessing or ensuring the quality of care delivered include (1) descriptions of peer review programs associated with specific hospitals, insurance carriers, state or national professional associations, or community health centers, and (2) the nature of mental health specialist and generalist physicians' prescribing practices for psychotropic medications. The implication is that those practices that conform to implicit or explicit criteria underlying a particular program's or facility's practice protocols reflect high-quality care.

Three other major sources of process criteria of the quality of mental health care include those designed and promulgated by (1) professional associations such as the American Psychiatric Association or American Psychological Association, (2) NIMH and NIH Consensus Conferences, and (3) program evaluation systems for community health centers (Wells & Brook, 1989).

Outcomes. As with general medical care delivery, these development activities in the area of structure and process standards have not adequately linked program guidelines to patient outcomes. Additional research is needed on the efficacy of clinical therapies or treatments, as well as on the effectiveness of the care delivered in specific delivery settings. Psychopharmacological treatment of mental disorders has been one of the major developments supportive of the deinstitutionalization of the mentally ill. Individual variations in compliance, absorption, metabolism, side effects, and the interpersonal aspects of medication management can, however, greatly influence the overall effectiveness of these regimens.

Studies examining the effectiveness of specific therapies for both adults and children, such as psychotherapy, behavioral or cognitive individual therapy, group or family therapy, or crisis intervention, show promise of success with specific populations or problem areas, though no overall assessments of which therapies are most effective are available. Evaluations of inpatient care, alternatives to hospitalization, and aftercare services — such as residential treatment, day treatment, outpatient treatment, and case management — have also been conducted. These evaluations have shown mixed results with respect to improved patient functioning (little or no versus some improvement) or variations depending on the type, combination, or intensity of services provided (no versus extensive aftercare services postdischarge).

A RAND Corporation randomized trial showed no statistically significant or clinically meaningful differences in outcomes between families in a fee-for-service insurance plan and those in a prepaid group practice HMO, in which a less intensive style of mental health treatment was practiced (Wells, Manning, & Valdez, 1989; Wells, Keeler, & Manning, 1990).

As with outcomes and effectiveness research on medical care in general, improved specification is needed of the desired outcomes themselves, the precise treatment or program elements expected to affect these outcomes, and the costs of the therapies or interventions relative to any benefits achieved (Gottlieb, 1989; Hargreaves & Shumway, 1989; OTA, 1986; Wells & Brook, 1989).

Alcohol or Substance Abusers

Quality assurance and assessment procedures in the field of alcohol and substance abuse are either nonexistent, implicit, or very limited in application. As mentioned in previous chapters, the fragmentation of treatment for these disorders across a variety of clients, settings, providers, and modalities exacerbates and compounds the problems in setting uniform and systematic standards for structural, process, and outcome indicators of quality. To better reflect the state of the art of substance abuse treatment, an Institute of Medicine report on the treatment of alcohol problems, for example, suggested that the question, "Does treatment work?" should actually be rephrased, "Which kinds of individuals, with what kinds of . . . problems, are likely to respond to what kinds of treatments by achieving what kinds of goals when delivered by what types of practitioners?" (IOM, 1990, p. 143).

Structure/Process. A major problem in setting uniform and systematic standards within this field is the fact that there are a diverse array of practitioners providing services, with widely varying professional norms and expectations regarding the appropriate focus and outcomes of care. Alcohol and drug abuse counselors are, for example, an important component of treatment in many settings. In some programs (particularly methadone maintenance or residental therapeutic community treatment programs), former or recovering addicts or alcoholics serve as the principal caregivers or counselors. In other instances (such as private chemical dependency programs), master's-level or Ph.D.-trained therapists or M.D.s may be the principal providers or overseers of care. Further, for many individuals in recovery, volunteer self-help programs (such as Alcoholics Anonymous or Narcotics Anonymous) or those sponsored by community service agencies (such as the Salvation Army)—each of which has its own unique treatment or rehabilitation philosophy—may be important components of the aftercare process.

To the extent that certain institutions, agencies, or professionals engaged in substance abuse treatment seek to obtain either licensing, accreditation, or third-party reimbursement from relevant public or private agencies, they are likely to undertake efforts to conform to those groups' standards. Interest in and compliance with such standards are, however, quite variable across types of providers and settings (Gerstein & Harwood, 1990; IOM, 1990).

Not only are there widely varying structural norms for organizing substance abuse treatment services, but few explicit process measures of quality exist. Evaluations of the effectiveness of selected drug treatment programs have, for example, indicated that differing program outcomes may be a function of aspects of the treatment process: the dosages of methadone or psychoactive medications provided, the relative emphasis on medical versus social interventions, the length of time the client remains in the program, the quality of the relationships between counselors and clients, and staff turnover, among other factors. No systematic empirical research has been conducted to assist in the formulation of treatment standards in this area, however (Gerstein & Harwood, 1990).

Outcomes. A particularly problematic issue in outcomes-oriented assessments of substance abuse services is that, as with the mental health area, the desired outcomes are not well defined, and the match according to which programs will best achieve what outcomes is not clearly articulated. Alternative outcomes include primary aims, such as reducing or eliminating the actual intake of the substance or diminishing the prospect of death or disability or associated social costs (such as substance abuse–related crime or motor vehicle deaths). Outcomes also include secondary aims, such as improving individual or family social functioning, locating employment, or attaining educational or job-related skills. Neither the priorities nor the means for achieving them are well defined. Further, those clients with the most difficulties in all of these areas of functioning are most likely to be served by programs in the public or voluntary service sector—which tend to have the smallest per capita levels of investment (Gerstein & Harwood, 1990; IOM, 1990).

Suicide- or Homicide-Prone

No well-developed or widely shared standards regarding appropriate and effective prevention- and treatment-oriented interventions to reduce suicide and homicide are available. This is principally because of the purported multifactorial etiology of these problems, and the corollary lack of integrated, multidisciplinary, theory-based research and evaluations of program effectiveness to guide the development of such standards.

Structure/Process. A major implicit structural consideration regarding quality in the areas of suicide and homicide prevention and treatment concerns the competency of gatekeepers and other personnel who might be in a position of identifying or treating at-risk individuals. Also crucial is the availability of case finding or outreach programs for particularly high-risk subgroups (such as the isolated or institutionalized elderly or teenage school dropouts). A further consideration is the adequacy and accessibility of treatment programs and services for the perpetrators, as well as survivors, of acts of intentional personal or interpersonal injury (such as suicidal attempters and their families or individuals incarcerated for assaultive violence).

However, what procedures and services might work best to prevent or attenuate violent behavior has not been clearly established. The prevention of such behavior may, in fact, lie in deeper changes in the social structure to address the differential social status and associated investments in social and human capital available to individuals and communities most vulnerable to such violence (Gurr, 1989; Osgood & McIntosh, 1986).

Outcomes. Major interventions to prevent youth suicide include (1) affective education, to help them understand and cope with problems that lead to suicide; (2) early identification and treatment of those most at risk; (3) school-based screening programs; (4) crisis centers and hotlines; (5) improved training of professionals; and (6) restriction of access to the three main methods of suicide (firearms, medications, and high places). A survey of experts in the field of youth suicide prevention failed to yield a consensus regarding which was the most effective intervention (Eddy, Wolpert, & Rosenberg, 1989).

Some evidence exists that those interventions that limit the availability of options to harm oneself (such as the regulation of handguns or prescription medications) may be more effective than those that rely primarily on individuals' deciding to change their behavior (education or counseling) (Starfield, 1989). There are no conclusive studies demonstrating that one type of treatment—psychotherapeutic, behavioral, or psychopharmacological—is clearly superior in treating adolescent suicide attempters (Trautman, 1989).

The major types of interventions to prevent or diminish the pursuit of "criminal careers" and associated crimes of violence include (1) strategies to prevent initial participation in such activities, (2) strategies to modify the criminal career once it begins, and (3) collective or selective incapacitation (incarceration) of serious or repeat offenders. More well-designed demonstrations and evaluations are required to fully assess the effectiveness of these alternatives.

Evidence from small-sample studies have, however, demonstrated that early childhood intervention and enrichment programs such as Head Start and programs to train parents and teachers in methods of communicating with and supervising children to modify antisocial behaviors resulted in lower rates of subsequent criminal activity.

Attempts to modify criminal careers through behavioral modification approaches have met with some success with small samples of delinquents followed for short periods of time. Indirect approaches to career modification through intensive drug abuse surveillance and treatment appear to be most successful in reducing the frequency of serious offenses by criminals addicted to hard drugs. Programs to upgrade employment skills have been documented to be successful in modifying offenders' careers in the United Kingdom, but not thus far in studies conducted in the United States.

Incapacitation (or incarceration) principally attempts to reduce crime by removing offenders from the community. Collective incapacitation seeks to lengthen the period of incarceration for groups of offenders (those who committed violent crime, for example), while selective incarceration focuses on individuals who are deemed to be at most risk of being continued offenders. Considerable ethical controversy surrounds the use of selective incapacitation. Major ethical questions are raised by the prospect of imposing a punishment on an individual before a crime is committed and by the fact that certain individuals or subgroups (such as racial/ethnic minorities) are more likely to be targeted for lengthened periods of imprisonment using this approach.

In either case, the impact of these methods is likely to be small relative to the number of individuals that would need to be imprisoned to offset criminal activity in the community. Further, these methods do not address the fundamental issue of whether "replacements" may continue to be produced for those who are removed from circulation, since the underlying sources of the problem remain unaddressed (Blumstein, Cohen, Roth, & Visher, 1986a).

Abusing Families

As with a number of other categories of vulnerable populations just reviewed, the standards of appropriate and efficacious care for victims of intimate abuse are not well developed.

Structure/Process. Structural considerations of quality focus on the training and availability of personnel to treat victims of abuse. Some Child Protective Services caseworkers, for example, have caseloads of thirty to fifty (or even more) families, though many experts believe that caseworkers can effectively serve no more than twenty such cases. In some states, these workers have fewer than forty hours of training, and a number of states do not require that they hold a professional degree (Gelles & Cornell, 1990, pp. 129–130).

The medical model of training tends to reinforce a detached stance that inhibits or prevents physicians from asking questions to determine whether injuries seen in their practice result from abuse (Randall, 1990). A study in one large metropolitan hospital documented that only one battered woman in twenty-five was diagnosed as such by the attending physician (PHS, 1990).

The development and promulgation of protocols for identifying, treating, and properly referring victims of abuse and neglect are intended to enhance the appropriateness of their care. The Year 2000 Objectives call for extending such protocols to at least 90 percent of hospital emergency rooms — where a substantial proportion of victims are seen. Following staff training and the introduction of a standard protocol in the emergency medical department at the Medical College of Pennsylvania, the percentage of women identified as battered increased from 5.6 to 30 percent (PHS, 1990).

Some researchers have suggested that the development of standards and educational interventions to teach general parenting and childrearing skills may be effective means of preventing child abuse and neglect — particularly among young parents (Browne, Davies, & Stratton, 1988; Knudsen, 1988).

Outcomes. Attempts to assess the desired outcomes of prevention and treatment programs in this area are plagued with a number of methodological difficulties. A major problem concerns the lack of a clear specification of the desired outcome of a given intervention: Is it increased knowledge on the part of the family regarding identifying events or actions that might precipitate violence and the means for dealing with them, behavioral evidence regarding changes in the family members' patterns of interaction, a reduction in the reported prevalence of abuse, or an increase in the reported rates of abuse that were previously unreported (Helfer, 1982; Leventhal, 1987)?

Other major methodological problems in documenting what is the best means to improve the outcomes for this population include the lack of well-developed theories for guiding the design of experimental interventions, the absence of randomized designs, and the lack of replicative evidence of program success across a variety of communities or population groups.

The Minneapolis Police Experiment (MPE) documented lower recidivism rates when mandatory (presumptive) arrest was used when abuse was suspected compared to other approaches to dealing with domestic disturbances (separation and advice and mediation). Major problems existed with the internal and external validity of the MPE study design, however, and a replication of the experiment in Omaha yielded more mixed results (Gelles & Cornell, 1990).

Federally funded evaluations of the National Demonstration Program in Child Abuse and Neglect (1974–1977), involving eleven treatment programs, and the Clinical Demonstration of Child Abuse and Neglect (1979–1981), in which nineteen clinical demonstration projects were assessed, yielded valuable information regarding the cost-effectiveness of different prevention and treatment alternatives. (This information was summarized in Chapter Eight.) Nonetheless, these major evaluation studies also suffered from serious methodological shortcomings: there was a lack of nonexperimental comparison groups, the assignment of clients to treatment alternatives was not random, the primary source of outcome data was from clinical staff who worked most closely with the patients, and no long-term outcome data were available posttreatment (Dubowitz, 1990).

Homeless

The problem of establishing quality-of-care norms for the homeless is exacerbated by the fact that most have inadequate access to care of any kind. Even when they do get care, it may be virtually impossible for them to carry through with recommended treatment or follow-up regimens given the circumstances of their lives on the street. Major publicly and privately supported projects concerned with the delivery of health care services for the homeless (RWJF-HCH, HRSA-HCH, VA-HCMI, among others) have attempted to tailor programs to take into account the unique needs and circumstances of the homeless.

Structure/Process. One focus of improving the quality of care to the homeless is more appropriate training for the personnel that care for them. This includes public and community health nurses; family physicians, pediatricians, and other physicians who see the homeless in their practices; and hospital emergency room or outpatient service providers. The important cadre of health professional volunteers, who provide care to the homeless in shelters, free clinics, or other places where the homeless gather, also require such training (Abdellah, Chamberlain, & Levine, 1986; Berne, Dato, Mason, & Rafferty, 1990; Bowdler, 1989; Weinreb & Bassuk, 1990). Case managers are an important component of the major health and mental health care programs serving the homeless described earlier. The roles and qualifications of these case managers are, however, neither clearly nor uniformly defined (IOM, 1988c; Stephens, Dennis, Toomer, & Holloway, 1991).

Studies conducted in connection with the Robert Wood Johnson Foundation Health Care for the Homeless program have provided invaluable data on the health and health care of the homeless (Brickner, Scharer, Conanan, Savarese, & Scanlan, 1990). The information gleaned from these and other studies provides an informational base for designing more targeted and effective interventions for addressing the unique and multifaceted needs of the homeless (Brickner, Scharer, Conanan, Elvy, & Savarese, 1985; Brickner, Scharer, Conanan, Savarese, & Scanlan, 1990; Wright & Weber, 1987).

Quality assurance activities for programs serving the homeless must take into account that different processes or procedures (additional follow-up activities) may be required to obtain desired standards, such as child immunization levels, that might be achieved with less effort in other types of practice (Altamore, Mitchell, & Weber, 1990).

Programs that incorporate outreach and case management components appear to have been successful in getting many of the homeless in for needed services. These are intensive and expensive services that are still largely unavailable to the homeless in most U.S. cities and localities, however. Adequate discharge planning and the availability of residential treatment options are significant gaps in addressing the long-term needs of the multiproblem homeless (Drake, Wallach, & Hoffman, 1989; IOM, 1988c). An evaluation of the VA-HCMI program showed that those veterans who completed a prescribed length of stay in residential treatment postdischarge had the best long-term mental and physical outcomes (Rosenheck, Gallup, Leda, Gorchov, & Errera, 1990).

Outcomes. As with other categories of vulnerable populations, the desired outcomes of "treating" the homeless are not well specified in a policy or program sense. Perhaps the best and most desirable outcome is for no one to be "homeless" in the first place.

Immigrants and Refugees

The quality of care obtained by immigrants and refugees is greatly affected by its accessibility, adequacy, and acceptability. That is, the quality of care is determined by (1) what type of care they are able to get, (2) whether it is enough as well as appropriate for their needs, and (3) whether they are able and/or willing to follow the plan recommended for treating their complaint.

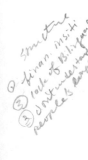

Structure/Process. The financial and institutional barriers that inhibit immigrant and refugee populations' seeking care were discussed in Chapter Seven. The lack of bilingual providers or translators can influence whether people feel comfortable going to a particular facility as well as the quality of the care they receive there. Sometimes impromptu interpreters, such as janitors or orderlies, are called on to translate, which may result in inaccurate information being conveyed and reluctance on the part of the patient to be forthcoming. Providers who do not clearly understand the symptoms or complaints being presented by patients are more likely to inaccurately diagnose the problem or prescribe inappropriate therapies. Similarly, patients may not fully understand what they are being told is wrong and the instructions they are subsequently given to treat it (Rumbaut, Chavez, Moser, Pickwell, & Wishik, 1988).

The delivery of high-quality medical care to immigrant and refugee populations is also inhibited by providers' limited knowledge of how to treat their special health problems and needs as well as by the patients' limited knowledge of public health or health promotion practices. Health care workers who are not aware of the higher prevalence of genetic-related disorders — such as Cooley's anemia, lactose intolerance, or other problems — among ethnic or racial subgroups are less likely to screen for them and more likely to misdiagnose or misprescribe as a result. Providers may also be unfamiliar with how to diagnose or treat diseases such as parasitic infestations or congenital malaria, which are common in certain foreign-born populations but relatively rare in general U.S. medical practice. The special anatomical and physiological characteristics (lighter body weight or eye conformation) of certain ethnic subgroups (Asians) may require adaptations of medications or surgical procedures (dosages or lens implantation in cataract surgery), which providers should take into account in treating these patients (Lin-Fu, 1988).

Cultural beliefs and practices affect immigrant and refugee populations' willingness to seek and/or comply with Western medical practices. Mexican immigrants, particularly those residing along the border, use folk healers (*curanderos*) who understand the folk illnesses and diagnoses common in Mexico. Many Hmong and Khmer refugees adhere to traditional healing methods, especially those practiced by shamans (the Hmong *txi neng*, the Khmer *krou*). A traditional home healing practice used in Southeast Asia called *kos khyal* ("coining" or applying warm coins) can create burns or bruises on a child's stomach, back, arms, and legs that look similar to those inflicted by intentional abuse. Toxic lead and arsenic are components of some Chinese folk remedies. The prevalence of smoking has been found to be high and the level of knowledge of the risk factors associated with cancer and heart disease low among Southeast Asian refugee and immigrant groups.

Religious and cultural beliefs and attitudes toward the unborn child, women's roles, and the role of family members in making decisions come into play as well in different groups' willingness to accept and/or adhere to Western medical practices. Many refugees suffer from serious mental health problems, which require a culturally sensitive process of diagnosis and treatment (Chen, Kuun, Guthrie, Li, & Zaharlick, 1991; Forbes & Wegner, 1987; Jenkins, McPhee, Bird, & Bonilla, 1990; Lee, 1988; Lin-Fu, 1988; Rumbaut, Chavez, Moser, Pickwell, & Wishik, 1988).

Outcomes. Knowledge of the social and cultural factors that play an important role in the life of foreign-born populations can facilitate the development of a more acceptable, adequate, and effective care plan — from both the provider's and the patient's point of view.

The next chapter reviews these and other questions that need to be addressed in more fully understanding, and addressing, the health and health care needs of vulnerable populations.

10

What Do We Still
Need to Know?

As with the system of providing and paying for services for the vulnerable, the conduct of research in this area is often categoric, fragmented, and not linked to other relevant bodies of research, and it fails to identify the issues that cut across different professional or service delivery domains. For example, policy makers, providers, and researchers concerned with the chronically ill elderly or chronically ill children or the mentally ill or persons with AIDS or the homeless may be interested in the utility of case management for improving the delivery of services to the population group of most concern to them. But they usually have little or no knowledge of the experiences in implementing particular case management models with other populations.

This book illuminates the cross-cutting insights that can be gained from reviewing the efforts and experiences in identifying, understanding, and addressing a wide array of vulnerable populations. As can be seen from the preceding chapters, much is known but much still needs to be learned in this area. This chapter highlights and critiques the existing body of knowledge on the health and health care needs of vulnerable populations.

Three major types of research needs and priorities can be identified. These include descriptive, analytical, and evaluative research. *Descriptive research* focuses on the methods and measures for identifying who are the vulnerable, how many there are, and who is most likely to be vulnerable. *Analytical research* is directed more toward understanding why some groups are more vulnerable than others and the program or policy alternatives that are, therefore, most relevant for preventing vulnerability or caring for those who are already in need. *Evaluative research* is concerned with assessing how well the programs and services that have been developed and implemented, based on previous descriptive and analytical research, have done in addressing or mitigating the needs of the groups they were most intended to serve.

Examples of descriptive, analytical, and evaluative research needed to identify, understand, and address the health and health care needs of vulnerable populations are highlighted in the discussion of each group, and in the summary of cross-cutting issues that follows.

Cross-Cutting Issues

The review confirms that further research is needed to more clearly characterize who the vulnerable are, to understand the origins of their vulnerability, and to evaluate which programs are most likely to be successful in either meeting or ameliorating their needs. Following is a summary of major cross-cutting research difficulties.

Descriptive Research

- Ambiguity in the definitions of the population
- Variability in the quality or completeness of information available on the population across data sources
- Changes in the definitions of the population or the availability of information on it over time
- Lack of demographic identifiers or detail (for example, race/ethnicity) for the comparison of subgroups within the population

Analytical Research

- Lack of well-developed, integrated, multidisciplinary theoretical perspectives and associated empirical research on the origins of the problem
- Paucity of longitudinal research — either within the life span of individuals or in the aggregate — on the origins, incidence, and consequences of the problem
- Paucity of comparative data — either on rare or hard-to-locate at-risk subpopulations or cross-nationally — on the origins, prevalence, and consequences of the problem

Evaluative Research

- Lack of well-articulated program and policy goals
- Lack of formal state-of-the-art review and assessment of existing research on program performance
- Lack of clearly articulated short-term and long-term research agendas for assessing probable program performance
- Lack of well-designed small-scale and large-scale demonstration projects for evaluating actual program performance
- Need to build the capacity and knowledge base through training researchers, replicating studies, and disseminating current research on program performance
- Need to develop comprehensive, coordinated interagency-oriented research agendas to address cross-cutting programmatic needs for vulnerable populations

Descriptive Research

A fundamental problem in identifying who and how many are vulnerable is ambiguity in the definitions of the vulnerable populations themselves. High-risk mothers and infants have been variously identified using predictors and indicators of both morbidity and mortality (such as rates of teen births, low- or very-low-birthweight infants, and maternal and infant deaths). The chronically ill and disabled have been defined based on diagnoses, disability, functional status, and quality-of-life measures. The case definition of AIDS has been revised three times since it was first published in 1982. At least four generations of studies in the mental health field can be identified in this century, all of which used either different approaches or different instruments for defining cases of mental illness.

The measurement of alcohol or substance abuse is made more difficult by the fact that there are different stages in the development of the addictive behaviors themselves: nonaddictive use, excessive use (abuse), addictive dependency, and recovery or relapse. Accurate reports of homicides and suicides depend on accurately discerning the intent of the perpetrators of the acts resulting in these deaths. Maltreatment can encompass both acts of commission (abuse) and omission (neglect), as well as a variety of types of harm or endangerment (physical, sexual, or emotional). The condition of homelessness can be assessed with respect to time (temporarily, episodically, or chronically homeless) or location (living on the streets, in temporary housing, or doubled up with relatives). Immigrants and refugees encompass those who are here legally as well as those who are not, and among the latter, settlers, sojourners, and commuters are all included.

Different studies tend to use different definitions or focus on different aspects of need for these groups. Often data are not available in a timely fashion or vary a great deal in quality and completeness across studies and sources. Cutbacks in funding, as well as changes in definitions of cases over time (which may be warranted to capture the changing dynamics of the problem, such as AIDS), can nonetheless jeopardize the availability of longitudinal data to trace changes in the incidence or prevalence of these problems. The lack of relevant demographic identifiers or detail (by race and ethnicity, for example) can also limit the ability to look at differences between groups for whom the risk or magnitude of problems is most likely to vary.

Researchers in a particular area need to work toward identifying common definitions of terms, the content and timing for collecting information for a minimum basic data set on a given population of interest, and uniform standards for evaluating and reporting data quality.

Analytical Research

A major limitation in adequately understanding the origins of many of the problems examined here is the absence of well-developed or integrated theoretical perspectives. Practitioners and researchers tend to focus on explanations rooted in their own disciplinary frameworks (of medicine, psychiatry, psychology, sociology, or social work, among others). Biological, psychological, and sociological explanations have all been used to understand the origins of suicide and interpersonal violence, for example. However, the complexity of these and other problems points to the need for broader, multidisciplinary theory development and research, and a corresponding expansion of the types of information gathered to adequately conduct research based on this perspective.

Longitudinal studies (over time) best illuminate the causes and consequences of vulnerability. For an individual, the development of chronic illness or suicidal tendencies or AIDS or substance abuse may be a product of a life course of experiences (being in a particular family, living a certain life-style, or working in a stressful or high-risk job). Similarly, at a national and local level, the magnitude and risks of these and other problems (such as homicide, family violence, or homelessness) may be affected by social, economic, or political changes (such as the loss of jobs in certain sectors of the economy, diminished federal or local commitments to maintaining the stock of low-income housing, or a declining tax base for the support of public education and related social services). Currently there is a paucity of longitudinal research looking at the correlates and consequences of vulnerability—either within the life span of individuals or in the aggregate, over time, at the local and national level.

Comparative studies are also useful in addressing the question of why some groups are more vulnerable than others. Collecting data on rare or hard-to-locate at-risk populations (such as drug users, runaways, pregnant homeless women, or elderly women living alone) is often costly and complex but provides valuable information for generating and/or testing hypotheses regarding the probable causes and consequences of vulnerability. Cross-national comparative studies are also useful in exploring the impact of political, social, cultural, economic, and related factors on the prevalence or incidence of addictive behavior or family abuse, for example.

Evaluative Research

As indicated in previous chapters, a limited amount of research has been conducted evaluating the costs and benefits of many programs and services designed to care for the vulnerable. The desired outcomes of these programs are often ambiguous or ill-defined, and the research that has been done has not been summarized or integrated in a coherent fashion.

A first step in developing a more solid foundation for designing new programs is to review and systematically evaluate research on the success or failures of existing programs and on how these outcomes were measured, based on formal meta-analysis procedures or consensus conferences of experts.

This process should lead to the formulation of a research agenda focusing on programs and services both to address immediate and pressing needs and to ameliorate or eliminate these problems over the long term. An aspect of the dilemma in dealing with certain issues (such as substance abuse or family violence) at present is the previous lack of investment or a diminished continuation of investment in research to understand what works and what does not work.

Given the paucity of funding for research in most areas, small-scale demonstration and evaluation studies could be conducted to establish a basis for deciding whether to proceed with larger-scale demonstration projects. Program evaluations should, however, attempt to apply sound tenets of experimental design, to maximize the internal validity (accuracy) and external validity (generalizability) of what is learned from these efforts.

An important aspect of this agenda-setting process would be to build the capacity and knowledge base in an area through providing support to train researchers, replicate previous studies, and integrate and disseminate findings.

Building a coordinated and comprehensive research agenda also requires cooperation between agencies in the design, implementation, and evaluation of programs, where none has traditionally existed. The multifaceted mosaic of needs of many of the vulnerable (such as those coping with homelessness, substance abuse, family abuse, and AIDS) does not fit neatly into existing agency or governmental divisions of categoric program responsibility.

Population-Specific Overview

The descriptive, analytical, and evaluative research priorities for vulnerable populations are summarized in the discussion that follows.

High-Risk Mothers and Infants

More information is needed to identify demographic (particularly ethnic) subgroups, behavioral risks, and appropriate care protocols for high-risk mothers and infants.

Descriptive Research. Birth and death certificates are the major sources of data on high-risk mothers and infants. The information recorded in these sources is often inaccurate or incomplete (Brunskill, 1990; Hexter et al., 1990; Lammer, Brown, Anderka, & Guyer, 1989). Particular problems with vital statistics data include the unavailability and/or misclassifications of detailed racial/ethnic group breakdowns. National data on births of Hispanic parentage were first available in 1978 in only seventeen states. In 1988, these data were available in only thirty states and the District of Columbia. Low birthweight on births of Asian parentage were first published in 1984. Data on Native American populations are limited to those who live in states with reservations. The "revolving door" of Mexico-U.S. migration patterns has also given rise to concerns about serious underreporting of Hispanic infant deaths in the border regions of the United States. Further, there is a three- to four-year time lag in the availability of national natality and mortality estimates (Kennedy & Deapen, 1991; Miller, Fine, & Adams-Taylor, 1989; Selby, Lee, Tuttle, & Loe, 1984).

Analytical Research. More analytical studies are needed to examine the risk factors associated with poor pregnancy outcomes. Data on income, behavioral and medical risks, program eligibility, and medical care use have not tradi- tionally been available from vital statistics sources. The National Center for Health Statistics has initiated a number of new activities to provide more comprehensive information on the correlates and outcomes of pregnancy. These include the development of expanded standardized birth, death, and fetal death certificates; linked birth and death record files, beginning with the 1983 birth cohort; and the 1988 National Maternal and Infant Health (NMIH) and 1990 Longitudinal Follow-up surveys.

Beginning in 1989, the expanded birth certificates collect additional information on the medical and behavioral risk factors associated with preg- nancy and the technologies used at birth. The revised death certificates col- lect more detailed information on causes of death. Linked birth and death records permit a direct examination of the association between infant mor- tality and various maternal risk factors, and whether these associations are changing over time.

The NMIH survey collects an array of risk factor and care data from mothers, hospitals, and prenatal care providers, based on national samples of death, birth, and fetal death certificates. The NMIH follow-up survey permits an examination of child development and outcomes for infants over time (Smith, 1989). An Infant Mortality Survey conducted by the Health Care Financing Administration Infant Health Task Force and the Centers for Disease Control Division of Reproductive Health provides newborn in- fant data from state Medicaid files, linked with other federal program, med- ical record, and vital statistics data (HCFA, 1990).

These data sources constitute rich mines of information for examin- ing the impact of risk and related care factors on pregnancy outcomes cross- sectionally and over time. However, there is a lag in the availability of these data as well—particularly the linked birth-death record sources.

Evaluative Research. Studies to examine the impact of particular programs on perinatal outcomes are often based on weak evaluation research designs. Shadish and Reis (1984) provide a critical review and synthesis of studies of the effectiveness of programs to improve pregnancy outcomes. They point out that in many of these studies, history, differential selection, and attri- tion are powerful alternatives to concluding that any particular program (such as WIC or MICP projects) had an impact on reducing infant mortality rates, for example.

There is also a paucity of research on the probable impact of many of the expanded components of prenatal care recommended by the PHS expert panel—such as preconception visits, behavioral risk assessment and intervention, and psychosocial counseling—on actual birth outcomes (PHS, 1989). Technology assessment studies are also needed to estimate the costs and effectiveness of high-technology prenatal care and birthing procedures, particularly for high-risk newborns.

The Institute of Medicine panel on prenatal care concluded that there is a surfeit of research documenting the financial and institutional barriers to prenatal care. Subsequent research should focus on the cost and effectiveness of mechanisms for removing these barriers to prenatal care (IOM, 1988d).

Chronically Ill and Disabled

Descriptive research should focus on the development of uniform definitions and data sets for identifying the chronically ill and disabled, and more analytic and evaluative research is needed to guide the formulation of cost-effective long-term care policy for this population.

Descriptive Research. One of the principal problems in conducting research on the chronically ill and disabled is the considerable variability that exists in the definitions and criteria that have been used to describe this population. Fundamental conceptual questions concern which type of indicators—diagnoses, disability, functional status, quality-of-life measures, or others—are most relevant for describing the chronically ill and disabled, and why (Bergner, 1989; Gallin & Given, 1976; Spilker, Molinek, Johnston, Simpson, & Tilson, 1990; Spitzer, 1987; Stein et al., 1987; Stewart et al., 1989; Thompson-Hoffman & Storck, 1991).

Disability and functional status–related measures, such as ADLs (Activities of Daily Living) and IADLs (Instrumental Activities of Daily Living), are often-used indicators of the chronically ill and disabled elderly, though the operational definitions of these measures vary a great deal across studies. This becomes particularly problematic in estimating the numbers of individuals in need of home care services and in establishing subsequent program eligibility. Very different magnitudes of those in need may be estimated depending on the criteria and cutting points applied (Interagency Forum on Aging-Related Statistics, 1989; Rowland, Lyons, Neuman, Salganicoff, & Taghavi, 1988; Spector, 1990; Stone & Murtaugh, 1990).

There are also a paucity of national data on certain categories of the chronically ill and disabled, such as children. The Census and the National Center for Health Statistics and other agencies within the Department of Health and Human Services are planning an array of surveys to monitor the impact of the Americans with Disabilities Act (ADA) and other disability-related programs (Hendershot, 1990). These studies should provide invaluable information on the characteristics of chronically ill and disabled children and nonelderly, as well as elderly, adults.

The long-term focus of care for the chronically ill and disabled compels a look at whether their status improves or declines over time. Longitudinal data from needs assessment and related studies of this population are needed to facilitate forecasting changes in the profile of needs and probable case mix of services (Habib et al., 1988).

Formal and informal caregivers are a particularly important component of care for the chronically ill and disabled. Barer and Johnson (1990) point out that the caregiving research has been plagued by inadequate attention to who exactly is included in the definition of *caregivers*. Other factors that have been neglected include the extent of patient needs as they influence variability in caregiver demands and the generalizability and representativeness of study samples. The omission of the patients' own perspectives on their functional ability is an obvious deficiency, as is the failure to consider the presence of an extended support network in addition to the primary providers of care.

Analytical Research. Analytical questions of interest with respect to the chronically ill and disabled include considerations of models to predict rates of utilization or expenditures for nursing home, home care, or related long-term care services. Such models are useful, for example, in computing the actuarial risk of service use in formulating long-term care insurance policies (Liu, Manton, & Liu, 1990; Williams, Phillips, Torner, & Irvine, 1990), determining the importance of knowledge or other access barriers to care seeking (McCaslin, 1988), and assessing the influence of community or political factors on public expenditures for long-term care (Lowe, 1988).

A number of federal agencies have formulated research agendas related to issues in caring for the chronically ill and disabled. The National Institute on Aging developed a conceptual framework that calls for a look at the characteristics of both the providers and recipients of long-term care and the assumptions that underlie and the factors that affect their interaction. It also recommends methodological approaches for studying these relationships. The major analytical questions it indicates should be addressed, based on this framework, include how to reduce the need for and associated costs of long-term care, how to improve the quality and efficiency of long-term care, how to monitor its changing supply and demand, and what the special problems of subpopulations, such as the oldest old, women, and older rural people are (NIA, 1989).

The National Center for Health Statistics established recommendations for the minimum basic data set and types of analyses needed to guide the development of long-term care and aging policy, based on large-scale surveys conducted under its auspices (NCHS, 1979, 1988b).

Evaluative Research. As mentioned in Chapters Eight and Nine, numerous studies have been conducted on the cost and effectiveness of alternative models of long-term care delivery. Investigations in this area have tended to suffer from deficiencies in the development of theory to guide the conduct of the research, the strength of the evaluation designs, and the specification and measurement of program outcomes (Hughes, 1985; Shaughnessy, 1985; Toseland & Rossiter, 1989).

Research is also needed that examines the impact of new policy initiatives, such as prevention-oriented programs and DRGs and related financing and cost-containment options, on the health and well-being of the chronically ill and disabled (NIA, 1989).

Persons with AIDS

Changes in definitions, the dynamic nature of the epidemic, and constrained research and service delivery funding have complicated efforts to understand the origins and consequences of AIDS.

Descriptive Research. Identifying who has AIDS, as well as who is likely to develop it, is one of the fundamental research questions in tracking the epidemiology of the epidemic. Since it was first published in 1982, the case definition for AIDS has been revised three times (in 1985, 1987, and 1993) (CDC, 1985, 1987a). The 1987 revision allowed for the presumptive diagnosis (without laboratory evidence of HIV infection) of AIDS-associated diseases and expanded the spectrum of HIV-associated diseases reportable as AIDS. These changes affected the comparability of case reports over time and differentially increased the rates and case-mix severity for certain subgroups (such as minorities and IV drug users), when compared with earlier definitions (Payne, Rutherford, Lemp, & Clevenger, 1990; Selik, Buehler, Karon, Chamberland, & Berkelman, 1990). A study of AIDS deaths in San Francisco found that the numbers of deaths for minorities (especially Hispanics) was even higher than reported due to the misclassification of Hispanics as non-Hispanic whites (Lindan et al., 1990). The Centers for Disease Control proposed another approach to identifying AIDS cases, based on whether a person had 200 or fewer CD4 cells per cubic milliliter of blood or an expanded set of HIV-associated illnesses, to take effect in 1993 (APHA, 1991b). This revised definition is likely to result in an earlier diagnosis of women and children who have AIDS. Careful consideration of the definitional and measurement issues in identifying persons with AIDS is essential in accurately describing and forecasting the future of this dynamic epidemic.

HIV seroprevalence surveys are a particularly important tool for this purpose, since they provide an idea of who and how many are likely to develop AIDS over time. The sensitivity and specificity (accuracy) of the HIV antibodies tests developed for population-based screening are generally very good, though the ethical implications of disclosing test results for any given individual — particularly inaccurate (either positive or negative) results — may be very problematic (Burke et al., 1988; Khabbaz, Hartley, Lairmore, & Kaplan, 1990; Meyer & Pauker, 1987). CDC is currently conducting a family of HIV seroprevalence surveys in selected, purposively selected, sentinel sites—STD clinics, drug treatment centers, and selected hospitals, among others (CDC, 1990g). These sites are, however, not representative of the population as a whole or of at-risk subgroups within it. Plans for a CDC national household seroprevalence survey were abandoned because of serious political opposition, as well as methodological problems with adequately capturing groups most at risk in the survey (APHA, 1991a).

The National Research Council Committee on AIDS Research and the Behavioral, Social, and Statistical Sciences and other groups have strongly endorsed the conduct of more extensive methodological research on designing high-quality seroprevalence and other surveys of persons most at risk of AIDS—who may also be the hardest to locate and interview (such as IV drug users). This research agenda includes approaches to designing probability samples of rare populations, reducing nonresponse bias, and enhancing the validity and reliability of the data obtained from these respondents (Laumann, Gagnon, Michaels, Michael, & Coleman, 1989; Miller, Turner, & Moses, 1990; Watters & Biernacki, 1989).

Analytical Research. Federal funding for AIDS has tended to focus on biomedical and clinic research, and more recently on educational and behavioral interventions to halt the spread of the disease (OTA, 1985, 1990a). An array of analytical epidemiological, behavioral, and social science research is needed, however, to better understand the correlates and consequences of the epidemic (Allen & Curran, 1988; Henry, 1988). An Institute of Medicine report on the AIDS Research Program of the National Institutes of Health called for the development of a five-year plan for its budget, as well as a better balance of priorities, including basic research on the biology of AIDS, behavioral studies of high-risk activities, and health services research on the care and quality of life of patients (IOM, 1991a).

Comprehensive and valid methodologies for estimating and projecting the rates of survival and costs of AIDS care are essential for evaluating the probable price tag and economic impact of the epidemic (Begley, Crane, & Perdue, 1990; Bilheimer, 1989; Scitovsky, 1988, 1989a, 1989b; Thompson & Meyer, 1989).

The Agency for Health Care Policy and Research convened a conference in June 1988 to consider the issues and methodologies for AIDS-related health services research (Sechrest, Freeman, & Mulley, 1989). Statistical models for estimating and comparing risks among groups, examining the prognosis at different stages of the disease, and projecting subsequent rates of survival post diagnosis would be useful in evaluating the process and outcome of care for persons with AIDS (Baltimore & Feinberg, 1989; Feinstein, 1989; Haseltine, 1989; Justice, Feinstein, & Wells, 1989; Redfield & Tramont, 1989).

Basic social and behavioral science research on the sexual behavior of subgroups who may be most at risk—homosexual and bisexual males, teenage heterosexuals, male and female prostitutes—or those for whom the risks may increase over the course of the epidemic, such as the elderly, is needed to assist in designing targeted interventions for these groups (Riley, Ory, & Zablotsky, 1989; Turner, Miller, & Moses, 1989).

Shadish (1989) has argued for the use of "critical multiplism" as a strategy in the design and conduct of research related to AIDS. Such an approach would employ a variety of contrasting (quantitative and qualitative) methods of sampling, data collection, and measurement, as well as protocols for evaluating the biases of each method throughout the course of the study.

Evaluative Research. Relatively little evaluative research exists on the cost and effectiveness of community-based and other models of care for persons with AIDS (AHCPR, 1990a). The NRC Committee on AIDS Research and the Behavioral, Social, and Statistical Sciences has developed a number of recommendations regarding how to improve the design of studies to evaluate AIDS health care and public health interventions (Coyle, Boruch, & Turner, 1991; Miller, Turner, & Moses, 1990; Turner, Miller, & Moses, 1989). The committee calls for a wider use of randomized field experiments. If randomization is not possible, it recommends the application of carefully conceived quasi-experimental or related designs to control for the array of alternative explanations besides the program itself (such as who chooses to use it, who drops out of it, what other things are going on in the community, and so on) that may account for any changes that are observed.

Evaluations of the major AIDS prevention programs—media campaigns, health education and risk reduction, and testing and counseling— should address the extent to which they become operational (formative evaluation), how well they work (process evaluation), and whether they achieve their intended goals (outcome evaluation). Better specification of the desired outcomes of these programs is also needed, particularly in terms of the behaviors they are intended to influence.

Mentally Ill and Disabled

Significant methodological issues surround how best to identify and collect data on the mentally ill and disabled.

Descriptive Research. The design of methodologies for studies of the prevalence and distribution of mental illness has been and continues to be a challenge for the field of psychiatric epidemiology. At least four generations of epidemiological studies, with varying methodologies, have been conducted or proposed. The first generation, prior to World War II, used record sources and key informants to define "cases." The second generation, post–World War II, typically used a single psychiatrist or a small team headed by a psychiatrist. Community residents were interviewed, and in some cases, standardized protocols were used. The Epidemiological Catchment Area program surveys, using lay interviewers and standardized survey sampling and data collection procedures, typify the third generation of studies (Dohrenwend & Dohrenwend, 1982; Klerman, 1990; Robins, 1990).

A continuing methodological concern in psychiatric surveys is the definition of *caseness* — that is, how individuals come to be classified as mentally ill. This problem is rooted in philosophical disputes regarding the appropriateness of assigning primacy to psychiatric diagnoses in making these judgments. Other questions pertain to the validity and reliability of specific instruments used for this purpose, such as the Diagnostic Interview Schedule (DIS) applied in the Epidemiological Catchment Area surveys (Anthony et al., 1985; Dingemans, 1990; Helzer, Spitznagel, & McEvoy, 1987; Klerman, 1989; Kovess & Fournier, 1990; Mirowsky & Ross, 1989a, 1989b; Robins, Helzer, Croughan, & Ratcliff, 1981; Swartz, Carroll, & Blazer, 1989; Tweed & George, 1989; Williams, Tarnopolsky & Hand, 1980).

A related problem is the design of culturally sensitive and appropriate approaches to measuring the prevalence of disorders in different racial/ethnic groups and cross-nationally (Marsella, 1978; Neighbors, Jackson, Campbell, & Williams, 1989; Robins, 1989; Rogler, 1989; Williams, 1986).

Further, the "need" for mental health services has variously been measured indirectly through social indicator–type community profiles reflecting correlated risks of mental illness (such as income and racial distribution), as well as rates of mental illness under treatment or the proportion of "cases" receiving or not receiving mental health services (Cleary, 1989; Goldsmith, Lin, Bell, & Jackson, 1988). Bebbington (1990) argued for a fourth generation of psychiatric surveys focusing more explicitly on the social functioning of those identified as mentally ill, as a more informed basis for planning programs to meet their needs.

Analytical Research. A recent reorganization and integration of health services research activities within NIMH, as well as a series of conferences and proceedings on methodologies for studying the operation and performance of the mental health care system, attest to the development of mental health services research as a field of study (AHSR, 1991; Fineberg, 1987; Jencks, Horgan, Goldman, & Taube, 1987; Taube, 1986; Taube & Burns, 1988; Taube, Mechanic, & Hohmann, 1989).

Priority health services research areas within NIMH include the crosscutting mental health needs of vulnerable populations (such as the chronically mentally ill, those with co-occurrence disorders such as alcohol or drug abuse, and violent behavior), particularly at-risk demographic subgroups (children and adolescents, minorities, and rural populations), and the financing and delivery of services (such as psychiatric rehabilitation), as well as agency and academic research partnerships for the conduct of mental health services research (through a public-academic liaison program).

The report *The Future of Mental Health Services Research* (Taube, Mechanic, & Hohmann, 1989) outlines a research agenda for addressing an array of unanswered analytical questions with respect to the structure and organization of systems of providing mental health services. It also makes suggestions for research dealing with the costs, financing, reimbursement, and regulation of these services; determinants and patterns of use; and the outcomes of mental health care. Analytical methods from general health services research — such as decision analysis, mathematical modeling, screening scale development, computer-assisted educational and decision-making aids, and prospective payment-setting methodologies — are also being increasingly applied in the conduct of mental health services research (Fineberg, 1987; Jencks, Horgan, Goldman, & Taube, 1987).

Evaluative Research. As mentioned in previous chapters, there is a paucity of systematic, well-designed evaluations of the operation and impact of mental health treatment and services delivery programs. A place to begin would be to conduct meta-analyses (that is, a systematic, quantitative synthesis and critique) of the findings from existing evaluations of various programs (such as case management or other aftercare options). This would then provide a foundation for understanding what can be validly concluded from existing research, as well as for formalizing and focusing an evaluative mental health services research agenda (Hargreaves & Shumway, 1989).

As with evaluations of the impact of health care programs in general, a better specification is needed of the outcomes the programs are expected to accomplish — such as those developed in the RAND Medical Outcomes Study (MOS) for comparing the physical, social, and role functioning of depressed patients seen in a variety of delivery settings (Ware, 1989; Wells & Brook, 1989).

The National Advisory Mental Health Council has formulated a research agenda for evaluating care for people with severe persistent disabling mental disorders. The three main areas this group identified in which research is needed are methods for (1) improving the quality of care being provided this population, (2) improving the organization and financing of services to facilitate the delivery of effective services, and (3) developing the capacity for doing and disseminating relevant research (NIMH, 1991).

Alcohol or Substance Abusers

The knowledge base on alcohol and substance abuse is characterized by considerable variability across data sources and disciplines.

Descriptive Research. A variety of data sources and approaches are used in estimating the prevalence and distribution of substance abuse problems. These include more behaviorally oriented social surveys, such as the National Household Survey on Drug Abuse and the Monitoring the Future survey of high school seniors; epidemiologically oriented studies of problem prevalence, such as the Epidemiological Catchment Area surveys; surveillance systems, such as the Drug Abuse Warning Network (DAWN); and facilities-based sources, such as the National Drug and Alcoholism Treatment Unit Survey (NDATUS).

These different types of studies measure different aspects of the problem or focus on different subgroups of the population. As a result, they may point to somewhat conflicting conclusions about the patterns of drug dependence — a decreased prevalence of the problem based on national household and school-based surveys, but higher rates of drug-related deaths reported through the routine surveillance systems. The data obtained from different sources may, however, be capturing different stages of the development of the addictive behavior: nonaddictive use, excessive use (abuse), addictive dependency, and recovery or relapse (Collins & Zawitz, 1990; NCHS, 1985b; Westermeyer, 1990).

A Public Health Task Force on Drug Abuse Data and a conference convened by the RAND Corporation's Drug Policy Research Center reviewed the current substance abuse–related data systems and made a number of recommendations for improving and enhancing the usefulness of these disparate data gathering activities (Haaga & Reuter, 1991; PHS Task Force on Drug Abuse Data, 1990).

The major areas of need included information on the nature and extent of drug abuse (particularly for at-risk populations such as pregnant women, persons with AIDS, prisoners, and the homeless), the morbidity and mortality associated with drug abuse, data on the capacity and utilization of the prevention and treatment systems, the costs and financing of care, and treatment outcomes. Better integration and validation of existing data gathering efforts is also needed — through, for example, using common core questionnaire items and determining the extent of overlap across sampling frames. In addition, more analytical and integrative analyses should be conducted across the array of existing data sets to address drug policy issues.

Analytical Research. The Institute of Medicine, the General Accounting Office, and the World Health Organization have undertaken a number of studies in recent years to develop and identify a research agenda for the prevention and treatment of alcohol and drug abuse problems (Board on Mental Health and Behavioral Medicine, Institute of Medicine, 1985; Fillmore, 1988; GAO, 1990b; Gerstein & Harwood, 1990; IOM, 1980, 1987, 1989c, 1990).

Conclusions that have emerged from these studies include the need for more theory-driven research and for the integration of the theoretical perspectives and findings of biomedical, social science, and behaviorally oriented research in understanding and designing interventions to address the multiplicity of causes of the disorders. Other themes include the following: the integration of long-term, life-span, and developmental as well as comparative (including cross-national) research perspectives; the clarification and quantification of desired treatment or prevention outcomes; the support of long-term community trials; and studies to evaluate both the cost and effectiveness of prevention and treatment-oriented interventions.

Evaluative Research. The support of federal research for mental and addictive disorders through the major constituent institutes of the Alcohol Drug Abuse and Mental Health Administration (ADAMHA) — NIMH, NIDA, and NIAA — declined in real purchasing power from 1966 to the mid 1980s (Board on Mental Health and Behavioral Medicine, Institute of Medicine, 1985).

No large-scale evaluations of drug abuse treatment programs have been completed in recent years. Two major long-term studies of treatment results — the Drug Abuse Reporting Program (DARP), which tracked a sample of clients in treatment from 1969 to 1973, and the Treatment Outcome Prospective Study (TOPS), which tracked clients from 1979 to 1981 — were terminated in the early 1980s with the advent of block grants. The Client Oriented Data Acquisition Process to collect data on clients in drug abuse treatment, begun in 1972, was effectively terminated with the 1981 Omnibus Reconciliation Act, in which states were no longer required to report these data. During the 1980s, when the drug problem was growing in importance, the availability of research funds for the generation of knowledge for addressing the problem was declining.

Since 1986, the research budgets of these agencies have begun to grow. NIDA and NIAAA are in the process of developing a Minimum Treatment Client Data Set (MTCDS), and a Drug Abuse Treatment Outcome Study (DATOS) has been developed to evaluate program effectiveness. A GAO study on the status of drug abuse treatment research provided the following recommendations regarding how best to allocate the new funds going into this area: NIDA should develop a long-term strategic plan for drug abuse research, more funds should be provided for training researchers in this area, the knowledge base should be extended by funding and evaluating large-scale treatment demonstrations and how best to match clients to programs, and the focus should shift from a long-standing emphasis on heroin and other opiate addiction to crack and cocaine addiction (GAO, 1990b; Haaga & Reuter, 1991).

A Report to Congress and the White House on the Nature and Effectiveness of Federal, State, and Local Drug Prevention/Education Programs concluded that existing knowledge about the prevention of alcohol and drug abuse is limited by several problems. These include a rush to pass judgment on a program before it is stable enough to be evaluated, weak or imprecise measures of program outcome, poor research designs, inadequate information about how the programs were implemented, and an emphasis on statistical significance to the neglect of policy or programmatic significance. The report also pointed out that, traditionally, most prevention programs have focused on educational or psychosocial interventions with individuals in an effort to remedy deficiencies of knowledge, coping skills, and behavior. The causes of substance abuse include a variety of social and environmental, in addition to individual, correlates. More recently, prevention has begun to focus on the individual in the context of peers, families, schools, and communities. The report concludes, "Comprehensive programs that address a number of factors influencing drug use are likely to hold the most promise for prevention. Prevention efforts that focus on only one or two factors are unlikely to be successful" (U.S. Department of Education and U.S. Department of Health and Human Services, 1987, p. i).

The research functions of the three ADAMHA agencies (NIAAA, NIDA, NIMH) have been incorporated in the National Institutes of Health (NIH) (Hooper, 1991). Treatment and service delivery programs remain within a new agency—Substance Abuse and Mental Health Services Administration. This reorganization may reduce the support of research that is more service delivery oriented, rather than principally clinical, in focus.

Suicide- or Homicide-Prone

Longitudinal studies and demonstration projects are needed to better understand the origins of violence and how best to prevent or ameliorate it.

Descriptive Research. Information on completed (and particularly attempted) suicides and homicides is variable and incomplete. No common definition of what constitutes a "suicide" exists, and because of the social stigma that often results from suicides, other causes of death may be assigned to save the family or other survivors embarrassment. A survey of 200 medical examiners yielded the estimate that the number of suicides reported may be half the "true" number. Further, attempted suicides are not currently reportable through any vital statistics or epidemiological surveillance system. There is also generally at least a two- to three-year lag in the availability of data on completed suicides and homicides through the vital statistics system (Jobes, Berman, & Josselson, 1987; Moscicki, 1989; O'Carroll, 1989; Rosenberg, Smith, Davidson, & Conn, 1987).

Major sources of data on homicide-related crime include the Federal Bureau of Investigation Uniform Crime Reports (UCR) (particularly its Supplementary Homicide Reports) and the National Crime Survey (NCS) of U.S. households. The UCR provides reports only on known assaults, and local police have a great deal of discretion with respect to whether and how to fill out such reports. Systematic and easy methods for amending or updating such reports once new information is obtained on the case are also not currently in place.

The National Crime Survey is intended to elicit information on crimes that might not be reported formally to local police authorities. The NCS was recently revised to correct the major problems that had previously characterized that study (anomalous findings, inadequate measurement of revictimization, and sample attrition). NCS results are nonetheless affected by the problems that usually attend surveys addressing such topics (such as greater noncoverage or nonresponse of particularly at-risk groups or the underreporting of sensitive or personally traumatic events). Neither of these data sources capture good information on a particularly important correlate of homicide—interpersonal family violence and abuse (Rokaw, Mercy, & Smith, 1990; Rosenberg & Mercy, 1986; Skogan, 1990; Taylor, 1989; Whitaker, 1989).

Analytical Research. No information is currently available on death certificates that would facilitate studies of the correlates and causes of violent deaths due to homicide or suicide—such as a previous history of suicide or mental illness, substance abuse, family structure, or socioeconomic status. Psychological autopsies have been used to assess the reasons why a particular individual may have chosen to commit suicide. This procedure involves an intensive interview or series of interviews with persons who knew the victim to determine the social and psychological circumstances surrounding the incident. This methodology, along with other types of data, may be useful in generating meaningful theories and hypotheses regarding the etiology of suicidal acts (Brent, 1989; Rosenberg, Smith, Davidson, & Conn, 1987).

Much more research is needed using life-span and developmental and/or causal approaches to understanding suicidal and homicidal behavior. Theories of suicide have tended to emphasize cross-sectional, not longitudinal, analyses. Studying individual suicide and criminal careers, as well as the experience of historical demographic (age-sex-race) cohorts, may, for example, provide a better understanding of the etiology and evolution of violent behaviors at both the individual and societal level. A better understanding is needed as well of the extent to which violent acts are contagious—or lead to other acts of individual or interpersonal violence.

There is also a paucity of multidisciplinary theory and research examining the array of biological, psychological, and social antecedents and correlates that have been identified from disparate bodies of research in this area—particularly for those groups who might be most at risk (the elderly and minorities, for example). An important ethical question posed in estimating the cost of violent deaths in terms of years lost of life is the implicit devaluing of the elderly, for whom suicide rates are highest, by focusing on the estimated years of productive life lost—that is, those up to age sixty-five (ADAMHA, 1989a, 1989b, 1989c, 1989d; Berlin, 1985, 1987; Blumstein, Cohen, Roth, & Visher, 1986a; Gibbs, 1988; Gould, Wallenstein, & Davidson, 1989; Grossman, Milligan, & Dayo, 1991; Hendin, 1986; Leenaars, 1989; Osgood & McIntosh, 1986; Rosenberg, Smith, Davidson, & Conn, 1987; Stack, 1987; Stafford & Weisheit, 1988; Stephens, 1987).

Evaluative Research. As mentioned in previous chapters, much more research is needed that evaluates the cost and effectiveness of prevention and treatment-oriented interventions to address problems of personal and interpersonal violence. Such evaluations should focus on what types of services in particular might work best (hotlines, therapy, outreach, and so on), and for what groups (adolescents, the elderly, minorities).

An important strategy for beginning to fill the substantial gaps in knowledge in this area is to support small-scale demonstration projects, along with well-designed independent program evaluations, to see what works best. Based on the results of these studies, models could be selected for larger-scale demonstration projects and subjected to rigorous external evaluation as a basis for developing better-informed programmatic and policy priorities in this area (ADAMHA, 1989a, 1989b, 1989c, 1989d; Blumstein, Cohen, Roth, & Visher, 1986a; Streiner & Adam, 1987).

Abusing Families

A deeper understanding of abusing families could be gained from more integrated, multidisciplinary theory development and research in this area.

Descriptive Research. Considerable variability exists in how abusing families are defined. Maltreatment can be designated by acts of commission (abuse) or omission (neglect); probable injury (endangerment) as well as actual injury (harm); professional reports of incidents of harm (cases) or family reports of actions that could result in harm (family violence); physical, as well as sexual or emotional, abuse; and by victim—child, wife, husband, sibling, parent, elderly, and so on. The terms *abuse* and *neglect* are often used interchangeably in the literature, though *maltreatment* is generally considered to encompass both (Cicchetti & Carlson, 1989; Gelles & Cornell, 1990; Pagelow, 1984).

These varying definitions, as well as the differing methodologies used to gather data, lead to varying estimates of the incidence and prevalence of the problem. The major types of studies (and examples of each) include clinical studies of victims or perpetrators of abuse (Clinical Demonstration of Child Abuse and Neglect), official reports to protective service agencies (National Study on Child Neglect and Abuse Reporting), interviews with abuse and neglect service providers (Study of the National Incidence and Prevalence of Child Abuse and Neglect), and surveys of U.S. families (National Crime Survey, National Surveys of Family Violence).

Clinical studies tend to be based on few cases and rely on clinician judgments of maltreatment. Official reports overrepresent certain groups (minorities, low income), double-count cases (due to more than one incident being reported), and may or may not be verified (substantiated) by a fuller investigation. Middle-class professionals tend to label certain incidents as abuse or neglect that others would not, as a function of their cultural referents and norms or particular disciplinary background. Family members may not feel comfortable in reporting sensitive events, such as acts of intrafamily violence or victimization, in surveys.

The relative advantages and disadvantages of these various data gathering approaches need to be weighed and understood in designing surveillance systems to monitor the prevalence and incidence of maltreatment (Cicchetti & Carlson, 1989; Eckenrode, Munsch, Powers, & Doris, 1988; Gelles & Cornell, 1990; Hampton & Newberger, 1985; Knudsen, 1989; Pagelow, 1984).

Numerous methodological difficulties surround correctly identifying incidents of child sexual abuse in particular—either through surveys (Edwards & Donaldson, 1989; Haugaard & Emery, 1989; Wyatt & Peters, 1986a, 1986b), the use of anatomical dolls in counseling or court (Freeman & Estrada-Mullaney, 1988), or medical examinations (Kleinman, Blackbourne, Marks, Karellas, & Belanger, 1989; Krugman, 1989). More research is needed to refine the reliability and validity of methods of detecting this particularly sensitive type of abuse. The moral and ethical implications of false positives or false negatives are substantial for both the suspected victim and perpetrator of such acts (Haugaard & Reppucci, 1988).

Analytical Research. A major limitation of analytical research on maltreatment is the absence of a well-developed theoretical foundation. As mentioned in Chapter Four, an array of micro- and macro-oriented theories have been utilized by investigators. The respective theories have tended to focus on discrete dynamics or explanations of causality (psychopathology, learning behavior, or status inequality, among others), or they have encompassed so many interacting components as to be virtually untestable empirically (systems theory). Further, research based on these theories has tended to utilize cross-sectional or retrospective study designs, with all the attendant weaknesses of trying to attribute the causes of events after their occurrence (Cicchetti & Carlson, 1989; Gelles & Cornell, 1990; Pagelow, 1984).

Subsequent research in this area should focus on developing a multidisciplinary theoretical foundation and prospective (or longitudinal) analytical (in addition to descriptive) data bases. Research should seek to uncover and understand the commonalities, as well as the discrete causes, of the array of acts encompassed within the concepts of maltreatment (or family violence). Professionals from different disciplines (psychiatry, psychology, sociology, and medicine, among others) must engage in dialogue that invites a multidisciplinary look at the problem. They should also be willing to discard disciplinary prejudices (or paradigms) when the empirical evidence consistently fails to support those perspectives.

Further, the problem must come to be viewed in a developmental context and the research designed accordingly to look over time (or longitudinally) at why and how these patterns emerge. This theory-building and associated research agenda is particularly important in developing a sound foundation for predicting who is most likely to be at risk and the design of prevention or treatment interventions that work because they fundamentally address the root causes of the problem (Browne, Davies, & Stratton, 1988; Cicchetti & Carlson, 1989; Finkelhor, Hotaling, & Yllö, 1988; Frieze, 1987; Gelles & Cornell, 1990; Helfer & Kempe, 1987; Hotaling, Finkelhor, Kirkpatrick, & Straus, 1988a, 1988b; Maiuro & Eberle, 1989; Pagelow, 1984; Schene & Bond, 1989; Straus, 1988).

Evaluative Research. Most large-scale demonstration projects and evaluations in this area have focused on child abuse and neglect. A number of reviews have been published summarizing the results and methodological problems associated with evaluations of primary prevention programs for child abuse and neglect in general (Fink & McCloskey, 1990; Garbarino, 1986; Helfer, 1982). Other reviews cover specific primary prevention programs focusing on hospital-based interventions during the perinatal period (Helfer, 1987) or school-based interventions for older children (Wurtele, 1987). Still others survey the evaluations of the overall effectiveness (Cohn & Daro, 1987; Lamphear, 1986) and cost-effectiveness of treatment programs for individuals and families in which maltreatment has already occurred (Daro, 1988; Dubowitz, 1990).

These reviews point to a number of steps that should be taken to improve the design and conduct of such evaluations. Program objectives should be clarified and clearly operationalized, and the theoretical underpinnings and key elements of the intervention—as well as the extent to which it was actually implemented—should be specified. Individuals and/or families should be randomly assigned to experimental and control groups (or at least the need for relevant comparison groups should be attended to). It is important to replicate the intervention across a number of different populations and/or communities and to select a sufficiently large sample size and relevant statistical procedures for ensuring the statistical conclusion validity of study results. The extent to which program effects are sustained over the long term should be assessed. Finally, investigators should be sensitive to the unintended negative consequences or side effects of the intervention as well (such as fear arousal in children regarding abuse).

The results of these child abuse and neglect evaluations suggest that prevention efforts to stop maltreatment before it begins are much more likely to be both effective and economical than the treatment of individuals or families for whom it has already emerged as a problem. Further, "total reform prevention" directed at underlying social and political inequities (structural unemployment, gender discrimination, and so on) may ultimately be more successful than "patchwork prevention" that attempts to categorically address discrete pieces of the problem (sex abuse education, violence prevention) (Garbarino, 1986). Thus far, no substantial social or political interventions have sought to adopt the total reform prevention approach to maltreatment (however maltreatment is defined), and patchwork prevention in this area remains just that.

Homeless

There is a paucity of data on the number and needs of the homeless throughout the nation, and insufficient attention to examining the deeper social and economic roots of homelessness.

Descriptive Research. Homelessness is a difficult and dynamic concept to define and measure. It is perhaps most appropriately considered as a point along a continuum defined by both time and space — ranging from a complete absence of shelter to the lack of a stable home environment (U.S. Commission on Security and Cooperation in Europe, 1990).

People may be temporarily, episodically, or chronically homeless. That is, they may be displaced from their homes temporarily because of an economic or natural calamity (such as a loss of a job or fire), they may go in and out of homelessness (due to intermittent bouts of family violence or unstable aftercare arrangements postinstitutionalization), or they may be without a stable residence for extended periods of time (because of the lack of ties to family or institutional care arrangements) (IOM, 1988c).

Homelessness may also be defined based primarily on the place where people usually live. The McKinney Act defined a homeless person as someone who (1) lacked a fixed, regular, and adequate nighttime residence, or (2) who had a primary nighttime residence that was a supervised shelter that provided temporary living accommodations, an institution that provided a temporary residence for individuals intended to be institutionalized, or a public or private place not designed for, or ordinarily used as, a regular sleeping accommodation for human beings.

Some individuals may not be literally without a roof over their heads but are still at considerable risk of being so. These include people who are doubled up with friends or family, those living in accommodations they are renting simply by the day or week, or those in jails or hospitals awaiting discharge but with no stable home to return to (National Alliance to End Homelessness, 1988).

The two major methods that have been employed in generating national estimates of the homeless include indirect estimation and one-time censuses. The former involves asking knowledgeable informants (such as shelter administrators or city officials) about the estimated number of homeless (IOM, 1988c). Examples include the U.S. Conference of Mayors Task Force on Hunger and Homelessness and the USDHUD National Survey of Shelters (U.S. Conference of Mayors, 1991; USDHUD, 1989c). The indirect estimation method is conducted at one point in time in a given area where the homeless are expected to gather, as did the 1990 U.S. Census Street and Shelter Night count and the Chicago Homeless Study (Rossi, 1989; Taeuber & Siegel, 1990).

The estimates yielded by these or other methods may differ as a function of when and where a particular study was done. Further, estimates of the prevalence of homelessness at one point in time may differ from the number of incidents (incidence) of people being homeless in the course of a year.

Estimates of categories of the homeless (such as the homeless mentally ill or substance abusers, among others) are equally or even more difficult to obtain (GAO, 1988a). The paucity of adequate state, local, and national data, and particularly the number and characteristics of subgroups of the homeless, complicates efforts to adequately plan programs and services to meet their needs.

Analytical Research. A place to start in designing the next generation of more explanatory studies of homelessness is to systematically synthesize what is known already. A 1986 NIMH conference attempted to synthesize the first generation of largely descriptive studies of the homeless mentally ill, to provide a foundation for subsequent analytical research in this area (Morrissey & Levine, 1987). A 1988 Institute of Medicine report provided an overview and synthesis of research on the health and health care of the homeless (IOM, 1988c). Some members of the Institute of Medicine panel that produced that report, however, filed a supplementary statement, asserting that the report did not go far enough in examining the deep political, social, and economic "root causes" of the problem (Holden, 1988).

There is a paucity of longitudinal research on the homeless that traces their movement in and out of homelessness and the physical, psychological, and social correlates and consequences of homelessness—particularly for the burgeoning number of children numbered among the homeless—however defined.

Evaluative Research. Wyatt (1986) cautioned that lessons for developing policies and programs to address homelessness should be drawn from the failures of deinstitutionalization, in which a large-scale social experiment was rapidly put into place in the absence of supporting scientific evidence of its likely consequences.

A number of the major programs to serve the homeless described earlier (such as the RWJF-HCH, VA-HCMI, and McKinney Act programs, among others) have had accompanying evaluations of their implementation, if not their impact. More interagency cooperation and coordination is needed in reviewing the results of evaluations conducted to date in this area, and in developing demonstrations and evaluations of alternatives for caring for particularly vulnerable subgroups of the homeless, such as the chronically and mentally ill and disabled, substance abusers, persons with AIDS, and children (USDHUD, 1988a, 1989a).

Both short-term alternatives for addressing the consequences of homelessness and long-term options for ameliorating its causes must be elements of research, demonstrations, *and* policy in this area.

Immigrants and Refugees

Research on immigrant and refugee populations presents special challenges regarding how to find hard-to-locate populations (particularly illegal aliens), designing culturally sensitive research protocols, and discerning the unintended and intended consequences of health and social policies.

Descriptive Research. No precise counts exist of the number of illegal aliens residing in the United States. Research to derive such estimates has been conducted by the Census Bureau, the Immigration and Naturalization Service, and the Program for Research on Immigration Policy (a joint effort of the RAND Corporation and the Urban Institute), among others. This research has been based on special surveys done expressly for that purpose or on projections derived from data on the number of illegals apprehended (Bean, Edmonston, & Passel, 1990; Bean, Vernez, & Keely, 1989).

Illegal aliens have been conceptualized as belonging to three major groups based on their intended duration of residence in the U.S.: settlers, sojourners, or commuters. Settlers are those who intend to reside in the United States permanently; sojourners plan to return to their country of origin; and commuters include those who live in Mexico or Canada, for example, and regularly cross the border to work in the United States. No precise estimates of the number in each group, much less their varying needs, demands, and contributions to U.S. society, exist (Bean, Edmonston, & Passel, 1990; Bean, Vernez, & Keely, 1989).

Individual case studies or local patient or community surveys have been conducted to document the needs of discrete categories of legal and illegal immigrants or refugees. The INS, Current Population Survey, and Census provide general demographic and/or socioeconomic status information on the foreign born. Annual surveys of refugees conducted by the Office of Refugee Resettlement have focused primarily on issues of their economic adjustment: employment and labor force participation and use of public assistance or services. No comprehensive data on the health and mental health needs of major categories of recent immigrants and refugees are available at the state or national level. The basis for the time-limited coverage of benefits and services for refugees is primarily bureaucratic and political, rather than empirical (Ahearn & Athey, 1991; Chavez, Cornelius, & Jones, 1985; Haines, 1989; Rumbaut, Chavez, Moser, Pickwell, & Wishik, 1988).

Analytical Research. More formalized epidemiological surveillance methods in refugee camps, as well as in immigrant and refugee communities in the United States, are needed to identify the reasons for and rates of illness outbreaks in these populations (Elias, Alexander, & Sokly, 1990; Rumbaut, Chavez, Moser, Pickwell, & Wishik, 1988).

As indicated in previous chapters, a variety of factors may influence whether immigrants and refugees go for medical care. More research is needed to understand the relative importance of the availability, affordability, and acceptability of services, among other factors, that affect different immigrant and refugee subgroups' access. This research needs to be designed in a culturally sensitive fashion — with keen attention to the beliefs and practices that are likely to influence their behavior, and to how best to design studies to accurately capture these influences.

Evaluative Research. Epidemiological as well as access data would be useful in evaluating the impact of public health or medical care interventions to address the needs of the foreign born.

Unintended, as well as intended, consequences have resulted from U.S. immigration policies and programs. For example, the Program for Research on Immigration Policy has suggested that the Immigration and Reform Control Act of 1986 will both reduce the immigration of the undocumented foreign born (intended) and will increase employer discrimination against the foreign born in general (unintended) (Bean, Edmonston, & Passel, 1990; Bean, Vernez, & Keely, 1989).

U.S. refugee resettlement policies have also had negative impacts on refugees' mental health, as a result of the scattering or separation of families. A kind of experiment occurs for refugees at the end of the eighteen- or thirty-six-month period for which Medicaid coverage is guaranteed. However, no research has been conducted that directly examines the health and mental health impact of what for some might be a precipitous loss of benefits (Rumbaut, Chavez, Moser, Pickwell, & Wishik, 1988; Westermeyer, 1987).

The final chapter reviews the principles and parameters of a community-oriented health policy to address the health and health care needs of vulnerable populations, based on the information and analyses presented in this and previous chapters.

11

What Programs and Policies
Are Needed?

A major recommendation emerges from the preceding analyses of the health and health care needs of vulnerable populations. To most clearly illuminate the origins and remedies of vulnerability, the "second" language of community (reciprocity, interdependence, and the common good), in addition to the "first" language of individualism (autonomy, independence, and individual rights), must come to be more widely understood and used in social and political discourse surrounding these issues.

Critics of the American political process have argued that developing the primordial (primary, personal), as well as purposive (secondary, task-oriented), ties between individuals in families and small social or community groups can be a powerful social and organizational alternative for enhancing individual *and* collective well-being. Dahl and Lindblom (1963, p. 520), for example, assert:

> In so far as it is attainable at all, for most people much of "the good life" is found in small groups. Family life, the rearing of children, love, friendship, respect, kindness, pity, neighborliness, charity: these are hardly possible except in small groups. . . . The nation-state can only provide the framework within which "the good life" is possible; it cannot fulfill the functions of the small groups that must make up the immediate environment of good living. To the extent that it attempts to do so, the nation-state must provide either an impoverished substitute for, or a grotesque perversion of, small-group functions. For it is on small groups that most people must rely for love, affection, friendship, "the sense of belonging," and respect.

Most large-scale contemporary institutions concerned with enhancing individual or community well-being (such as medical care, social services, and education, among others) are characterized by increasingly bureaucratized and centralized models of social organization, with hierarchical forms of management by specialized experts (or technocrats). This form of organization tends to mediate the interpersonal social ties between the individuals working within them, the intersectoral linkages and cooperation between the diverse institutions, and the interdisciplinary collaboration and communication among the dominant professional groups within each (Coleman, 1990).

Planners have elaborated the transformative organizational possibilities for enhancing individual and collective well-being that can emerge when local action groups — ordinary people directly involved in struggles close to their ordinary lives — come together to formulate shared goals and objectives and build networks and coalitions of empowerment to accomplish these goals. In such an arena, the knowledge and insight for defining and addressing problems emerge from the "participatory expertise" and "social learning" emanating from direct and nonhierarchical interaction with others, who may hold either similar or competing views. With such an approach, scientific or technocratic judgment may well provide input to, but does not dominate, the problem definition and decision-making process (Fischer, 1990; Friedmann, 1987; Lindblom, 1990; Lindblom & Cohen, 1979).

Social and Economic Policy: Investing in Individuals and the Ties Between Them

Community-oriented health policy focuses on the importance of local community involvement in the development and oversight of programs and resources to ameliorate the risks and/or consequences of vulnerability to poor physical, psychological, or social health. It acknowledges the central role that community-oriented social and economic, as well as medical care and public health, policies play in attenuating the risks and consequences of vulnerability through investing in individuals and the supportive ties between them (Figure 1.1).

Social Status

Employment opportunities and associated wage rates — particularly in the top-earning positions — continue to be more limited for women and minorities than for white males. Unlike adults, children are not in a position to organize and advocate for themselves. The overt or covert use of violence is sanctioned in many families to reinforce the power-dominance relationships between males and females or parents and children.

Social and economic policy to ameliorate vulnerability would focus on mitigating the socially and legally sanctioned power and status differentials, based on age, sex, and/or racial or ethnic group membership. In the absence of a responsive social and legal infrastructure for addressing these claims, community-oriented social action is likely to be manifested in grass-roots social movements (the civil rights and women's movements, for example), and related nonviolent (marches on Washington) and violent (the Los Angeles riots) public protests to bring attention to these claims (Piven & Cloward, 1971).

Social Capital

The increase in the number of families in which infants and children are being raised by a single parent, young and elderly adults living alone, and new (or at least increasingly visible) forms of emotional and sexual intimacy manifest in relationships between "mingles" or "long-time companions" calls for a renewed look at how social and economic policy might serve to enhance, rather than diminish, the prospect for social capital formation within such arrangements.

Family-centered policies represent a step toward this objective, where families could be defined to encompass the array of primary social units or households concerned with the mutual care and support of members. The strengthening of these units and the caring and nurturing functions they serve would be the focus of family-centered public policy. Recent state and federal legislation to promulgate parental leave, child care, family preservation–oriented child welfare legislation, family-centered care for children with special needs, and caregiver respite alternatives are examples of more family-oriented social and economic and associated health care policies.

Related community-based efforts include attempts to build cooperative bridges between the variety of human and social services agencies and programs (such as schools, child welfare agencies, adult protective services, correctional systems, mental health, drug or alcohol treatment, or related domains) to address the needs of multiproblem families. Such initiatives recognize the importance of a holistic and multifaceted approach to the multidimensional functions of the family unit.

Those local initiatives that offer the greatest promise of success are ones in which neighborhood residents are directly involved in the needs identification and program development process. Having this grass-roots investment is most likely to lead to programs that match community needs as well as catalyze the greatest measure of local ownership and participation. Perhaps equally or more important, the act of involvement itself may serve to generate or strengthen informal networks of support (for child care, transportation, or respite, for example) between neighborhood residents to lighten their individual and collective burdens.

Human Capital

The availability of social capital directly affects the level of investments in human capital. Family or other social support is important in encouraging children to stay in school or assisting with child care, to facilitate individual family members' participation in the workforce. Household and per capita incomes are directly affected by the number, as well as earning power, of the individuals contributing to those revenues. Families and intimate social networks help to ensure that members have a home or a place to live.

Community-oriented social and economic policy acknowledges the importance of investing in those community institutions and resources that are both indirectly and directly supportive of the generation of human capital. Recent decades have, however, seen a diminished, rather than enhanced, federal policy commitment in many of these domains, such as schools, jobs, housing, and associated family and individual economic safety nets.

Certain school-oriented investments may greatly increase both social and human capital generation. Early childhood education programs, particularly those such as Head Start that encourage parental involvement and skills development have demonstrated significant short-term and long-term successes. This has been the case both educationally and socially (for instance, in terms of better school performance, reduced dropout rates, and fewer teen pregnancies). School-based clinics and associated parent- and family-oriented multiservice programs (where mothers can get parenting or family planning advice or earn their GED, for example) offer opportunities to support young and/or single-parent families in developing parenting, educational, and job-related skills. The reform of federal, state, and local financing of public education could help to minimize the widely varying levels of investments in children in different communities. Per capita expenditures tend to be the least in those economically and socially segregated neighborhoods in which the children (low-income minorities) can least afford the diminished opportunities resulting from poor educational preparation.

Well-paying jobs sufficient to support themselves and their families are an increasingly elusive possibility for many Americans. Young, single-parent families and minority males have been most adversely affected by these trends. However, the experience of college-educated married couples, both of whom must work to fulfill the American dream their parents accomplished on a single breadwinner's salary, as well as the high-school graduate working full-time whose earnings still fail to lift his family out of poverty, also provides pervasive evidence of the impact of the nation's changing economy on U.S. families. A national public and private commitment to full employment and targeted interventions in particularly economically depressed neighborhoods are approaches to mitigating these impacts. States and municipalities could be encouraged to forge and strengthen partnerships for economic development among neighborhood organizations, local businesses, and governmental agencies. With support from federal and state sources, depressed communities and neighborhoods could organize local community improvement and development councils to attract and retain new businesses.

Social and economic trends and policies have served to increase rather than diminish disparities in the distribution of income and wealth in U.S.

society. As has been discussed, economic development efforts and initiatives
to create new jobs would assist in remedying these disparities. The reduction of blocked opportunities to equal pay and positions in higher-paying
sectors on the part of women and minorities could also be undertaken, as
could human capital investments in education and jobs training for particularly at-risk groups. The minimum wage, unemployment, and transfer program benefits must be more directly tied to inflation if they are to provide
a stronger economic safety for individuals and families. Expanding the Earned
Income Credit for families based on family size, as well as improving the
enforcement of child support payments, would also contribute directly to
enhancing the economic well-being of families with dependent children.

Renewed federal, state, and local governmental support, as well as encouragement of private sector involvement in developing low-income housing alternatives, would help to ameliorate the burgeoning crisis of homelessness. Local community involvement is essential in planning such initiatives,
so that the integrity of existing neighborhoods, as well as the cooperation of
adjoining ones, is assured. Tearing down buildings in deteriorating areas
by eminent domain and constructing either expensive high-rise middle-class
or public welfare brick-and-mortar ghettos in their place will not necessarily
solve the problem of affordable and habitable domiciles for low-income community residents. Supportive housing alternatives for many of the vulnerable populations examined here, such as the chronically ill elderly, the mentally ill, persons with AIDS, and the homeless, are urgently needed in many
U.S. communities. Both local advocates and opponents must be encouraged
to engage in dialogue about these options around the norm of community
responsibility, to balance the voices of "nimby"-ism (not-in-my-backyard) that
are likely to characterize the response of residents in many U.S. neighborhoods.

Medical Care and Public Health Policy: Paying for the Future—A Shared Responsibility

The current array of programs and services to address the health and health
care needs of vulnerable populations (such as high-risk mothers and infants,
persons with AIDS, substance abusers, and victims of family abuse, among
others) is underdeveloped and poorly integrated and poses substantial organizational and financial barriers to access in many U.S. communities. Further, current methods of private and public third-party reimbursement tend
to exacerbate rather than ameliorate these difficulties.

Sharply divided tiers of service exist for the vulnerable and can be seen
in publicly versus privately supported service sectors. This is particularly the
case in the mental health and substance abuse fields, but it is also increasingly
the experience of persons with AIDS and others. Distinctly different doors
are opened (or closed), based on how they intend (or more important, whether
they can afford) to pay for care.

Many face an imposing jungle of conflicting requirements and application procedures to establish eligibility for needed programs and services. Categoric funding streams and related financial incentives have tended to encourage the formation of competitive agencies or programs operating in discrete noncollaborating sectors, rather than an integrated system of care for individuals in need of services from a variety of agencies or institutions.

A more community-oriented set of norms would attempt to encourage interagency cooperation around population- or client-centered goals. A number of programs focusing on different groups of the vulnerable (such as the RWJF and HRSA Health Care for the Homeless projects, NIMH Community Support Program and Child and Adolescent Service System Program, and RWJF AIDS Health Services Program, among others) have encouraged the formation of community consortia of agencies and providers to facilitate the development of more integrated systems of caring for the most vulnerable. These initiatives may be viewed as bureaucratic surrogates, or in some cases, as catalysts for the development of local grass-roots efforts to assist and support vulnerable community members. These consortia and related programs and experiences should be evaluated with respect to their success in developing these formal and informal community arrangements. More important, they should be evaluated in terms of whether outcomes were improved for the populations they were intended to serve.

The contemporary policy debate regarding reform of the U.S. medical care system focuses on alternatives for covering and paying for services. A plethora of proposals has emerged in recent years. They all attempt to enhance near-universal coverage but differ primarily in the means for doing so. They may be broadly grouped into three main types based on the nature of the changes proposed: (1) reform-oriented *private market–based proposals* to create options and incentives for consumers to be more prudent purchasers of care in the medical care marketplace or to develop managed care arrangements to encourage the more cost-effective practice of medicine; (2) *employer-based* ("play-or-pay") *proposals* that build on the present system whereby employers either provide insurance to employees or pay taxes to finance an alternative public system; and (3) reform-oriented *government-sponsored single-payer plans* modeled after the Canadian system.

These initiatives are primarily lodged in the individual perspective on vulnerability to poor physical, psychological, and/or social health. Specific proposals should, however, be evaluated with respect to the incentives or disincentives they provide for (1) reducing or eliminating existing financial barriers to access, as well as for (2) developing a more universal community-oriented continuum of programs and services to address the health and health care needs of vulnerable populations. Selected criteria proposed here relate to features of the (1) plan itself, as well as the distribution of benefits and burdens between (2) patients and (3) providers.

Plan

Criteria for evaluating features of the plans include (1) the universality of coverage, (2) the provision of a decent basic minimum set of covered services, (3) minimization of disparities between public and private tiers of payers, and (4) the use of community rating as a basis for determining premiums.

Those plans that cover everyone in a similar fashion and use a broad, rather than a narrow, actuarial base in computing risks are most likely to ensure equity of access. The former minimizes the disparities in the type or extent of coverage provided, and the latter ensures that the burdens and benefits are spread more widely and evenly.

Need and effectiveness norms focus on whether certain procedures or services have been demonstrated, in the aggregate, to improve patient functioning or well-being. Such a perspective would underlie the entire range of prevention-oriented, treatment-oriented, and long-term care services for vulnerable populations. Existing and proposed models for providing and paying for care for the vulnerable should be evaluated in the context of their adequacy in providing a decent basic minimum set of services across this caregiving continuum.

Community rating refers to the fact that computation of actuarial risks and the attendant impact on premiums rests on broad, rather than narrow, population groupings. Experience rating, in contrast, bases the rate setting on a narrowly defined group of eligibles. This latter strategy provides incentives to limit eligibility and enrollment to those who are likely to require the least or least expensive care, to keep the price of premiums down. The result is that those most in need (those with serious health problems or at risk of developing them, such as persons who are HIV positive) are likely to be excluded or charged very high rates for coverage.

Patients

The features to consider in minimizing financial barriers to access from the point of view of the patients include (1) the use of progressive (rather than regressive) methods for determining their contributions, and (2) limiting the amount patients have to pay out of pocket. These are quite intimately linked, rather than discrete, criteria.

Health insurance premiums are relatively regressive methods of paying for medical care, in that they do not take into account the varying incomes or resources available to enrollees. Progressive taxation or related means of financing tied to ability to pay provide a more equitable basis for distributing the cost of coverage. The burden of out-of-pocket costs for medical care has traditionally fallen most heavily on low-income individuals, for whom even a relatively small dollar outlay comprises a substantial proportion of their financial resources. Evidence from the RAND Health Insurance Experiment suggests that increased cost sharing does reduce consumers' utilization of services (Brook et al., 1983). The findings also suggest that increased cost sharing may serve to ration more effective (prevention-related) rather than less effective (hospitalized) care and also differentially affects the access of those who either need care most or can least afford it as a result.

Providers

Plan features that reduce the disincentives for providers to treat certain types of patients include (1) using the same reimbursement rate regardless of who pays for the care (private versus public insurer, for example), and (2) limiting or capping reimbursement across all providers.

One of the major dilemmas that has emerged with the current multitiered system of financing care is the widely varying rates of reimbursement to providers by different payers. As has been documented in previous chapters, the rates of Medicaid reimbursement in some states are much lower than those of private insurers, which has resulted in a dramatic reduction in the number of providers who are willing to see Medicaid-eligible clients.

The maintenance of the usual and customary fee arrangements under Medicare and Medicaid have contributed significantly to the spiraling costs of medical care in the decades that followed. Diagnosis-related groups (DRGs) and physician relative value–based reimbursement under Medicare are the major policy instruments that have been developed to deal with this issue in the public sector. Medical care systems in other countries, such as Canada, use more macro- rather than micro-oriented approaches to limiting reimbursement, through negotiating global budgets and fee schedules with providers.

The assumption underlying these or other methods of capping provider reimbursement, however, is that providers, not patients, are the main generators of demand for costly medical care services (hospitalizations, high-technology procedures, tests, pharmaceuticals, and so on). Cost-containment incentives need to be developed for these important medical care "consumers" as well. However, if these incentives are to be implemented fairly, they must be applied across all the payers (or players) that reimburse providers for care. Otherwise, the incentives remain, as they do now, for providers to serve those who can pay their full asking price and to refuse to provide care for the rest — many of whom are the sickest and most vulnerable.

Community-Oriented Health Policy: Building a Community-Oriented Continuum of Care

Community-oriented health policy acknowledges that individuals' health and well-being are affected by the communities and families into which they are born and spend their lives, and it is to these social arrangements that people return after being discharged from the medical care system. It attempts to bridge both the individual and community perspectives on vulnerability, and to design programs and services to ameliorate the risks and consequences of poor physical, psychological, and/or social health.

A community-oriented health policy would encourage intersectoral linkages between the medical care and other human and social service resource development programs and services within a community, as well as interdisciplinary collaboration between and among professionals in these institutions. It would also encourage local leadership in developing and implementing programs to address the complex medical, psychological, social, and economic needs of the community.

Features of such a policy are, for example, manifest in the "town meetings" being held in different states and localities to debate universal health insurance options. They are also reflected in the formation of community-based organizations (CBOs) and consortia to develop programs and services for vulnerable populations, such as the homeless, persons with AIDS, and/or the chronically mentally ill. Other relevant measures include the promulgation of models of community organization and action for implementing the Year 2000 Public Health Objectives for the Nation, and the development of community or neighborhood health centers and community-oriented primary care models of service delivery. Client- or family-centered case management may also be a useful program component or complement to facilitate individuals' seeking and using relevant programs and services encompassed within a community-oriented continuum of care. Tables 5.1 through 5.9 in Chapter 5 summarized the major types of programs and services that could be incorporated in such a continuum—including primary prevention-oriented, treatment-oriented, and long-term care services. Such a continuum provides a means for mitigating the risks that give rise to, as well as those that result from, being in poor health.

Primary prevention efforts include both community and public health programs and services. The risk of illness is greatest for those who have the fewest material and nonmaterial resources. Poverty and its associated deprivations and risks is a major correlate of poor birth outcomes in minority populations. The dramatic diminishment of low-income housing stock in many U.S. cities due to the combined policies of gentrification and the withdrawal of federal financial support is a major contributor to homelessness. Lack of adequate family or social support compromises the ability of the chronically ill elderly to continue to live on their own. Addressing these fundamental correlates and consequences of vulnerability lies outside the traditional domain of medical care practice and policy. Their contribution to understanding the root causes of vulnerability, however, points to the broader policy and social context in which vulnerability must be addressed.

The public health system has been the traditional focus of community interventions—particularly primary prevention–oriented programs (in the areas of lead paint abatement, AIDS education, and smoking cessation, among others)—to address the health and health care needs of vulnerable populations. The Public Health Service's 1990 and Year 2000 Health Objectives for the Nation define a comprehensive public health agenda that deals with a number of the vulnerable populations that have been the explicit focus of this book. These populations include high-risk mothers and infants, the chronically ill and disabled, alcohol or substance abusers, and suicide and homicide victims, as well as those subgroups most likely to be at risk (children, adolescents, the elderly, and minorities).

Primary prevention efforts at the beginning of the care continuum are small relative to the resources devoted to the treatment of the physical, mental, and social consequences of poor pregnancy outcomes, chronic physical or mental illness, AIDS, alcohol and substance abuse, violence, and the conditions prevalent in particularly at-risk homeless and refugee populations. Similarly, at the other end of the continuum, long-term institutional and home and community-based care for vulnerable populations is an important, but undeveloped and underfinanced, component of needed programs and services.

The arguments and evidence presented throughout the book pose the question of what allocation of medical and nonmedical investments may be most beneficial for enhancing Americans' health and well-being.

The answer provided here from the point of view of community-oriented health policy is that human and social capital and the families and communities in which these resources are both generated and consumed should be the primary focus of public and private investments in Americans' individual and collective well-being. It compels inviting, asking, listening to, and empowering U.S. families and communities to be full participants in shaping their collective welfare. This perspective considers the universal investments needed to facilitate this developmental process, as well as the specific entitlements required to open more windows of opportunity for the most vulnerable. A community-oriented point of view reconsiders the extent to which hierarchical, bureaucratic, professionally dominated forms of organization are the best or most effective methods for addressing multifaceted human and social needs. It calls for an evaluation of needed preventive medical care and public health investments and scrutinizes the incentives and disincentives built into existing and proposed systems of organizing and financing medical care in the United States for reducing the risk of poor physical, psychological, and social health.

Ultimately, this perspective argues that the remedies for our individual and collective vulnerability are found in the bonds of caring human communities.

RESOURCES

Resource A: National Data Sources on Vulnerable Populations.

Agency and data source	Universe/sample	Vulnerable populations								
		MCH	CHR	PWA	MEN	SAB	S&H	FAB	HOM	REF
Agency for Health Care Policy and Research										
AIDS Cost and Service Utilization Survey (ACSUS)	Sample of AIDS providers and patients in different geographical locations (1991)			X						
National Medical Care Expenditure Survey (NMCES)	Sample of U.S. civilian noninstitutionalized population, plus physicians, facilities, and employers providing them care or coverage (1977–1979)		X		X					
National Medical Expenditure Survey (NMES)	Sample of U.S. civilian noninstitutionalized population, American Indians and Alaskan Natives, plus physicians, facilities, and insurers providing them care or coverage (1987)		X		X					
American Humane Association and National Center on Child Abuse and Neglect										
National Study on Child Neglect and Abuse Reporting	Child maltreatment reports from state Child Protective Service personnel (1976–1987)							X		
Centers for Disease Control										
AIDS Surveillance System	All AIDS cases and deaths reported in 50 states, D.C., U.S. dependencies and possessions (1981–present)			X		X				
Behavioral Risk-Factor Surveillance System (BRFSS)	Sample of populations in selected states and D.C. with phones (1981–present)					X				
HIV Seroprevalence Surveys	HIV seroprevalence tests in sentinel sites (such as STD clinics, drug treatment centers, women's health centers, and others) throughout the U.S. (1989–present)			X						

Note: MCH = high-risk mothers and infants; CHR = chronically ill and disabled; PWA = persons with AIDS; MEN = mentally ill and disabled; SAB = alcohol or substance abusers; S&H = suicide- or homicide-prone; FAB = abusing families; HOM = homeless; REF = immigrants and refugees.

Resource A: National Data Sources on Vulnerable Populations, Cont'd.

Agency and data source	Universe/sample	MCH	CHR	PWA	MEN	SAB	S&H	FAB	HOM	REF
Health Care Financing Administration										
National Long-Term Care Survey (NLTCS)	Sample of disabled Medicare population (baseline–1982; follow-up–1984, 1988)		X		X					
Health Care Financing Administration and Centers for Disease Control										
Infant Mortality Data Survey	Sample of Medicaid mothers and infants in 47 states and D.C. (1989)	X				X				
International Center for the Disabled (ICD)	Sample of U.S. civilian noninstitutionalized disabled population 16+ (1986)		X							
National Aging Resource Center on Elder Abuse										
Survey of the States on the Incidence of Elder Abuse	Survey of Adult Protective Service and State Units on Aging in 50 states, D.C., Guam, Puerto Rico, and Virgin Islands (1988)							X		
National Center on Child Abuse and Neglect										
Study of National Incidence and Prevalence of Child Abuse and Neglect	Child maltreatment reports from community professionals in state Child Protective Service and other agencies in sample of 29 U.S. counties (1980, 1986)							X		
National Center for Health Statistics/ Centers for Disease Control										
Hispanic Health and Nutrition Examination Survey (HHANES)	Sample of Hispanics 6 months–74 years in 5 states and 2 localities with large Hispanic populations (1982–1984)		X		X	X				
Linked Birth and Infant Death Record Project (NCHS)	Linked birth and death records (1983–1987)	X	X							

Survey	Description				
National Ambulatory Medical Care Survey (NAMCS)	Sample of nonfederal office-based physicians and visits in 48 contiguous states (1973–1981 annually; 1985 to present triennially)		X	X	X
National Health (and Nutrition) Examination Survey (HANES)	Survey of selected age groups of U.S. civilian noninstitutionalized population (1959–1962, 1963–1965, 1966–1970, 1971–1975, 1976–1980) and follow-up (1982–1984)		X	X	X
National Health Interview Survey	Sample of U.S. civilian noninstitutionalized population (annual)		X	X	
Alcohol–Health Practices Supplement	(1983)				X
Child Health Supplement	(1981,1988)		X	X	
Health Habits (Health Promotion and Disease Prevention) Supplement	(1976, 1977, 1985, 1990)				X
Home Care Supplement	(1979–1980)		X	X	
Smoking Supplement	(1970, 1978–1980)				X
Supplement on Aging	(Baseline–1984; follow-up–1986, 1988)		X	X	
National Center for Health Statistics/Centers for Disease Control					
National Hospital Discharge Survey	Sample of discharges from U.S. hospitals (1965–present)		X	X	X
National Infant Mortality Surveillance Project (CDC)	Linked birth and death records (1980)	X		X	

Note: MCH = high-risk mothers and infants; CHR = chronically ill and disabled; PWA = persons with AIDS; MEN = mentally ill and disabled; SAB = alcohol or substance abusers; S&H = suicide- or homicide-prone; FAB = abusing families; HOM = homeless; REF = immigrants and refugees.

Resource A: National Data Sources on Vulnerable Populations, Cont'd.

Agency and data source	Universe/sample	Vulnerable populations								
		MCH	CHR	PWA	MEN	SAB	S&H	FAB	HOM	REF
National Maternal and Infant Health Survey and Longitudinal Follow-up Survey	Sample of death, birth, and fetal death records (1988) and follow-up (1990)	X	X			X				
National Natality Survey (NNS) and National Fetal Mortality Survey (NFMS)	Sample of 1963–1969, 1972, and 1980 birth cohorts plus late fetal deaths (1980)	X	X			X				
National Nursing Home Survey	Sample of nursing homes, residents, and employees (1973–1974, 1977, 1985)		X		X	X				
National Survey of Family Growth	Sample of women 14–45 years of age—U.S. civilian noninstitutionalized population (1973, 1976, 1982, 1988)	X				X				
National Survey of Personal Health Practices and Consequences (NSPHPC)	Sample of U.S. adults 20–64 years of age—in households with phones (1979, 1980)				X	X				
National Vital Statistics System										
Mortality Statistics	State death certificates	X	X	X	X	X	X			
Natality Statistics	State birth certificates	X								
National Center for Health Statistics/Centers for Disease Control and Health Care Financing Administration										
National Medical Care Utilization and Expenditure Survey (NMCUES)	Sample of U.S. civilian noninstitutionalized population and Medicaid enrollees in California, Michigan, New York, and Texas (1980–1981)		X		X					
National Institute on Alcohol Abuse and Alcoholism, Division of Biometry and Epidemiology										
Alcohol Epidemiologic Data System (AEDS)	Surveillance data on alcohol consumption, alcohol-related conditions and deaths (1970–present)					X				

National Institute on Drug Abuse

Community Epidemiology Work Group (CEWG)	Surveillance of patterns and trends in drug abuse in 19 major U.S. cities (1976–present)	X
Monitoring the Future: A Continuing Study of the Lifestyles and Values of Youth	National sample of high school seniors and follow-up of subsamples as young adults (1975–present)	X
National Household Survey on Drug Abuse	Sample of U.S. civilian noninstitutionalized population, 12+ (1972–present)	X

National Institute on Drug Abuse and Drug Enforcement Agency (DEA)

Drug Abuse Warning Network (DAWN)	Panel of hospital ERs in 21 Primary Metropolitan Statistical Areas (PMSAs), medical examiners/coroners in 27 PMSAs, plus selected hospitals outside PMSAs (1972–present)	X

National Institute on Drug Abuse and National Institute on Alcohol Abuse and Alcoholism

National Drug and Alcoholism Treatment Unit Survey (NDATUS)	Sample of alcohol and/or drug treatment and prevention programs in 50 states, D.C., and U.S. territories (1974, 1979, 1984, 1987, 1989)	X
State Alcohol and Drug Abuse Profile (SADAP)	Sample of alcohol and/or drug treatment programs in 50 states, D.C., and U.S. territories (1982–present)	X

Note: MCH = high-risk mothers and infants; CHR = chronically ill and disabled; PWA = persons with AIDS; MEN = mentally ill and disabled; SAB = alcohol or substance abusers; S&H = suicide- or homicide-prone; FAB = abusing families; HOM = homeless; REF = immigrants and refugees.

Resource A: National Data Sources on Vulnerable Populations, Cont'd.

Agency and data source	Universe/sample	MCH	CHR	PWA	MEN	SAB	S&H	FAB	HOM	REF
National Institute on Drug Abuse and National Institute of Justice										
Treatment Outcome Prospective Study (TOPS)	Sample of individuals entering public drug abuse treatment programs and follow-up 5 years later in 10 cities (1979, 1980, 1981)					X	X			
National Institute of Mental Health										
Client/Patient Sample Survey of Inpatient, Outpatient, and Partial Care Programs	Sample of clients admitted, readmitted, discharged, and transferred into and out of organized mental health settings (1986), plus those under active care as of April 1, 1986				X	X				
Epidemiological Catchment Area (ECA) Program Surveys	Sample of population in mental health service catchment areas in New Haven, Conn. (1980–1981), Baltimore (1981–1982), St. Louis (1981–1982), Durham, N.C. (1982–1983), Los Angeles (1983–1984)				X	X	X	X		
Inventory of Mental Health Organizations and General Hospital Mental Health Services (IMHO/IGHMHS)	Complete enumeration surveys of all specialty mental health organizations (Biennially, 1986–present)				X	X				
Inventory of Community Mental Health Centers (ICMHC)	(Biennially, 1968–1981)									
IMHO	(Biennially, 1968–1986)									
IGHMHS	(Biennially, 1968–1986)									
National Surveys of Family Violence	Sample of members of U.S. families (1976, 1986)							X		
National Institute of Mental Health and National Institute on Drug Abuse										
National Youth Survey	National sample of juveniles 11-17 and their parents (1976) plus follow-up (1986)				X	X	X			

Organization / Survey	Description	MCH	CHR	PWA	MEN	SAB	S&H	FAB	HOM	REF
National Public Health and Hospital Institute										
U.S. Hospital AIDS Survey	Sample of U.S. hospitals (1986–present)			X						
Office of Refugee Resettlement										
Annual Survey of Refugees	Sample of U.S. refugees (1975–present)									X
Partnership for the Homeless										
City Surveys on the Homeless	Surveys of agencies addressing homelessness in largest U.S. cities and localities (1985–present)			X	X				X	
Public Health Service, Office of Disease Prevention and Health Promotion, Centers for Disease Control, and National Institute on Drug Abuse										
National Adolescent Student Health Survey (NASHS)	National sample of eighth- and tenth-grade students from public and private schools (1987)					X	X			
RAND Corporation										
Medical Outcomes Study (MOS)	Sample of physicians in 4 regions plus patients seen in 5-day screening period and those with tracer conditions (1986–1989)		X	X						
U.S. Bureau of the Census										
Census Count of the Homeless	Counts and characteristics of people at pre-identified selected locations, where "homeless persons" usually gather, on "Shelter and Street Night" (March 20/21, 1990)								X	

Note: MCH = high-risk mothers and infants; CHR = chronically ill and disabled; PWA = persons with AIDS; MEN = mentally ill and disabled; SAB = alcohol or substance abusers; S&H = suicide- or homicide-prone; FAB = abusing families; HOM = homeless; REF = immigrants and refugees.

Resource A: National Data Sources on Vulnerable Populations, Cont'd.

Agency and data source	Universe/sample	MCH	CHR	PWA	MEN	SAB	S&H	FAB	HOM	REF
					Vulnerable populations					
Current Population Survey (CPS)	Longitudinal monthly survey of sample of U.S. civilian noninstitutionalized population	X								
Survey of Income Program Participation (SIPP)	Longitudinal panel survey of U.S. civilian noninstitutionalized population (1984–present)		X		X					
U.S. Conference of Mayors										
City Surveys of Hunger and Homelessness	Surveys of city officials in cities on U.S. Conference of Mayors Task Force on Hunger and Homelessness (1985–present)			X	X	X			X	
U.S. Department of Defense										
Worldwide Survey of Substance Abuse and Health Behaviors among Military Personnel	Sample of active duty military personnel in the Army, Navy, Marines, and Air Force (1980, 1982, 1985, 1988)			X		X				
U.S Department of Housing and Urban Development										
National Survey of Shelters for the Homeless	National sample of shelter managers and program administrators (1984, 1988)		X	X	X	X		X	X	
U.S. Department of Justice, Bureau of Justice Statistics										
National Crime Survey (NCS)	Sample of U.S. civilian noninstitutionalized population, 12+ (1973–present)					X	X	X		
Survey of Inmates of Local Jails	National sample of inmates in local jails (1972, 1978, 1983, 1989)					X	X			
Survey of Inmates of State Correctional Facilities	National sample of inmates in state prisons (1974, 1979, 1986, 1991)					X	X			
Survey of Youth in Custody	National sample of youth in long-term, state-operated juvenile institutions (1987)					X	X	X		

Source and survey	Description	MCH	CHR	PWA	MEN	SAB	HOM	S&H	FAB	REF
U.S. Department of Justice, Federal Bureau of Investigation — Uniform Crime Reports (UCR)/Supplementary Homicide Report	Arrest data from city, county, state law enforcement agencies (1930–present)				X		X	X		
U.S. Department of Justice Immigration and Naturalization Service — *Statistical Yearbook of the Immigration and Naturalization Service*	Compilation of immigration statistics from entry visas and change-of-immigration-status forms (annual)									X
U.S. Department of Justice National Institute of Justice, Bureau of Justice Assistance — Drug Use Forecasting (DUF)	Quota of male and female arrestees and juvenile detainees in 23 cities (1986–present)				X	X				
U.S. Department of Labor — National Longitudinal Survey of Youth	Longitudinal panel survey of national household sample of youth 14–22 in 1979									
Drug use (1984, 1988)					X					
Alcohol use (1982–1985, 1988)					X					
Urban Institute — National Survey of Urban Homeless Adults	Nationally representative sample of homeless adults who used soup kitchens and shelters in cities of 100,000+ (1987)	X		X	X				X	

Note: MCH = high-risk mothers and infants; CHR = chronically ill and disabled; PWA = persons with AIDS; MEN = mentally ill and disabled; SAB = alcohol or substance abusers; S&H = suicide- or homicide-prone; FAB = abusing families; HOM = homeless; REF = immigrants and refugees.

RESOURCE B:
SOURCE NOTES ON THE DATA TABLES

Table 2.1

1. *1970, 1975, 1980–1987:* NCHS, 1990f, Table 7 (pp. 97–98).
   1988: NCHS, 1990h, Table 1-81 (p. 241).
   1989: NCHS, 1991a, Table 13 (pp. 28–29).
2. *1970, 1975, 1980–1987:* NCHS, 1990f, Table 15 (p. 107).
   1988: NCHS, 1990a, Table E (p.9).
   1989: NCHS, 1992a, Table E (p.9).
3. *1970, 1975, 1980–1987:* NCHS, 1990f, Table 7 (pp. 97–98).
   1988: NCHS, 1990h, Table 1-44 (p. 74).
   1989: NCHS, 1991a, Table 29 (pp. 43–44).
4. *1970, 1975, 1980–1987:* NCHS, 1990f, Table 2 (p. 92).
   1988: NCHS, 1990h, Table 1-6 (p. 7).
   1989: NCHS, 1991a, Table 4 (pp. 20–21).
5. *1970, 1980, 1983–1987:* NCHS, 1990f, Table 31 (p. 136).
   1975, 1981, 1982: NCHS, 1986f, Table 1-15 (p. 65).
   1988: NCHS, 1990a, Table F (p. 11).
   1989: NCHS, 1992a, Table F (p. 11).

Table 2.2

1. *1970, 1980, 1983–1987:* NCHS, 1990f, Table 23 (pp. 121–122);
   NCHS, 1990g, Table 1-8 (p. 1-12).
   1975: NCHS, 1983, Table 15 (pp. 105–106).
   1981, 1982: NCHS, 1986d, Table 21 (pp. 98–99).
   1988: NCHS, 1991c, Table 24 (pp. 78–79).
   1989: NCHS, 1992a, Table 5 (pp. 17–19).
2. *1982:* NCHS, 1985a, Table 57 (pp. 81–82).
   1983: NCHS, 1986a, Table 57 (pp. 80–81).
   1984: NCHS, 1986b, Table 57 (pp. 81–82).
   1985: NCHS, 1986c, Table 57 (pp. 82–83).
   1986: NCHS, 1987, Table 57 (pp. 85–86).
   1987: NCHS, 1988a, Table 57 (pp. 84–85).
   1988: NCHS, 1989a, Table 57 (pp. 84–85).
   1989: NCHS, 1990e, Table 57 (pp. 83–84).
3. *1975, 1980.:* NCHS, 1982, Table 27 (p. 80).
   1981: NCHS, 1983, Table 27 (p. 126).
   1983: NCHS, 1990f, Table 50 (p. 162).
   1984, 1989: NCHS, 1991c, Table 52 (p. 121).
   1985: NCHS, 1986d, Table 38 (p. 123).
   1986: NCHS, 1988c, Table 43 (p. 89).
   1987: NCHS, 1989c, Table 48 (p. 93).
   1988: NCHS, 1990f, Table 50 (p. 162).

4. *1987:* Leon & Lair, 1990, Table 3 (p. 9), Table 4 (p. 11).
5. *1985:* NCHS, 1989d, Table 28 (p. 38).

Table 2.3

1. *1984–1989:* NCHS, 1992b, Table 51 (p. 188), Table 53 (pp. 190–191). *1990, 1991, Cumulative Total:* CDC, 1992a, Table 3 (p. 9).
2. NCHS, 1992b, Table 52 (p. 189), Table 54 (pp. 192–193).
3. *1989:* CDC, 1990g, pp. 6, 8, 10, 12, 14, 15, 19, 20, 22, 23. *1990:* CDC, 1992c, pp. 7, 9, 12, 14, 19, 22, 23, 24, 26, 27.

Table 2.4

1. Regier et al., 1988, Table 3 (p. 980), Table 4 (p. 981).

Table 2.5

1. Rosenstein, Milazzo-Sayre, & Manderscheid, 1990, Tables 2.6, 2.7 (p. 159).

Table 2.6

1. Rosenstein, Milazzo-Sayre, & Manderscheid, 1990, Tables 2.13, 2.14 (p. 165).

Table 2.7

1. Strahan, 1990, Table A (p. 228).

Table 2.8

1. *1974–*1990: NIDA, 1991d, Table 2.6 (p. 24), Table 2.7 (p. 25), Table 2.8 (p. 26), Table 2.10 (p. 28), Table 2.11 (p. 29), Table 2.12 (p. 30). *1991:* NIDA, 1991f.
2. *1980–1990:* University of Michigan, 1991, Tables 11, 12, 13. *1991:* University of Michigan, 1992, Tables 2, 3, 4.
3. *1980–1988:* IHS, 1991, Table 4.23 (p. 49).
4. *1988–1991:* NIDA, 1992.

Table 2.9

1. *1950, 1960, 1970, 1980–1983:* NCHS, 1986d, Table 31 (pp. 114–115), Table 32 (pp. 116–117). *1984–1988:* NCHS, 1991c, Table 34 (pp. 97–98), Table 35 (pp. 99–100). *1989:* NCHS, 1992a, Table 5 (pp. 17–19).

Table 2.10

1. American Humane Association, 1989, Figure 1 (p. 5), Figure 2 (p. 6).

2. Sedlak, 1991, Table 3-1 (p. 3–3).
3. Tatara, 1990, pp. 9–10.
4. Gelles & Straus, 1988, Figure 1 (p. 249), Figure 2 (p. 250), Figure 3 (p. 251).

Table 2.12

1. U.S. Bureau of the Census, 1991c, Table 7 (p. 10), Table 10 (p. 11).

Table 3.1

1. *1980:* NCHS, 1984b, Table 1-39 (p. 1-64), Table 1-76 (p. 1-268); NCHS, 1991c, Table 6 (pp. 56–57); NCHS, 1992b, Table 7 (pp. 128–129). *1989:* NCHS, 1991a, Table 13 (pp. 28–29), Table 26 (p. 40), Table 28 (p. 42); NCHS, 1992b, Table 7 (pp. 128–129).
2. *1980:* NCHS, 1992b, Table 18 (pp. 141–142). *1989:* NCHS, 1992a, Table E (p. 9), Table 26 (p. 46). *Race (Native American)* IHS, 1991, Table 3.7 (p. 28).
3. *1980:* NCHS, 1984b, Table 1-44 (pp. 1-69–1-70); NCHS, 1992b, Table 8 (pp. 130–131). *1989:* NCHS, 1991a, Table 26 (p. 40), Table 29 (pp. 43–44).
4. *1980:* NCHS, 1984b, Table 1-6 (pp. 1-11–1-12). *1989:* NCHS, 1991a, Table 4 (pp. 20–21).
5. *Race (White, Black)* *1980:* NCHS, 1985c, Table 1-15 (p. 1-65); NCHS, 1992b, Table 38 (p. 172). *1989:* NCHS, 1992a, Table F (p. 11). *Race (Native American)* IHS, 1991, Table 3.5 (p. 26).

Table 3.2

1. *Age, Race by Sex (White, Black)* *1980:* NCHS, 1991c, Table 27 (pp. 85–86), Table 28 (pp. 87–88), Table 29 (pp. 89–90). *1989:* NCHS, 1992a, Table 5 (pp. 17–19), Table 12 (pp. 30–31). *Race (Native American)* *1988:* IHS, 1991, Table 4.9 (p. 38).
2. *1982:* NCHS, 1985a, Table 57 (pp. 81–82), Table 58 (pp. 83–84), Table 59 (pp. 85–86). *1989:* NCHS, 1990e, Table 57 (pp. 83–84), Table 58 (pp. 85–86), Table 59 (pp. 87–88).
3. *1983:* NCHS, 1990f, Table 50 (p. 162). *1989:* NCHS, 1991c, Table 52 (p. 121).

Race (Hispanic)
1979–1980: NCHS, 1984a, Table 13 (pp. 50–51), Table 14 (pp. 52–53).
4. *1987:* Leon & Lair, 1990, Table 3 (p. 9), Table 4 (p. 11).
5. *1985:* NCHS, 1989d, Table 28 (p. 38).

Table 3.3

1. *Percent distribution of total number*
    Sex: CDC, 1992a, Table 8 (p. 14).
    Race: CDC, 1992a, Table 4 (p. 10).
    Percent distribution by transmission category
    Sex: Under 13: Not available.
            13+ : CDC, 1992a, Table 5 (p. 11).
    Race: CDC, 1992a, Table 4 (p. 10).
2. CDC, 1992a, Table 13 (p. 18).
3. CDC, 1992c, pp. 7, 9, 12, 13, 14, 19, 22, 23, 24, 26, 27.

Table 3.4

1. *Age, Sex*
    Regier et al., 1988, Table 5 (pp. 982–983).
2. *Race (New Haven, Baltimore, St. Louis)*
    Robins et al., 1984, Table 7 (p. 956).
    Race (Los Angeles)
    Karno et al., 1987, Table 1 (p. 696).

Table 3.5

1. Rosenstein, Milazzo-Sayre, & Manderscheid, 1990, Table 2.2 (p. 155), Table 2.3 (p. 156), Table 2.4 (p. 157), Table 2.5 (p. 158).

Table 3.6

1. Rosenstein, Milazzo-Sayre, & Manderscheid, 1990, Table 2.9 (p. 161), Table 2.10 (p. 162), Table 2.11 (p. 163), Table 2.12 (p. 164).

Table 3.7

1. Strahan, 1990, Table 6.1 (p. 234).

Table 3.8

1. *1985:* NIDA, 1988, Table 21 (p. 36), Table 22 (p. 37), Table 29 (p. 47), Table 30 (p. 48), Table 40 (p. 60), Table 41 (p. 61).
    1990: NIDA, 1991e, Tables 2-A–2-D (pp. 17–19), Tables 3-A–3-D (pp. 23–25), Tables 4-A–4-D (pp. 29–31), Tables 5-A–5-D (pp. 35–37),

Tables 7-A–7-D (pp. 47–49), Tables 13-A–13-D (pp. 83–85), Tables 14-A–14-D (pp. 89–91).
Education:
NIDA, 1991d, Table 2.14 (p. 32), Table 3.2 (p. 39), Table 3.3 (p. 40), Table 4.2 (p. 53), Table 4.3 (p. 54), Table 4.9 (p. 60), Table 5.5 (p. 68), Table 7.2 (p. 89), Table 7.3 (p. 90), Table 8.2 (p. 102), Table 8.3 (p. 103).
2. Bachman, Wallace, Kurth, Johnston, & O'Malley, 1991, Tables 14–16 (pp. 52–54); Tables 3–5 (pp. 20–22).
3. IHS, 1991, Table 4.23 (p. 49), Table 4.24 (p. 50).
4. NIDA, 1991a, Table 2.11 (p. 43), Table 2.12 (p. 44), Table 4.01 (p. 85).

Table 3.9

1. *Age, Race by Sex (White, Black)*
   NCHS, 1992a, Table 5 (pp. 17–19), Table 12 (pp. 30–31).
2. *Native American*
   IHS, 1991, Table 4.19 (p. 45), Table 4.21 (p. 47).

Table 3.10

1. American Humane Association, 1988, Table 4 (p. 20), Table 5 (p. 21), Table 10.1 (p. 28).

Table 3.12

1. U.S. Bureau of the Census, 1991c, Table 7 (p. 10), Table 10 (p. 11).

REFERENCES

Abdellah, F. G., Chamberlain, J. G., & Levine, I. S. (1986). Role of nurses in meeting needs of the homeless: Summary of a workshop for providers, researchers, and educators. *Public Health Reports, 101,* 494–498.

Achté, K. (1988). Suicidal tendencies in the elderly. *Suicide and Life-Threatening Behavior, 18,* 55–65.

Adams, G. R., Gullotta, T., & Clancy, M. A. (1985). Homeless adolescents: A descriptive study of similarities and differences between runaways and throwaways. *Adolescence, 20,* 715–724.

Aday, L. A., Aitken, M. J., & Wegener, D. H. (1988). *Pediatric home care: Results of a national evaluation of programs for ventilator assisted children.* Chicago: Pluribus Press.

Agency for Health Care Policy and Research [AHCPR]. (1990a). *AHCPR conference proceedings: Community-based care of persons with AIDS: Developing a research agenda* (DHHS Publication No. PHS 90-3456). Washington, DC: U.S. Government Printing Office.

Agency for Health Care Policy and Research. (1990b). *AHCPR program note: Health services research on HIV/AIDS-related illnesses.* Washington, DC: U.S. Government Printing Office.

Agency for Health Care Policy and Research. (1990c). *AHCPR program note: Selected bibliography on AIDS for health services research.* Washington, DC: U.S. Government Printing Office.

Ahearn, F. L., Jr., & Athey, J. L. (Eds.). (1991). *Refugee children: Theory, research, and services.* Baltimore, MD: Johns Hopkins University Press.

Alan Guttmacher Institute. (1987). *Blessed events and the bottom line: Financing maternity care in the United States.* New York: Author.

Albrecht, G. L. (Ed.). (1976). *The sociology of physical disability and rehabilitation.* Pittsburgh, PA: University of Pittsburgh Press.

Alcohol, Drug Abuse, and Mental Health Administration [ADAMHA]. (1989a). *Report of the Secretary's Task Force on Youth Suicide: Vol. 1. Overview and recommendations* (DHHS Publication No. ADM 89-1621). Washington, DC: U.S. Government Printing Office.

Alcohol, Drug Abuse, and Mental Health Administration. (1989b). *Report of the Secretary's Task Force on Youth Suicide: Vol. 2. Risk factors for youth suicide* (DHHS Publication No. ADM 89-1622). (L. Davidson & M. Linnoila, Eds.). Washington, DC: U.S. Government Printing Office.

Alcohol, Drug Abuse, and Mental Health Administration (1989c). *Report of the Secretary's Task Force on Youth Suicide: Vol. 3. Prevention and interventions in youth suicide* (DHHS Publication No. ADM 89-1623). (M. R. Feinleib, Ed.). Washington, DC: U.S. Government Printing Office.

Alcohol, Drug Abuse, and Mental Health Administration. (1989d). *Report of the Secretary's Task Force on Youth Suicide: Vol. 4. Strategies for the prevention of youth suicide* (DHHS Publication No. ADM 89-1624). (M. L. Rosenberg & K. Baer, Eds.). Washington, DC: U.S. Government Printing Office.

Alcohol, Drug Abuse, and Mental Health Administration (1990). *Alcohol and health: Seventh special report to the U.S. Congress from the Secretary of Health and Human Services* (DHHS Publication No. ADM 90-1656). Washington, DC: U.S. Government Printing Office.

Allen, J. R., & Curran, J. W. (1988). Prevention of AIDS and HIV infection: Needs and priorities for epidemiologic research. *American Journal of Public Health, 78,* 381–386.

Alperstein, G., & Arnstein, E. (1988). Homeless children: A challenge for pediatricians. *Pediatric Clinics of North America, 35,* 1413–1425.

Alperstein, G., Rappaport, C., & Flanigan, J. M. (1988). Health problems of homeless children in New York City. *American Journal of Public Health, 78,* 1232–1233.

Altamore, R., Mitchell, M., & Weber, C. M. (1990). Assuring good-quality care. In P. W. Brickner, L. K. Scharer, B. A. Conanan, M. Savarese, & B. C. Scanlan (Eds.), *Under the safety net: Health and social welfare of the homeless in the United States* (pp. 371–383). New York: Norton.

American Academy of Pediatrics, Committee on Community Health Services. (1988). Health needs of homeless children. *Pediatrics, 82,* 938–940.

American Association of Retired Persons [AARP]. (1989). *Options for the public financing of long-term care.* Washington, DC: Author.

American Association of Retired Persons. (1991a). *Nursing home reform* (FS4-2/91). Public Policy Institute Fact Sheet. Washington, DC: Author.

American Association of Retired Persons. (1991b). *The role of the Older Americans Act in providing long-term care* (FS1-1/91). Public Policy Institute Fact Sheet. Washington, DC: Author.

American Humane Association [AHA]. (1984). *Trends in child abuse and neglect: A national perspective.* Denver, CO: Author.

American Humane Association. (1988). *Highlights of official child neglect and abuse reporting, 1986.* Denver, CO: Author.

American Humane Association. (1989). *Highlights of official aggregate child neglect and abuse reporting, 1987.* Denver, CO: Author.

American Medical Association [AMA]. (1989). Health care needs of homeless and runaway youths. *Journal of the American Medical Association, 262,* 1358–1361.

American Psychiatric Association [APA]. (1980). *Diagnostic and statistical manual of mental disorders* (3rd ed.). Washington, DC: Author.

American Public Health Association [APHA]. (1989). Senate passes landmark rights bill. *Nation's Health, 19*(10,11), 4.

American Public Health Association. (1990a). Appropriations panel rejects AIDS support for cities, states. *Nation's Health, 20*(10), 5.

American Public Health Association. (1990b). Home care standards need improving, GAO says. *Nation's Health, 20*(2), 5.

American Public Health Association. (1991a). CDC abandons plan for national HIV-infection rate survey. *Nation's Health, 21*(2), 4.

American Public Health Association. (1991b). CDC announces expanded definition of AIDS. *Nation's Health, 21*(12), 4.

American Public Health Association. (1991c). Health groups seek $3 billion AIDS budget. *Nation's Health, 21*(5,6), 7.

American Public Health Association. (1992). Case focuses on Medicaid rights of pregnant, alien women. *Nation's Health, 22*(2), 1, 12.

Anderson, S. C., Boe, T., & Smith, S. (1988). Homeless women. *Affilia, 3*(2), 62–70.

Andrulis, D. P., Weslowski, V. B., & Gage, L. S. (1989). The 1987 U.S. Hospital AIDS Survey. *Journal of the American Medical Association, 262,* 784–794.

Anthony, J. C., Folstein, M., Romanoski, A. J., Von Dorff, M. R., Nestadt, G. R., Chahal, R., Merchant, A., Brown, D. H., Shapiro, S., Kramer, M., & Gruenberg, E. M. (1985). Comparison of the lay diagnostic interview schedule and a standardized psychiatric diagnosis. *Archives of General Psychiatry, 42,* 667–675.

Aoun, H. (1989). When a house officer gets AIDS. *New England Journal of Medicine, 321,* 693–696.

Araki, S., & Murata, K. (1986). Social life factors affecting suicide in Japanese men and women. *Suicide and Life-Threatening Behavior, 16,* 458–468.

Araki, S., & Murata, K. (1987). Suicide in Japan: Socioeconomic effects on its secular and seasonal trends. *Suicide and Life-Threatening Behavior, 17,* 64–71.

Archambault, D. (1989). Adolescence: A physiological, cultural, and psychological no man's land. In G. W. Lawson & A. W. Lawson (Eds.), *Alcoholism and substance abuse in special populations.* Rockville, MD: Aspen.

Aruffo, J. F., Coverdale, J. H., & Vallbona, C. (1991). AIDS knowledge in low-income and minority populations. *Public Health Reports, 106,* 115–119.

Asarnow, J. R., & Carlson, G. (1988). Suicide attempts in preadolescent child psychiatry inpatients. *Suicide and Life-Threatening Behavior, 18,* 129–136.

Asen, K., George, E., Piper, R., & Stevens, A. (1989). A systems approach to child abuse: Management and treatment issues. *Child Abuse and Neglect, 13,* 45–57.

Association for Health Services Research [AHSR]. (1991, January). NIMH reorganizes mental health services research programs. *Health Services Report,* pp. 4–5.

Austin, G. A., Johnson, B. D., Carroll, E. E., & Lettieri, D. J. (Eds.). (1977). *Drugs and minorities.* National Institute on Drug Abuse, Research Issues Series. Washington, DC: U.S. Government Printing Office.

Babor, T. F., & Mendelson, J. H. (1986). Ethnic/religious differences in the manifestation and treatment of alcoholism. *Annals of the New York Academy of Sciences, 472,* 46–59.

Bachman, J. G., Wallace, J. M., Jr., Kurth, C. L., Johnston, L. D., & O'Malley, P. M. (1991). *Drug use among black, white, Hispanic, Native American, and Asian American high school seniors (1976–1989): Prevalence, trends, and correlates* (Monitoring the Future, Occasional Paper No. 30). Ann Arbor, MI: University of Michigan, Institute for Social Research.

Bachrach, L. L. (1976). *Deinstitutionalization: An analytical review and sociological perspective* (DHEW Publication No. ADM 76-351). National Institute of Mental Health, Series D, No. 4. Washington, DC: U.S. Government Printing Office.

Bachrach, L. L. (1985). Chronic mentally ill women: Emergence and legitimation of program issues. *Hospital and Community Psychiatry, 36,* 1063–1069.

Bachrach, L. L. (1987). Homeless women: A context for health planning. *Milbank Quarterly, 65,* 371–396.

Bailey, S. L., & Hubbard, R. L. (1990). Developmental variation in the context of marijuana initiation among adolescents. *Journal of Health and Social Behavior, 31,* 58–70.

Baily, M. A., Bilheimer, L., Wooldridge, J., Langwell, K., & Greenberg, W. (1990). Economic consequences for Medicaid of human immunodeficiency virus infection. *Health Care Financing Review, Annual Supplement,* 97–108.

Baker, F. M. (1987). The Afro-American life cycle: Success, failure, and mental health. *Journal of the National Medical Association, 79,* 625–633.

Baltimore, D., & Feinberg, M. B. (1989). HIV revealed: Toward a natural history of the infection. *New England Journal of Medicine, 321,* 1673–1675.

Bangert-Drowns, R. L. (1988). The effects of school-based substance abuse education: A meta-analysis. *Journal of Drug Education, 18,* 243–264.

Barber-Madden, R., & Kotch, J. B. (1990). Maternity care financing: Universal access or universal care? *Journal of Health Politics, Policy and Law, 15,* 797–814.

Barer, B. M., & Johnson, C. L. (1990). A critique of the caregiving literature. *Gerontologist, 30,* 26–29.

Barrett, M. E., Simpson, D. D., & Lehman, W.E.K. (1988). Behavioral changes of adolescents in drug abuse intervention programs. *Journal of Clinical Psychology, 44,* 461–473.

Baruffi, G., Strobino, D. M., & Paine, L. L. (1990). Investigation of institutional differences in primary cesarean birth rates. *Journal of Nurse Midwifery, 35,* 274–281.

Bassuk, E., & Rubin, L. (1987). Homeless children: A neglected population. *American Journal of Orthopsychiatry, 57,* 279–286.

Baughan, D. M., White-Baughan, J., Pickwell, S., Bartlome, J., & Wong, S. (1990). Primary care needs of Cambodian refugees. *Journal of Family Practice, 30,* 565–568.

Bauman, K. E., LaPrelle, J., Brown, J. D., Koch, G. G., & Padgett, C. A. (1991). The influence of three mass media campaigns on variables related to adolescent cigarette smoking: Results of a field experiment. *American Journal of Public Health, 81,* 597–604.

Bayer, R. (1989). *Private acts, social consequences: AIDS and the politics of public health.* New York: Free Press.

Bayer, R. (1991). AIDS: The politics of prevention and neglect. *Health Affairs, 10*(1), 87–97.

Beachler, M. (1990). The mental health services program for youth. *Journal of Mental Health Administration, 17,* 115–121.

Bean, F. D., Edmonston, B., & Passel, J. S. (Eds.). (1990). *Undocumented migration to the United States: IRCA and the experience of the 1980s.* Santa Monica, CA: RAND Corporation.

Bean, F. D., Vernez, G., & Keely, C. B. (1989). *Opening and closing the doors: Evaluating immigration reform and control.* Santa Monica, CA: RAND.

Beauchamp, D. E. (1988). *The health of the republic: Epidemics, medicine, and moralism as challenges to democracy.* Philadelphia: Temple University Press.

Beauvais, F., Oetting, E. R., Wolf, W., & Edwards, R. W. (1989). American Indian youth and drugs, 1976–87: A continuing problem. *American Journal of Public Health, 79,* 634–636.

Bebbington, P. E. (1990). Population surveys of psychiatric disorder and the need for treatment. *Social Psychiatry and Psychiatric Epidemiology, 25,* 33–40.

Becker, M. H., & Joseph, J. G. (1988). AIDS and behavioral change to reduce risk: A review. *American Journal of Public Health, 78,* 394–410.

Beers, M. H., Fink, A., & Beck, J. C. (1991). Screening recommendations for the elderly. *American Journal of Public Health, 81,* 1131–1140.

Begley, C. E., Crane, M. M., & Perdue, G. (1990). Estimating the mortality cost of AIDS: Do estimates of earnings differ? *American Journal of Public Health, 80,* 1268–1270.

Behrman, R. E. (1987). Premature births among black women. *New England Journal of Medicine, 317,* 763–765.

Bell, C. S., & Battjes, R. J. (Eds.). (1990). *Prevention research: Deterring drug abuse among children and adolescents* (DHHS Publication No. ADM 90-1334). National Institute on Drug Abuse, Research Monograph Series, No. 63. Washington, DC: U.S. Government Printing Office.

Bellah, R. N., Madsen, R., Sullivan, W. M., Swidler, A., & Tipton, S. M. (1985). *Habits of the heart: Individualism and commitment in American life.* Berkeley: University of California Press.

Benjamin, A. E. (1988). Long-term care and AIDS: Perspectives from experience with the elderly. *Milbank Quarterly, 66,* 415–443.

Benjamin, A. E. (1989). Perspectives on a continuum of care for persons with HIV illnesses. In W. N. LeVee (Ed.), *Conference Proceedings: New Perspectives on HIV-related Illnesses: Progress in Health Services Research* (DHHS Publication No. PHS 89-3449, pp. 145–158). Washington, DC: U.S. Government Printing Office.

Benjamin, A. E., Lee, P. R., & Solkowitz, S. N. (1988). Case management of persons with acquired immunodeficiency syndrome in San Francisco. *Health Care Financing Review, Annual Supplement,* 69–74.

Bennett, C. L. (1990). Quality of medical care for patients with AIDS and cancer. *Dissertation Abstracts International, 50,* 5566B. (University Microfilms No. AAD90-12735).

Bennett, M.B.H. (1988). Afro-American women, poverty, and mental health: A social essay. *Women and Health, 12,* 213–228.

Bergner, M. (1989). Quality of life, health status, and clinical research. *Medical Care, 27*(Suppl.), S148–S156.

Berlin, I. N. (1985). Prevention of adolescent suicide among some Native American tribes. *Adolescent Psychiatry, 12,* 77–93.

Berlin, I. N. (1987). Suicide among American Indian adolescents: An overview. *Suicide and Life-Threatening Behavior, 17,* 218–232.

Berne, A. S., Dato, C., Mason, D. J., & Rafferty, M. (1990). A nursing model for addressing the health needs of homeless families. *Image: Journal of Nursing Scholarship, 22,* 8–13.

Beschner, G., & Thompson, P. (1981). *Women and drug abuse treatment: Needs and services* (DHHS Publication No. ADM 81-1057). National Institute on Drug Abuse, Services Research Monograph Series. Washington, DC: U.S. Government Printing Office.

Bilheimer, L. (1989). AIDS cost modeling in the U.S.: A pragmatic approach. *Health Policy, 11,* 147–168.

Binder, R. L., & McNiel, D. E. (1987). Evaluation of a school-based sexual abuse prevention program: Cognitive and emotional effects. *Child Abuse and Neglect, 11,* 497–506.

Bingham, R. D., Green, R. E., & White, S. B. (Eds.). (1987). *The homeless in contemporary society.* Newbury Park, CA: Sage.

Blazer, D. G. (1989). The epidemiology of depression in late life. *Journal of Geriatric Psychiatry, 22,* 35–52.

Blumstein, A., Cohen, J., Roth, J. A., & Visher, C. A. (Eds.). (1986a). *Criminal careers and "career criminals"* (Vol. 1). Washington, DC: National Academy Press.

Blumstein, A., Cohen, J., Roth, J. A., & Visher, C. A. (Eds.). (1986b). *Criminal careers and "career criminals"* (Vol. 2). Washington, DC: National Academy Press.

Board on Mental Health and Behavioral Medicine, Institute of Medicine. (1985). Research on mental illness and addictive disorders: Progress and prospects. *American Journal of Psychiatry, 142*(Suppl.), 1–41.

Boone, M. S. (1985). Social and cultural factors in the etiology of low birthweight among disadvantaged blacks. *Social Science and Medicine, 20,* 1001–1011.

Boone, M. S. (1989). *Capital crime: Black infant mortality in America.* Newbury Park, CA: Sage.

Bowdler, J. E. (1989). Health problems of the homeless in America. *Nurse Practitioner, 14*(7), 44, 47, 50–51.

Bowering, J., Clancy, K. L., & Poppendieck, J. (1991). Characteristics of a random sample of emergency food program users in New York: II. Soup kitchens. *American Journal of Public Health, 81,* 914–917.

Bowlyow, J. E. (1990). Acute and long-term care linkages: A literature review. *Medical Care Review, 47,* 75–103.

Boyer, C. A. (1987). Obstacles in urban housing policy for the chronically mentally ill. In D. Mechanic (Ed.), *Improving mental health services: What the social sciences can tell us* (pp. 71–81). New Directions for Mental Health Services, No. 36. San Francisco: Jossey-Bass.

Brady, J., Sharfstein, S. S., & Muszynski, I. L., Jr. (1986). Trends in private insurance coverage for mental illness. *American Journal of Psychiatry, 143,* 1276–1279.

Braveman, P., Oliva, G., Miller, M. G., Reiter, R., & Egerter, S. (1989). Adverse outcomes and lack of health insurance among newborns in an eight-county area of California, 1982 to 1986. *New England Journal of Medicine, 321,* 508–513.

Brent, D. A. (1989). The psychological autopsy: Methodological considerations for the study of adolescent suicide. *Suicide and Life-Threatening Behavior, 19,* 43–57.

Brickner, P. W., Scanlan, B. C., Conanan, B. A., Elvy, A., McAdam, J., Scharer, L. K., & Vicic, W. J. (1986). Homeless persons and health care. *Annals of Internal Medicine, 104,* 405–409.

Brickner, P. W., Scharer, L. K., Conanan, B. A., Elvy, A., & Savarese, M. (Eds.). (1985). *Health care for homeless people.* New York: Springer.

Brickner, P. W., Scharer, L. K., Conanan, B. A., Savarese, M., & Scanlan, B. C. (Eds.). (1990). *Under the safety net: Health and social welfare of the homeless in the United States.* New York: Norton.

Brody, B. E. (1988). Employee assistance programs: An historical and literature review. *American Journal of Health Promotion, 2*(3), 13–19.

Brook, R. H., Ware, J. E., Jr., Rogers, W. H., Keeler, E. B., Davies, A. R., Donald, C. A., Goldberg, G. A., Lohr, K. N., Masthay, P. C., & Newhouse, J. P. (1983). Does free care improve adults' health? Results from a randomized controlled trial. *New England Journal of Medicine, 309,* 1426–1434.

Broughton, C. (1989, September-October). Serving refugee children and families in Head Start. *Children Today,* pp. 6–10.

Brown, D. R., Eaton, W. W., & Sussman, L. (1990). Racial differences in prevalence of phobic disorders. *Journal of Nervous and Mental Disease, 178,* 434–441.

Brown, F., & Tooley, J. (1989). Alcoholism in the black community. In G. W. Lawson & A. W. Lawson (Eds.), *Alcoholism and substance abuse in special populations* (pp. 115–137). Rockville, MD: Aspen.

Browne, K., Davies, C., & Stratton, P. (Eds.). (1988). *Early prediction and prevention of child abuse.* New York: Wiley.

Brunskill, A. J. (1990). Some sources of error in the coding of birth weight. *American Journal of Public Health, 80,* 72–73.

Buchanan, R. J. (1988). State Medicaid coverage of AZT and AIDS-related policies. *American Journal of Public Health, 78,* 432–436.

Bureau of Maternal and Child Health and Resources Development [BMC-HRD]. (1987). *Surgeon General's workshop on violence and public health: Report* (DHHS Publication No. HRS-D-MC 86-1). Washington, DC: U.S. Government Printing Office.

Bureau of Maternal and Child Health and Resources Development. (1988). *Continuity of care for at-risk infants and their families: Opportunities for maternal and child health programs and programs for children with special health needs.* Washington, DC: U.S. Government Printing Office.

Burke, D. S., Brundage, J. F., Redfield, R. R., Damato, J. J., Schable, C. A., Putman, P., Visintine, R., & Kim, H. I. (1988). Measurement of the false rate in a screening program for human immunodeficiency virus infections. *New England Journal of Medicine, 319,* 961–964.

Burke, K. C., Burke, J. D., Jr., Regier, D. A., & Rae, D. S. (1990). Age at onset of selected mental disorders in five community populations. *Archives of General Psychiatry, 47,* 511–518.

Burke, T. R. (1988). Long-term care: The public role and private initiatives. *Health Care Financing Review, Annual Supplement,* 1–5.

Burkhauser, R. V., & Duncan, G. J. (1988). Life events, public policy, and the economic vulnerability of children and the elderly. In J. L. Palmer, T. Smeeding, & B. B. Torrey (Eds.), *The Vulnerable* (pp. 55–88). Washington, DC: Urban Institute Press.

Burt, M. R. (1986). Estimating the public costs of teenage childbearing. *Family Planning Perspectives, 18,* 221–226.

Burt, M. R., & Cohen, B. E. (1989). *America's homeless: Numbers, characteristics, and programs that serve them.* Urban Institute Report No. 89-3. Washington, DC: Urban Institute Press.

Butter, I. H., & Kay, B. J. (1988). State laws and the practice of lay midwifery. *American Journal of Public Health, 78,* 1161–1169.

Caetano, R. (1988). Alcohol use among Hispanic groups in the United States. *American Journal of Drug and Alcohol Abuse, 14,* 293–308.

Cameron, J. M. (1989). A national community mental health program: Policy initiation and progress. In D. A. Rochefort (Ed.), *Handbook on mental health policy in the United States* (pp. 121–142). Westport, CT: Greenwood Press.

Capitman, J. A. (1988). Case management for long-term and acute medical care. *Health Care Financing Review, Annual Supplement,* 53–55.

Carcagno, G. J., & Kemper, P. (1988). The evaluation of the national long term care demonstration. *Health Services Research, 23,* 1–22.

Cargill, V. A., & Smith, M. S. (1990). HIV disease and the African-American community. In Maxwell Communications Corporation (Ed.), *San Francisco General Hospital AIDS Knowledge Base Text* (pp. 1–15). San Francisco: Maxwell Communications Corporation.

Carney, T. (1989). A fresh approach to child protection practice and legislation in Australia. *Child Abuse and Neglect, 13,* 29–39.

Caro, F. G., Marshall, E., Carter, A. B., Kalmuss, D., Fennelly, K., & Lopez, I. (1988). *Barriers to prenatal care: An examination of use of prenatal care among low-income women in New York City.* New York: Community Service Society of New York.

Carpenter, L. (1988). Special report: Medicaid eligibility for persons in nursing homes. *Health Care Financing Review, 10*(2), 67–77.

Casement, M. R. (1987). Economic research and prevention. *Alcohol Health and Research World, 12,* 16.

Caton, C.L.M. (1990). *Homeless in America.* New York: Oxford University Press.

Center for Health Policy Studies. (1989). *Assessment of the implementation of grants to provide health services to the homeless.* Washington, DC: Health Resources and Services Administration.

Center for Health Promotion and Education. (1990). *Aggressors, victims, and bystanders: An assessment-based middle school violence prevention curriculum: Project description.* Newton, MA: Education Development Center.

Centers for Disease Control [CDC]. (1985). Revision of the case definition of acquired immunodeficiency syndrome for national reporting—United States. *Morbidity and Mortality Weekly Report, 34,* 373–375.

Centers for Disease Control. (1987a). Revision of the CDC surveillance case definition for acquired immunodeficiency syndrome. *Morbidity and Mortality Weekly Report, 36*(Suppl. 1S), 3S–15S.

Centers for Disease Control. (1987b). Sudden unexplained death syndrome in Southeast Asian refugees: A review of CDC surveillance. *Morbidity and Mortality Weekly Report, 36*(No. 1SS), 43SS–53SS.

Centers for Disease Control. (1987c). Tuberculosis among Asians/Pacific Islanders—United States, 1985. *Morbidity and Mortality Weekly Report, 36,* 331–334.

Centers for Disease Control. (1988a). HIV-related beliefs, knowledge, and behaviors among high school students. *Morbidity and Mortality Weekly Report, 37,* 717–721.

Centers for Disease Control. (1988b). *Injury control: A review of the status and progress of the injury control program at the Centers for Disease Control.* Washington, DC: National Academy Press.

Centers for Disease Control. (1988c). Premature mortality due to homicides—United States, 1968–1985. *Journal of the American Medical Association, 260,* 2021–2033.

Centers for Disease Control. (1988d). Update: Sudden unexplained death syndrome among Southeast Asian refugees—United States. *Morbidity and Mortality Weekly Report, 37,* 568–570.

Centers for Disease Control. (1990a). AIDS in women. *Morbidity and Mortality Weekly Report, 39,* 845–846.

Centers for Disease Control. (1990b). Childhood injuries in the United States. *American Journal of Diseases of Children, 144,* 627–646.

Centers for Disease Control. (1990c). *Disease prevention and health promotion: Adolescent and school health resources: HIV and AIDS: A cumulation of the AIDS school health education database.* Atlanta, GA: Author.

Centers for Disease Control. (1990d). HIV prevalence estimates and AIDS case projections for the United States: Report based upon a workshop. *Morbidity and Mortality Weekly Report, 39*(No. RR-16), 1–31.

Centers for Disease Control. (1990e). HIV-related knowledge and behaviors among high school students—selected U.S. sites, 1989. *Morbidity and Mortality Weekly Report, 39,* 385–389, 396–397.

Centers for Disease Control. (1990f). Homicide among young black males: 1978–1987. *Morbidity and Mortality Weekly Report, 39,* 869–873.

Centers for Disease Control. (1990g). *National HIV seroprevalence surveys: Summary of results: Data from serosurveillance activities through 1989* (HIV-CID-9-90-006). Atlanta, GA: Author.

Centers for Disease Control. (1990h). State coalitions for prevention and control of tobacco use. *Morbidity and Mortality Weekly Report, 39,* 476–485.

Centers for Disease Control. (1991). Mortality attributable to HIV infection/AIDS—United States, 1981–1990. *Morbidity and Mortality Weekly Report, 40,* 41–44.

Centers for Disease Control. (1992a). *HIV/AIDS surveillance report: U.S. AIDS cases reported through December 1991.* Atlanta, GA: Author.

Centers for Disease Control. (1992b). *HIV/AIDS surveillance report: U.S. AIDS cases reported through March 1992.* Atlanta, GA: Author.

Centers for Disease Control. (1992c). *National HIV serosurveillance summary: Results through 1990* (HIV-NCID-11-91-011). Atlanta, GA: Author.

Champion, H. R., Copes, W. S., Buyer, D., Flanagan, M. E., Bain, L., & Sacco, W. J. (1989). Major trauma in geriatric patients. *American Journal of Public Health, 79,* 1278–1282.

Chavez, L. R., Cornelius, W. A., & Jones, O. W. (1985). Mexican immigrants and the utilization of U.S. health services: The case of San Diego. *Social Science and Medicine, 21,* 93–102.

Chen, M. S., Jr., Kuun, P., Guthrie, R., Li, W., & Zaharlick, A. (1991). Promoting heart health for Southeast Asians: A database for planning interventions. *Public Health Reports, 106,* 304–309.

Chenoweth, K., & Free, C. (1990). Homeless children come to school. *American Educator, 14*(3), 28–33.

Chicago Tribune Staff. (1986). *The American millstone: An examination of the nation's permanent underclass*. Chicago: Contemporary Books.

Children's Defense Fund [CDF]. (1990). *S.O.S. America! A children's defense fund budget*. Washington, DC: Author.

Children's Defense Fund. (1991a). *Child poverty in America*. Washington, DC: Author.

Children's Defense Fund. (1991b). Homelessness in rural America. *CDF Reports, 12*(7), 1, 2, 7.

Children's Defense Fund. (1991c). New report examines homelessness among children and families. *CDF Reports, 12*(7), 3.

Chirikos, T. N. (1986). Accounting for the historical rise in work-disability prevalence. *Milbank Quarterly, 64,* 271–301.

Ciardiello, J. A., & Bell, M. D. (Eds.). (1988). *Vocational rehabilitation of persons with prolonged psychiatric disorders*. Baltimore, MD: Johns Hopkins University Press.

Cicchetti, D., & Carlson, V. (1989). *Child maltreatment: Theory and research on the causes and consequences of child abuse and neglect*. Cambridge, England: Cambridge University Press.

Clancy, K. L., Bowering, J., & Poppendieck, J. (1991). Characteristics of a random sample of emergency food program users in New York: I. Food pantries. *American Journal of Public Health, 81,* 911–914.

Cleary, P. D. (1989). The need and demand for mental health services. In C. A. Taube, D. Mechanic, & A. A. Hohmann (Eds.), *The future of mental health services research* (DHHS Publication No. ADM 89-1600, pp. 161–184). National Institute of Mental Health. Washington, DC: U.S. Government Printing Office.

Cleary, P. D., Hitchcock, J. L., Semmer, N., Flinchbaugh, L. J., & Pinney, J. M. (1988). Adolescent smoking: Research and health policy. *Milbank Quarterly, 66,* 137–171.

Cleland, J. G., & van Ginneken, J. K. (1988). Maternal education and child survival in developing countries: The search for pathways of influence. *Social Science and Medicine, 27,* 1357–1368.

Coate, D., & Grossman, M. (1987). Change in alcoholic beverage prices and legal drinking ages: Effects on youth alcohol use and motor vehicle mortality. *Alcohol Health and Research World, 12*(1), 22–25, 59.

Cohen, L. H., & Stricker, G. (1983). Mental health quality assurance: Development of the American Psychological Association/CHAMPUS Program. *Evaluation & the Health Professions, 6,* 327–338.

Cohn, A. H. (1982). Stopping abuse before it occurs: Different solutions for different population groups. *Child Abuse and Neglect, 6,* 473–483.

Cohn, A. H., & Daro, D. (1987). Is treatment too late: What ten years of evaluative research tell us. *Child Abuse and Neglect, 11,* 433–442.

Cohn, A. H., & Lee, R. A. (1988). Child abuse and neglect. In H. M. Wallace, G. Ryan, Jr., & A. C. Oglesby (Eds.), *Maternal and Child Health Practices* (3rd ed., pp. 497–503). Oakland, CA: Third Party.

Coleman, J. S. (1990). *Foundations of social theory.* Cambridge, MA: Harvard University Press.

Collins, J. J., & Zawitz, M. W. (1990). *Federal drug data for national policy.* Washington, DC: U.S. Department of Justice, Office of Justice Programs, Bureau of Justice Statistics, Drugs and Crime Data.

Collins, J. W., Jr., & David, R. J. (1990). The differential effect of traditional risk factors on infant birthweight among blacks and whites in Chicago. *American Journal of Public Health, 80,* 679–681.

Combs-Orme, T., Reis, J., & Ward, L. D. (1985). Effectiveness of home visits by public health nurses in maternal and child health: An empirical review. *Public Health Reports, 100,* 490–499.

Commonwealth Fund Commission on Elderly People Living Alone. (1987). *Old, alone, and poor: A plan for reducing poverty among elderly people living alone.* Baltimore, MD.: Author.

Commonwealth Fund Commission on Elderly People Living Alone. (1988). *Aging alone: Profiles and projections.* Baltimore, MD.: Author.

Commonwealth Fund Commission on Elderly People Living Alone. (1989). *Help at home: Long-term care assistance for impaired elderly people.* Baltimore, MD.: Author.

Cooke, M., & Sande, M. A. (1989). The HIV epidemic and training in internal medicine: Challenges and recommendations. *New England Journal of Medicine, 321,* 1334–1337.

Cooney, J. P. (1985). What determines the start of prenatal care? Prenatal care, insurance, and education. *Medical Care, 23,* 986–997.

Coyle, S. L., Boruch, R. F., & Turner, C. F. (Eds.). (1991). *Evaluating AIDS prevention programs.* Washington, DC: National Academy Press.

Craig, R. T. (1988a). Community care for persons with serious mental illness: Removing barriers and building supports. *National Conference of State Legislatures: State Legislative Report, 13*(35), 1–8.

Craig, R. T. (1988b). Mental health services for children and youth: Strengthening the promise of the future. *National Conference of State Legislatures: State Legislative Report, 13*(25), 1–10.

Cramer, J. C. (1987). Social factors and infant mortality: Identifying high-risk groups and proximate causes. *Demography, 24,* 299–322.

Crocker, A. C. (1990). Medical care in the community for adults with mental retardation. *American Journal of Public Health, 80,* 1037–1038.

Crystal, S., & Dejowski, E. (1987). Substituted judgment and protective intervention. In D. Mechanic (Ed.), *Improving mental health services: What the social sciences can tell us* (pp. 83–91). New Directions for Mental Health Services, No. 36. San Francisco: Jossey-Bass.

Cunningham, P. J., & Monheit, A. C. (1990). Insuring the children: A decade of change. *Health Affairs, 9*(4), 76–90.

Dahl, R. A., & Lindblom, C. E. (1963). *Politics, economics, and welfare: Planning and politico-economic systems resolved into basic social processes.* New York: HarperCollins.

Daniels, N. (1990). Insurability and the HIV epidemic: Ethical issues in underwriting. *Milbank Quarterly, 68,* 497–524.

Daniels, N. (1991). Duty to treat or right to refuse? *Hastings Center Report, 21*(2), 36–46.

Daro, D. (1988). *Confronting child abuse: Research for effective program design.* New York: Free Press.

Davis, R. A. (1988). Adolescent pregnancy and infant mortality: Isolating the effects of race. *Adolescence, 23,* 899–908.

Davis, R. M. (1987). Current trends in cigarette advertising and marketing. *New England Journal of Medicine, 316,* 725–732.

Dean, A., & Ensel, W. M. (1983). Socially structured depression in men and women. *Research in Community and Mental Health, 3,* 113–139.

Dear, M. J., & Wolch, J. R. (1987). *Landscapes of despair: From deinstitutionalization to homelessness.* Princeton, NJ: Princeton University Press.

DeJong, W., & Winsten, J. A. (1990). The use of mass media in substance abuse prevention. *Health Affairs, 9*(2), 31–46.

Dengelegi, L., Weber, J., & Torquato, S. (1990). Drug users' AIDS-related knowledge, attitudes, and behaviors before and after AIDS education sessions. *Public Health Reports, 105,* 504–510.

Dennis, E. (1989). Mobile outreach program provides health services to sheltered homeless children in New York City. *Public Health Reports, 104,* 405.

Densen, P. M. (1991). *Tracing the elderly through the health care system: An update.* Rockville, MD: U.S. Department of Health and Human Services, Agency for Health Care Policy and Research.

Dent, C. W., Sussman, S., Johnson, C. A., Hansen, W. B., & Flay, B. R. (1987). Adolescent smokeless tobacco incidence: Relations with other drugs and psychosocial variables. *Preventive Medicine, 16,* 422–431.

Dickey, B., Binner, P. R., Leff, S., Uyda, M. K., Schlesinger, M. J., & Gudeman, J. E. (1989). Containing mental health treatment costs through program design: A Massachusetts study. *American Journal of Public Health, 79,* 863–867.

DiClemente, R. J., Boyer, C. B., & Morales, E. S. (1988). Minorities and AIDS: Knowledge, attitudes, and misconceptions among black and Latino adolescents. *American Journal of Public Health, 78,* 55–57.

DiClemente, R. J., Lanier, M. M., Horan, P. F., & Lodico, M. (1991). Comparison of AIDS knowledge, attitudes, and behaviors among incarcerated adolescents and a public school sample in San Francisco. *American Journal of Public Health, 81,* 628–630.

Diehr, P., Williams, S. J., Martin, D. P., & Price, K. (1984). Ambulatory mental health services utilization in three provider plans. *Medical Care, 22,* 1–13.

Dill, A.E.P. (1987). Issues in case management for the chronically mentally ill. In D. Mechanic (Ed.), *Improving mental health services: What the social sciences can tell us* (pp. 61–70). New Directions for Mental Health Services, No. 36. San Francisco: Jossey-Bass.

Dingemans, P. M. (1990). ICD-9-CM classification coding in psychiatry. *Journal of Clinical Psychology, 46,* 161–168.

Division of Maternal and Child Health. (1987). *Report of the Surgeon General's workshop on children with HIV infection and their families* (DHHS Publication No. HRS-D-MC 87-1). Washington, DC: U.S. Government Printing Office.

Division of Special Populations Program Development [DSPPD]. (1990a). *Comprehensive perinatal care program.* Rockville, MD: U.S. Department of Health and Human Services, Bureau of Health Care Delivery and Assistance.

Division of Special Populations Program Development. (1990b). *Health care for the homeless.* Rockville, MD: U.S. Department of Health and Human Services, Bureau of Health Care Delivery and Assistance.

Division of Special Populations Program Development. (1990c). *Health care services for the elderly.* Rockville, MD: U.S. Department of Health and Human Services, Bureau of Health Care Delivery and Assistance.

Division of Special Populations Program Development. (1990d). *Health services in the home.* Rockville, MD: U.S. Department of Health and Human Services, Bureau of Health Care Delivery and Assistance.

Division of Special Populations Program Development. (1990e). *HIV services and treatment program.* Rockville, MD: U.S. Department of Health and Human Services, Bureau of Health Care Delivery and Assistance.

Division of Special Populations Programs Development. (1991). *Health care for the homeless: Report to the Congress on the utilization and costs of health care services: Calendar year 1989.* Rockville, MD: U.S. Department of Health and Human Services, Bureau of Health Care Delivery and Assistance.

Dohrenwend, B. P. (1990). Socioeconomic status (SES) and psychiatric disorders: Are the issues still compelling? *Social Psychiatry and Psychiatric Epidemiology, 25,* 41–47.

Dohrenwend, B. P., & Dohrenwend, B. S. (1982). Perspectives on the past and future of psychiatric epidemiology. *American Journal of Public Health, 72,* 1271–1279.

Donabedian, A. (1980). *Explorations in quality assessment and monitoring: The definition of quality and approaches to its assessment* (Vol. 1). Ann Arbor, MI: Health Administration Press.

Dooley, D., Catalano, R., Rook, K., & Serxner, S. (1989a). Economic stress and suicide: Multilevel analyses: Part 1. Aggregate time-series analyses of economic stress and suicide. *Suicide and Life-Threatening Behavior, 19,* 321–336.

Dooley, D., Catalano, R., Rook, K., & Serxner, S. (1989b). Economic stress and suicide: Multilevel analyses: Part 2. Cross-level analyses of economic stress and suicidal ideation. *Suicide and Life-Threatening Behavior, 19,* 337–351.

Doty, P., Liu, K., & Wiener, J. M. (1985). An overview of long-term care. *Health Care Financing Review, 6*(3), 69–78.

Dowell, D. A., & Ciarlo, J. A. (1989). An evaluative overview of the community mental health centers program. In D. A. Rochefort (Ed.), *Hand-*

book on mental health policy in the United States (pp. 195–236). Westport, CT: Greenwood Press.

Drake, R. D., Wallach, M. A., & Hoffman, J. S. (1989). Housing instability and homelessness among aftercare patients of an urban state hospital. *Hospital and Community Psychiatry, 40,* 46–51.

Dryfoos, J. G. (1990). *Adolescents-at-risk: Prevalence and prevention.* New York: Oxford University Press.

Dubowitz, H. (1990). Costs and effectiveness of interventions in child maltreatment. *Child Abuse and Neglect, 14,* 177–186.

Dukes, R. L., & Lorch, B. D. (1989). The effects of school, family, self-concept, and deviant behaviour on adolescent suicide ideation. *Journal of Adolescence, 12,* 239–251.

DuPont, R. L. (Ed.). *Stopping alcohol and other drug use before it starts: The future of prevention* (DHHS Publication No. ADM 89-1645). Office for Substance Abuse Prevention, Prevention Monograph No. 1. Washington, DC: U.S. Government Printing Office.

Eckenrode, J., Munsch, J., Powers, J., & Doris, J. (1988). The nature and substantiation of official sexual abuse reports. *Child Abuse and Neglect, 12,* 311–319.

Eddy, D. M., Wolpert, R. L., & Rosenberg, M. L. (1989). Estimating the effectiveness of interventions to prevent youth suicides: A report to the Secretary's Task Force on Youth Suicide. In M. L. Rosenberg & K. Baer (Eds.), *Report of the Secretary's Task Force on Youth Suicide: Vol. 4. Strategies for the prevention of youth suicide* (DHHS Publication No. ADM 89-1624, pp. 37–81). Alcohol, Drug Abuse, and Mental Health Administration. Washington, DC: U.S. Government Printing Office.

Eden, S. L., & Aguilar, R. J. (1989). The Hispanic chemically dependent client: Considerations for diagnosis and treatment. In G. W. Lawson & A. W. Lawson (Eds.), *Alcoholism and substance abuse in special populations* (pp. 205–222). Rockville, MD: Aspen.

Edwards, P. W., & Donaldson, M. A. (1989). Assessment of symptoms in adult survivors of incest: A factor analytic study of the responses to childhood incest questionnaire. *Child Abuse and Neglect, 13,* 101–110.

Eggert, G. M., & Friedman, B. (1988). The need for special interventions for multiple hospital admission patients. *Health Care Financing Review, Annual Supplement,* 57–67.

Ehrlich, P., & Anetzberger, G. (1991). Survey of state public health departments on procedures for reporting elder abuse. *Public Health Reports, 106,* 151–154.

Eisenstaedt, R. S., & Getzen, T. E. (1988). Screening blood donors for human immunodeficiency virus antibody: Cost-benefit analysis. *American Journal of Public Health, 78,* 450–454.

Ekstrand, M. L., & Coates, T. J. (1990). Maintenance of safer sexual behaviors and predictors of risky sex: The San Francisco Men's Health Study. *American Journal of Public Health, 80,* 973–977.

Elias, C. J., Alexander, B. H., & Sokly, T. (1990). Infectious disease control in a long-term refugee camp: The role of epidemiologic surveillance and investigation. *American Journal of Public Health, 80,* 824–828.

Ellickson, P. L., & Bell, R. M. (1990a). Drug prevention in junior high: A multi-site longitudinal test. *Science, 247,* 1299–1305.

Ellickson, P. L., & Bell, R. M. (1990b). *Prospects for preventing drug use among young adolescents* (R-3896-CHF). Santa Monica, CA: RAND Corporation.

Ellwood, D. T. (1988). *Poor support: Poverty in the American family.* New York: Basic Books.

Ellwood, M. R., & Burwell, B. (1990). Access to Medicaid and Medicare by the low-income disabled. *Health Care Financing Review, Annual Supplement,* 133–148.

Elpers, J. R. (1987). Are we legislating reinstitutionalization? *American Journal of Orthopsychiatry, 57,* 441–446.

Emanuel, E. J. (1988). Do physicians have an obligation to treat patients with AIDS? *New England Journal of Medicine, 318,* 1686–1690.

Epstein, M. R. (1990). Networking in a rural community focuses on at-risk children. *Public Health Reports, 105,* 428–430.

Ernst, T. N., Philip, M., Viken, R. M., & Blaisdell, M. F. (1988). The effect of Southeast Asian refugees on medical services in a rural county. *Family Medicine, 20,* 141–142.

Escobedo, L. G., Anda, R. F., Smith, P. F., Remington, P. L., & Mast, E. E. (1990). Sociodemographic characteristics of cigarette smoking initiation in the United States: Implications for smoking prevention policy. *Journal of the American Medical Association, 264,* 1550–1555.

Eskander, G. S., Jahan, M. S., & Carter, R. A. (1990). AIDS: Knowledge and attitudes among different ethnic groups. *Journal of the National Medical Association, 82,* 281–286.

Faden, R. R., & Kass, N. E. (1988). Health insurance and AIDS: The status of state regulatory activity. *American Journal of Public Health, 78,* 437–438.

FAIR. (1986). *Fact Sheet.* No. 3. Washington, DC: Federation for American Immigration Reform.

Farkas, M. D., & Anthony, W. A. (1989). *Psychiatric rehabilitation programs: Putting theory into practice.* Baltimore, MD.: Johns Hopkins University Press.

Feder, J. (1990). Health care of the disadvantaged: The elderly. *Journal of Health Politics, Policy, and Law, 15,* 259–269.

Feinson, M. C. (1989). Are psychological disorders most prevalent among older adults? Examining the evidence. *Social Science and Medicine, 29,* 1175–1181.

Feinstein, A. R. (1989). Evaluation of prognosis and transitions: General strategic principles and applications to AIDS. In L. Sechrest, H. Freeman, & A. Mulley (Eds.), *Conference proceedings: Health Services Research Methodology: A Focus on AIDS* (DHHS Publication No. PHS 89-3439, pp. 189–195). Washington, DC: U.S. Government Printing Office.

Fellios, P. G. (1989). Alcoholism in women: Causes, treatment, and prevention. In G. W. Lawson & A. W. Lawson (Eds.), *Alcoholism and substance abuse in special populations* (pp. 11–34). Rockville, MD: Aspen.

Fernandez-Pol, B. (1986). Characteristics of 77 Puerto Ricans who attempted suicide. *American Journal of Psychiatry, 143,* 1460–1463.

Fiedler, J. L., & Wight, J. B. (1989). *The medical offset effect and public health policy: Mental health industry in transition.* New York: Praeger.

Filinson, R., & Ingman, S. R. (Eds.). (1989). *Elder abuse: Practice and policy.* New York: Human Sciences Press.

Fillmore, K. M. (1988). *Alcohol use across the life course: A critical review of 70 years of international longitudinal research.* Toronto: Addiction Research Foundation.

Fineberg, H. V. (1987). Foreword: Invitational conference on applications of analytic methods to mental health: Practice, policy, research. *Medical Care, 25*(Suppl.), S53.

Fingerhut, L. A., & Kleinman, J. C. (1989). *Firearm mortality among children and youth* (DHHS Publication No. PHS 90-1250). National Center for Health Statistics, Advance Data No. 178. Washington, DC: U.S. Government Printing Office.

Fingerhut, L. A., Kleinman, J. C., Godfrey, E., & Rosenberg, H. (1991). *Firearm mortality among children, youth, and young adults 1–34 years of age, trends and current status: United States, 1979–88.* National Center for Health Statistics, Monthly Vital Statistics Report, Vol. 39, No. 11. Washington, DC: U.S. Government Printing Office.

Fingerhut, L. A., Makuc, D., & Kleinman, J. C. (1987). Delayed prenatal care and place of first visit: Differences by health insurance and education. *Family Planning Perspectives, 19,* 212–234.

Fink, A., & McCloskey, L. (1990). Moving child abuse and neglect prevention programs forward: Improving program evaluations. *Child Abuse and Neglect, 14,* 187–206.

Finkhelhor, D., Hotaling, G. T., & Yllö, K. (1988). *Stopping family violence: Research priorities for the coming decade.* Newbury Park, CA: Sage.

Finn, P., & Colson, S. (1990). *Civil protection orders: Legislation, current court practice, and enforcement.* Washington, DC: U.S. Department of Justice, Office of Justice Programs, National Institute of Justice.

Fiore, M. C., Novotny, T. E., Pierce, J. P., Hatziandreu, E. J., Patel, K. M., & Davis, R. M. (1989). Trends in cigarette smoking in the United States: The changing influence of gender and race. *Journal of the American Medical Association, 261,* 49–55.

Firman, J. (1983). Reforming community care for the elderly and disabled. *Health Affairs, 1,* 66–82.

First, R. J., Roth, D., & Arewa, B. D. (1988). Homelessness: Understanding the dimensions of the problem for minorities. *Social Work, 33,* 120–124.

Fischer, F. (1990). *Technocracy and the politics of expertise.* Newbury Park, CA: Sage.

Fitzpatrick, S., Johnson, J., Shragg, P., & Felice, M. E. (1987). Health care needs of Indochinese refugee teenagers. *Pediatrics, 79,* 118–124.

Flanagan, T. J., & Maguire, K. (Eds.). (1990). *Sourcebook of criminal justice statistics 1989* (NCJ-124224). Washington, DC: U.S. Department of Justice, Office of Justice Programs, Bureau of Justice Statistics.

Fleishman, J. A., Mor, V., & Piette, J. (1991). AIDS management: The client's perspective. *Health Services Research, 26,* 447–470.

Flinn Foundation. (1989). *Dealing with teen pregnancy: A multi-faceted dilemma.* Phoenix, AZ: Flinn Foundation.

Forbes, K. R., & Wegner, E. L. (1987). Compliance by Samoans in Hawaii with service norms in pediatric primary care. *Public Health Reports, 102,* 508–511.

Ford, D. E., Kamerow, D. B., & Thompson, J. W. (1988). Who talks to physicians about mental health and substance abuse problems? *Journal of General Internal Medicine, 3,* 363–369.

Fossett, J. W., Perloff, J. D., Peterson, J. A., & Kletke, P. R. (1990). Medicaid in the inner city: The case of maternity care in Chicago. *Milbank Quarterly, 68,* 111–141.

Fox, D. M. (1986). AIDS and the American health polity: The history and prospects of a crisis of authority. *Milbank Quarterly, 64*(Suppl. 1), 7–33.

Fox, D. M., & Thomas, E. H. (Eds.). (1989). *Financing care for persons with AIDS: The first studies, 1985–1988.* Frederick, MD: University Publishing Group.

Fox, H. B., & Newacheck, P. W. (1990). Private health insurance of chronically ill children. *Pediatrics, 85,* 50–57.

Francis, M. B. (1987). Long-term approaches to end homelessness. *Public Health Nursing, 4,* 230–235.

Frank, R. G. (1989). The medically indigent mentally ill: Approaches to financing. *Hospital and Community Psychiatry, 40,* 9–12.

Frank, R. G., & Kamlet, M. S. (1985). Direct costs and expenditures for mental health care in the United States in 1980. *Hospital and Community Psychiatry, 36,* 165–168.

Frank, R. G., & Kamlet, M. S. (1990). Economic aspects of patterns of mental health care: Cost variation by setting. *General Hospital Psychiatry, 12,* 11–18.

Frank, R. G., & McGuire, T. G. (1986). A review of studies of the impact of insurance on the demand and utilization of specialty mental health services. *Health Services Research, 21*(2, P. II), 241–265.

Franklin, J. L., Solovitz, B., Mason, M., Clemons, J. R., & Miller, G. E. (1987). An evaluation of case management. *American Journal of Public Health, 77,* 674–678.

Franks, A. L., Berg, C. J., Kane, M. A., Browne, B. B., Sikes, R. K., Elsea, W. R., & Burton, A. H. (1989). Hepatitis B virus infection among children born in the United States to Southeast Asian refugees. *New England Journal of Medicine, 321,* 1301–1305.

Freeman, H. E., & Levine, S. (Eds.). (1989). *Handbook of medical sociology* (4th ed.). Englewood Cliffs, NJ: Prentice-Hall.

Freeman, K. R., & Estrada-Mullaney, T. (1988). *Using dolls to interview child victims: Legal concerns and interview procedures.* Washington, DC: U.S. Department of Justice, Office of Justice Programs, National Institute of Justice.

Freeman, R. B., & Hall, B. (1986). *Permanent homelessness in America?* Working Paper No. 2013. Cambridge, MA: National Bureau of Economic Research.

Freiman, M. P., Arons, B. S., Goldman, H. H., & Burns, B. J. (1990). Nursing home reform and the mentally ill. *Health Affairs, 9*(4), 47–60.

Friedman, A. S., & Beschner, G. M. (Eds.). (1985). *Treatment services for adolescent substance abusers* (DHHS Publication No. ADM 89-1342). National Institute on Drug Abuse, Treatment Research Monograph Series. Washington, DC: U.S. Government Printing Office.

Friedman, S. R., Sotheran, J. L., Abdul-Quader, A., Primm, B. J., Des Jarlais, D. C., Kleinman, P., Mauge, C., Goldsmith, D. S., El-Sadr, W., & Maslansky, R. (1987). The AIDS epidemic among blacks and Hispanics. *Milbank Quarterly, 65*(Suppl. 2), 455–499.

Friedmann, J. (1987). *Planning in the public domain.* Princeton, NJ: Princeton University Press.

Fries, J. F. (1989). The compression of morbidity: Near or far? *Milbank Quarterly, 67,* 208–232.

Frieze, I. H. (1987). Editorial. *Violence and Victims, 2,* 83–87.

Frisman, L. K., & McGuire, T. G. (1989). The economics of long-term care for the mentally ill. *Journal of Social Issues, 45,* 119–130.

Fritz, M. E. (1989). Full circle or forward. *Child Abuse and Neglect, 13,* 313–318.

Gallin, R. S., & Given, C. W. (1976). The concept and classification of disability in health interview surveys. *Inquiry, 13,* 395–407.

Garbarino, J. (1986). Can we measure success in preventing child abuse? Issues in policy, programming, and research. *Child Abuse and Neglect, 10,* 143–156.

Garner, J., & Clemmer, E. (1980). *Danger to police in domestic disturbances: A new look.* Washington, DC: U.S. Department of Justice, Office of Justice Programs, National Institute of Justice.

Gelles, R. J. (1987a). *Family violence* (2nd ed.). Sage Library of Social Research, No. 84. Newbury Park, CA: Sage.

Gelles, R. J. (1987b). *The violent home* (rev. ed.). Sage Library of Social Research, No. 13. Newbury Park, CA: Sage.

Gelles, R. J., & Cornell, C. P. (1990). *Intimate violence in families* (2nd ed.). Family Studies Text Series, No. 2. Newbury Park, CA: Sage.

Gelles, R. J., & Straus, M. A. (1988). *Intimate violence: Causes and consequences of abuse in the American family.* New York: Simon & Schuster.

General Accounting Office [GAO]. (1985). *Homelessness: A complex problem and the federal response* (GAO-HRD-85-40). Washington, DC: U.S. Government Printing Office.

General Accounting Office. (1986). *Special education: Financing health and educa-*

tional services for handicapped children (GAO-HRD-86-62BR). Washington, DC: U.S. Government Printing Office.

General Accounting Office. (1987a). *Posthospital care: Discharge planners report increasing difficulty in placing Medicare patients* (GAO-PEMD-87-5BR). Washington, DC: U.S. Government Printing Office.

General Accounting Office. (1987b). *Prenatal care: Medicaid recipients and uninsured women obtain insufficient care* (GAO-HRD-87-137). Washington, DC: U.S. Government Printing Office.

General Accounting Office. (1988a). *Homeless mentally ill: Problems and options in estimating numbers and trends* (GAO-PEMD-88-24). Washington, DC: U.S. Government Printing Office.

General Accounting Office. (1988b). *Long-term care for the elderly: Issues of need, access, and cost* (GAO-HRD-89-4). Washington, DC: U.S. Government Printing Office.

General Accounting Office. (1989a). *AIDS: Delivering and financing health services in five communities* (GAO-HRD-89-120). Washington, DC: U.S. Government Printing Office.

General Accounting Office. (1989b). *AIDS forecasting: Undercount of cases and lack of key data weaken existing estimates* (GAO-PEMD-89-13). Washington, DC: U.S. Government Printing Office.

General Accounting Office. (1989c). *Board and care: Insufficient assurances that residents' needs are identified and met* (GAO-HRD-89-50). Washington, DC: U.S. Government Printing Office.

General Accounting Office. (1989d). *Children and youths: About 68,000 homeless and 186,000 in shared housing at any given time* (GAO-PEMD-89-14). Washington, DC: U.S. Government Printing Office.

General Accounting Office. (1989e). *Health care: Home care experiences of families with chronically ill children* (GAO-HRD-89-73). Washington, DC: U.S. Government Printing Office.

General Accounting Office. (1989f). *Homelessness: Homeless and runaway youth receiving services at federally funded shelters* (GAO-HRD-90-45). Washington, DC: U.S. Government Printing Office.

General Accounting Office. (1989g). *Mental health: Prevention of mental disorders and research on stress-related disorders* (GAO-HRD-89-97). Washington, DC: U.S. Government Printing Office.

General Accounting Office. (1989h). *Respite care: Insights on federal, state, and private sector involvement* (GAO-T-HRD-89-12). Washington, DC: U.S. Government Printing Office.

General Accounting Office. (1990a). *AIDS education: Programs for out-of-school youth slowly evolving* (GAO-HRD-90-111). Washington, DC: U.S. Government Printing Office.

General Accounting Office. (1990b). *Drug abuse: Research on treatment may not address current needs* (GAO-HRD-90-114). Washington, DC: U.S. Government Printing Office.

General Accounting Office. (1990c). *Homelessness: Access to McKinney Act pro-*

grams improved but better oversight needed (GAO-RCED-91-29). Washington, DC: U.S. Government Printing Office.

General Accounting Office. (1990d). *Home visiting: A promising early intervention strategy for at-risk families* (GAO-HRD-90-83). Washington, DC: U.S. Government Printing Office.

General Accounting Office. (1990e). *Medicaid: Sources of information on mental health services* (GAO-HRD-90-100). Washington, DC: U.S. Government Printing Office.

General Accounting Office. (1991a). *Drug abuse: The crack cocaine epidemic: Health consequences and treatment* (GAO-HRD-91-55FS). Washington, DC: U.S. Government Printing Office.

General Accounting Office. (1991b). *Trauma care: Lifesaving system threatened by unreimbursed costs and other factors* (GAO-HRD-91-57). Washington, DC: U.S. Government Printing Office.

Gerbert, B., & Maguire, B. T. (1989). Public acceptance of the Surgeon General's brochure on AIDS. *Public Health Reports, 104,* 130–133.

Gerbert, B., Maguire, B. T., & Coates, T. J. (1990). Are patients talking to their physicians about AIDS? *American Journal of Public Health, 80,* 467–469.

Geronimus, A. T., & Bound, J. (1990). Black/white differences in women's reproductive-related health status: Evidence from vital statistics. *Demography, 27,* 457–466.

Gerstein, D. R., & Harwood, H. J. (Eds.). (1990). *Treating drug problems* (Vol. 1). Washington, DC: National Academy Press.

Gibbs, J. T. (1988). Conceptual, methodological, and sociocultural issues in black youth suicide: Implications for assessment and early intervention. *Suicide and Life-Threatening Behavior, 18,* 73–89.

Gibney, F., Jr. (1987, June 8). In Texas, a grim new Appalachia: Desperate lives in the nation's poorest region. *Newsweek,* pp. 27–28.

Gibson, R. C., & Jackson, J. S. (1987). The health, physical functioning, and informal supports of the black elderly. *Milbank Quarterly, 65*(Suppl. 2), 421–454.

Glantz, M. D., Peterson, D. M., & Whittington, F. J. (Eds.). (1983). *Drugs and the elderly adult* (DHHS Publication No. ADM 83-1269). National Institute on Drug Abuse, Research Issues Series, No. 32. Washington, DC: U.S. Government Printing Office.

Glynn, T. J. (Ed.). (1980). *Drugs and the family.* National Institute on Drug Abuse. Washington, DC: U.S. Government Printing Office.

Glynn, T. J., Pearson, H. W., & Sayers, M. (Eds.). (1983). *Women and drugs* (DHHS Publication No. ADM 83-1268). National Institute on Drug Abuse, Research Issues Series, No. 31. Washington, DC: U.S. Government Printing Office.

Goedert, J. J. (1987). What is safe sex? Suggested standards linked to testing for human immunodeficiency virus. *New England Journal of Medicine, 316,* 1339–1342.

Gold, R. B., & Kenney, A. M. (1985). Paying for maternity care. *Family Planning Perspectives, 17,* 103–111.

Gold, R. B., Kenney, A. M., & Singh, S. (1987). Paying for maternity care in the United States. *Family Planning Perspectives, 19,* 190–206.

Golding, J. M., & Lipton, R. I. (1990). Depressed mood and major depressive disorder in two ethnic groups. *Journal of Psychiatric Research, 24,* 65–82.

Goldman, H. H., & Manderscheid, R. W. (1987). Chronic mental disorder in the United States. In R. W. Manderscheid & S. A. Barrett (Eds.), *Mental health, United States, 1987* (DHHS Publication No. ADM 87-1518). National Institute of Mental Health. Washington, DC: U.S. Government Printing Office.

Goldsmith, H. F., Lin, E., Bell, R. A., & Jackson, D. J. (Eds.). (1988). *Needs assessment: Its future.* (DHHS Publication No. ADM 88-1550). National Institute of Mental Health, Series BN, No. 8. Washington, DC: U.S. Government Printing Office.

Goodman, E., & Cohall, A. T. (1989). Acquired immunodeficiency syndrome and adolescents: Knowledge, attitudes, beliefs, and behaviors in a New York City adolescent minority population. *Pediatrics, 84,* 36–42.

Goolkasian, G. A. (1986). *Confronting domestic violence: The role of criminal court judges.* Washington, DC: U.S. Department of Justice, Office of Justice Programs, National Institute of Justice.

Goplerud, E. N. (Ed.). (1990). *Breaking new ground for youth at risk: Program summaries* (DHHS Publication No. ADM 89-1658). Office for Substance Abuse Prevention, Technical Report No. 1. Washington, DC: U.S. Government Printing Office.

Gordis, E. (1987–88). The genetic paradigm: Implications for research and treatment. *Alcohol Health and Research World, 12,* 96–97.

Gore, S. (1989). Social networks and social supports in health care. In H. E. Freeman & S. Levine (Eds.), *Handbook of medical sociology* (4th ed., pp. 306–331). Englewood Cliffs, NJ: Prentice-Hall.

Gorsky, R. D., & Colby, J. P., Jr. (1989). The cost effectiveness of prenatal care in reducing low birth weight in New Hampshire. *Health Services Research, 24,* 583–598.

Gortmaker, S. L., Clark, C.J.G., Graven, S. N., Sobol, A. M., & Geronimus, A. T. (1989). Reducing infant mortality in rural America: Evaluation of the rural infant care program. In G. H. DeFriese, T. C. Ricketts III, & J. S. Stein (Eds.), *Methodological Advances in Health Services Research* (pp. 91–116). Ann Arbor, MI: Health Administration Press.

Gottlieb, G. L. (1989). Diversity, uncertainty, and variations in practice: The behaviors and clinical decisionmaking of mental health care providers. In C. S. Taube, D. Mechanic, & A. A. Hohmann (Eds.), *The future of mental health services research* (DHHS Publication No. ADM 89-1600, pp. 225–251). National Institute of Mental Health. Washington, DC: U.S. Government Printing Office.

Gould, M. S., Wallenstein, S., & Davidson, L. (1989). Suicide clusters: A critical review. *Suicide and Life-Threatening Behavior, 19,* 17–29.

Gould, M. S., Wallenstein, S., Kleinman, M. H., O'Carroll, P., & Mercy, J. A. (1990). Suicide clusters: An examination of age-specific effects. *American Journal of Public Health, 80,* 211–212.

Graham, J. W., Johnson, C. A., Hansen, W. B., Flay, B. R., & Gee, M. (1990). Drug use prevention programs, gender, and ethnicity: Evaluation of three seventh-grade project SMART cohorts. *Preventive Medicine, 19,* 305–313.

Graitcer, P. L. (1989). Evaluating community interventions to reduce drunken driving. *American Journal of Public Health, 79,* 271.

Grazier, K. L. (1989). Long-term care services for the chronically mentally ill: Reimbursement system structure, effects, and alternatives. *Medical Care Review, 46,* 45–73.

Griss, B. (1988). Measuring the health insurance needs of persons with disabilities and persons with chronic illness. *Access to Health Care, 1*(1,2), 1–63.

Griss, B. (1989). Strategies for adapting the private and public health insurance systems to the health related needs of persons with disabilities or chronic illness. *Access to Health Care, 1*(3,4), 1–91.

Grob, G. N. (1987). Mental health policy in post–World War II America. In D. Mechanic (Ed.), *Improving mental health services: What the social sciences can tell us* (pp. 15–32). New Directions for Mental Health Services, No. 36. San Francisco: Jossey-Bass.

Grossman, D. C., Milligan, B. C., & Deyo, R. A. (1991). Risk factors for suicide attempts among Navajo adolescents. *American Journal of Public Health, 81,* 870–874.

Gurr, T. R. (Ed.). (1989). *Violence in America: The history of crime* (Vol. 1). Newbury Park, CA: Sage.

Gust, S. W., & Walsh, J. M. (Eds.). (1989). *Drugs in the workplace: Research and evaluation data* (DHHS Publication No. ADM 89-1612). National Institute on Drug Abuse, Research Monograph Series, No. 91. Washington, DC: U.S. Government Printing Office.

Guttmacher, S. (1984). Immigrant workers: Health, law, and public policy. *International Journal of Health Services, 14,* 503–514.

Gwinn, M., Pappaioanou, M., George, J. R., Hannon, W. H., Wasser, S. C., Redus, M. A., Hoff, R., Grady, G. F., Willoughby, A., Novello, A. C., Peterson, L. R., Dondero, T. J., Jr., & Curran, J. W. (1991). Prevalence of HIV infection in childbearing women in the United States: Surveillance using newborn blood samples. *Journal of the American Medical Association, 265,* 1704–1708.

Haaga, J., & Reuter, P. (Eds.). (1991). *Improving data for federal drug policy decisions: A RAND note.* Santa Monica, CA: RAND, Drug Policy Research Center.

Habib, J., Manton, K., Danon, D., Dowd, J. E., Galinsky, D., Kovar, M. G., Olshansky, S. J., & Suzman, R. (1988). Workshop: Forecasting the care needs of the elderly: Methodology and limitations. *Public Health Reports, 103,* 541–543.

Hagen, J. L., & Ivanoff, A. M. (1988). Homeless women: A high-risk population. *Affilia, 3*(1), 19–33.

Haines, D. W. (Ed.). (1989). *Refugees as immigrants: Cambodians, Laotians, and Vietnamese in America.* Totowa, NJ: Rowman and Littlefield.

Hamilton, J. M. (Ed.). (1985). *Psychiatric peer review: Prelude and promise.* Washington, DC: American Psychiatric Press.

Hamilton, V. L., Broman, C. L., Hoffman, W. S., & Renner, D. S. (1990). Hard times and vulnerable people: Initial effects of plant closing on autoworkers' mental health. *Journal of Health and Social Behavior, 31,* 123–140.

Hampton, R. L., & Newberger, E. H. (1985). Child abuse incidence and reporting by hospitals: Significance of severity, class, and race. *American Journal of Public Health, 75,* 56–60.

Hankin, J., & Oktay, J. S. (1979). *Mental disorder and primary medical care: An analytical review of the literature* (DHEW Publication No. ADM 78-661). National Institute of Mental Health, Series D, No. 5. Washington, DC: U.S. Government Printing Office.

Harder, W. P., Gornick, J. C., & Burt, M. R. (1986). Adult day care: Substitute or supplement? *Milbank Quarterly, 64,* 414–441.

Hardy, A. M. (1990). National Health Interview Survey data on adult knowledge of AIDS in the United States. *Public Health Reports, 105,* 629–634.

Hargreaves, W. A., & Shumway, M. (1989). Effectiveness of mental health services for the severely mentally ill. In C. A. Taube, D. Mechanic, & A. A. Hohmann (Eds.), *The future of mental health services research* (DHHS Publication No. ADM 89-1600, pp. 253–286). National Institute of Mental Health. Washington, DC: U.S. Government Printing Office.

Harrington, C., & Newcomer, R. J. (1983). *Social/health maintenance organizations: A new policy option for the aged and disabled.* San Francisco: Institute for Health and Aging.

Harrington, C., & Newcomer, R. J. (1991). Social health maintenance organizations' service use and costs, 1985–89. *Health Care Financing Review, 12*(3), 37–52.

Haseltine, W. A. (1989). Silent HIV infections. *New England Journal of Medicine, 320,* 1487–1489.

Haug, M., Belgrave, L. L., & Gratton, B. (1984). Mental health and the elderly: Factors in stability and change over time. *Journal of Health and Social Behavior, 25,* 100–115.

Haugaard, J. J., & Emery, R. E. (1989). Methodological issues in child sexual abuse research. *Child Abuse and Neglect, 13,* 89–100.

Haugaard, J. J., & Reppucci, N. D. (1988). *The sexual abuse of children: A comprehensive guide to current knowledge and intervention strategies.* San Francisco: Jossey-Bass.

Hayes, C. D. (Ed.). (1987). *Risking the future: Adolescent sexuality, pregnancy, and childbearing.* Washington, DC: National Academy Press.

Health Care Financing Administration [HCFA]. (1989). *Economic consequences of HIV (human immunodeficiency virus) infection for Medicaid and Medicare programs: An exploratory study.* Washington, DC: U.S. Government Printing Office.

Health Care Financing Administration. (1990). HCFA news briefs: Results of infant mortality survey available. *Health Care Financing Review, 11,* 203.

Health Insurance Association of America [HIAA]. (1989a). *AIDS case management: What health insurance companies are doing.* Washington, DC: Author.

Health Insurance Association of America. (1989b). *The cost of maternity care and childbirth in the United States, 1989* (R1589). Washington, DC: Author.

Health Resources and Services Administration [HRSA]. (1986). *Healthy mothers, healthy babies: A compendium of program ideas for serving low-income women* (DHHS Publication No. PHS 86-50209). Washington, DC: U.S. Government Printing Office.

Health Resources and Services Administration. (1988). *Managing AIDS: Services and resources.* Washington, DC: U.S. Government Printing Office.

Health Resources and Services Administration. (1989). *HRSA AIDS activities.* Washington, DC: U.S. Government Printing Office.

Health Resources and Services Administration. (1990). *AIDS service demonstration programs: 3 year report, 1987–1989.* Washington, DC: U.S. Government Printing Office.

Heath, L., Kruttschnitt, C., & Ward, D. (1986). Television and violent criminal behavior: Beyond the bobo doll. *Victims and Violence, 1,* 177–190.

Hedrick, S. C., & Inui, T. S. (1986). The effectiveness and cost of home care: An information synthesis. *Health Services Research, 20,* 851–880.

Hedrick, S. C., Koepsell, T. D., & Inui, T. S. (1989). Meta-analysis of home-care effects on mortality and nursing-home placement. *Medical Care, 27,* 1015–1026.

Hedrick, S. C., Rothman, M. L., Chapko, M., Inui, T. S., Kelly, J. R., Ehreth, J., & the Adult Day Health Care Evaluation Development Group. (1991). Adult day health care evaluation study: Methodology and implementation. *Health Services Research, 25,* 935–960.

Helfer, R. E. (1982). A review of the literature on the prevention of child abuse and neglect. *Child Abuse and Neglect, 6,* 251–261.

Helfer, R. E. (1987). The perinatal period, a window of opportunity for enhancing parent-infant communication: An approach to prevention. *Child Abuse and Neglect, 11,* 565–579.

Helfer, R. E., & Kempe, R. S. (Eds.). (1987). *The battered child* (4th ed.). Chicago: University of Chicago Press.

Hellinger, F. J. (1988a). Forecasting the personal medical care costs of AIDS from 1988 through 1991. *Public Health Reports, 103,* 309–319.

Hellinger, F. J. (1988b). National forecasts of the medical care costs of AIDS: 1988–1992. *Inquiry, 25,* 469–484.

Hellinger, F. J. (1990). Updated forecasts of the costs of medical care for persons with AIDS, 1989–1993. *Public Health Reports, 105,* 1–12.

Hellinger, F. J. (1991). Forecasting the medical care costs of the HIV epidemic: 1991–1994. *Inquiry, 28,* 213–224.

Helzer, J. E., Spitznagel, E. L., & McEvoy, L. (1987). The predictive validity of lay diagnostic interview schedule diagnoses in the general population. *Archives of General Psychiatry, 44,* 1069–1077.

Hendershot, G. E. (1990, November). *National health interview survey: Capabilities and constraints.* Paper presented at the meeting on the technical feasibility of a national health interview survey on disability. National Center for Health Statistics, Hyattsville, MD.

Henderson, D. C., & Anderson, S. C. (1989). Adolescents and chemical dependency. *Social Work in Health Care, 14,* 87–105.

Hendin, H. (1986). Suicide: A review of new directions in research. *Hospital and Community Psychiatry, 37,* 148–154.

Hendin, H. (1987). Youth suicide: A psychosocial perspective. *Suicide and Life-Threatening Behavior, 17,* 151–165.

Henry, K. (1988). Setting AIDS priorities: The need for a closer alliance of public health and clinical approaches toward the control of AIDS. *American Journal of Public Health, 78,* 1210–1212.

Hermann, R. C. (1988). Center provides approach to major social ill: Homeless urban runaways, "throwaways." *Journal of the American Medical Association, 260,* 311–312.

Hexter, A. C., Harris, J. A., Roeper, P., Croen, L. A., Krueger, P., & Gant, D. (1990). Evaluation of the hospital discharge diagnoses index and the birth certificate as sources of information on birth defects. *Public Health Reports, 105,* 296–307.

Hill, A. (1989). Treatment and prevention of alcoholism in the Native American family. In G. W. Lawson & A. W. Lawson (Eds.), *Alcoholism and substance abuse in special populations* (pp. 247–272). Rockville, MD: Aspen.

Hill, I. T. (1990). Improving state Medicaid programs for pregnant women and children. *Health Care Financing Review, Annual Supplement,* 75–87.

Hing, E., & Bloom, B. (1991). Long-term care for the functionally dependent elderly. *American Journal of Public Health, 81,* 223–225.

Ho, M. M. (1987). New horizons for home health care: Responses to prospective payment. *Public Health Nursing, 4,* 219–223.

Holden, C. (1988). Health problems of the homeless. *Science, 242,* 188–189.

Holder, H. D. (1987). Alcoholism treatment and potential health care cost saving. *Medical Care, 25,* 52–71.

Holinger, P. C., & Offer, D. (1981). Perspectives on suicide in adolescence. *Research in Community and Mental Health, 2,* 139–157.

Holzer, C. E., Shea, B. M., Swanson, J. W., Leaf, P. J., Myers, J. K., George, L., Weissman, M. M., & Bednarski, P. (1986). The increased risk for specific psychiatric disorders among persons of low socioeconomic status: Evidence from the epidemiologic catchment area surveys. *American Journal of Social Psychiatry, 4,* 59–71.

Hombs, M. E., & Snyder, M. (1982). *Homelessness in America: Forced march to nowhere.* Washington, DC: Community for Creative Non-Violence.

Hombs, M. E., & Snyder, M. (1983). *Homelessness in America: Forced march to nowhere* (2nd ed.). Washington, DC: Community for Creative Non-Violence.

Honigfeld, L. S., & Kaplan, D. W. (1987). Native American postneonatal mortality. *Pediatrics, 80,* 575–578.

Hooper, C. (1991). NIH, ADAMHA research may wed. *Journal of NIH Research, 3,* 38–40.

Hope, M., & Young, J. (1986). *The faces of homelessness.* Lexington, MA: Heath.

Hoppe, S. K., & Martin, H. W. (1986). Patterns of suicide among Mexican Americans and anglos, 1960–1980. *Social Psychiatry, 21,* 83–88.

Hotaling, G. T., Finkelhor, D., Kirkpatrick, J. T., & Straus, M. A. (Eds.). (1988a). *Coping with family violence: Research and policy perspectives.* Newbury Park, CA: Sage.

Hotaling, G. T., Finkelhor, D., Kirkpatrick, J. T., & Straus, M. A. (Eds.). (1988b). *Family abuse and its consequences: New directions in research.* Newbury Park, CA: Sage.

Hough, R. L., Landsverk, J. A., Karno, M., Burnam, M. A., Timbers, D. M., Escobar, J. I., & Regier, D. A. (1987). Utilization of health and mental health services by Los Angeles Mexican Americans and non-Hispanic whites. *Archives of General Psychiatry, 44,* 702–709.

Houk, V. N., & Thacker, S. B. (1989). The Centers for Disease Control program to prevent primary and secondary disabilities in the United States. *Public Health Reports, 104,* 226–230.

Hu, D. J., Covell, R. M., Morgan, J., & Arcia, J. (1989). Health care needs for children of the recently homeless. *Journal of Community Health, 14,* 1–8.

Hughes, S. L. (1985). Apples and oranges? A review of evaluations of community-based long-term care. *Health Services Research, 20,* 461–488.

Iglehart, J. K. (1987). Financing the struggle against AIDS. *New England Journal of Medicine, 317,* 180–184.

Immigration and Naturalization Service [INS]. (1990). *Statistical Yearbook of the Immigration and Naturalization Service.* Washington, DC: U.S. Government Printing Office.

Indian Health Service [IHS]. (1991). *Trends in Indian health 1991.* Washington, DC: U.S. Government Printing Office.

Infant Health and Development Program. (1990). Enhancing the outcomes of low-birth-weight, premature infants: A multisite, randomized trial. *Journal of the American Medical Association, 263,* 3035–3042.

Institute of Medicine [IOM]. (1980). *Alcoholism, alcohol abuse, and related problems: Opportunities for research.* Washington, DC: National Academy Press.

Institute of Medicine. (1985). *Preventing low birthweight.* Washington, DC: National Academy Press.

Institute of Medicine. (1986). *Confronting AIDS: Directions for public health, health care, and research.* Washington, DC: National Academy Press.

Institute of Medicine. (1987). *Causes and consequences of alcohol problems: An agenda for research.* Washington, DC: National Academy Press.

Institute of Medicine. (1988a). *Confronting AIDS: Update 1988*. Washington, DC: National Academy Press.

Institute of Medicine. (1988b). *The future of public health*. Washington, DC: National Academy Press.

Institute of Medicine. (1988c). *Homelessness, health, and human needs*. Washington, DC: National Academy Press.

Institute of Medicine. (1988d). *Prenatal care: Reaching mothers, reaching infants* (S. S. Brown, Ed.). Washington, DC: National Academy Press.

Institute of Medicine. (1989a). *Medical professional liability and the delivery of obstetrical care* (Vol. 1). Washington, DC: National Academy Press.

Institute of Medicine. (1989b). *Medical professional liability and the delivery of obstetrical care* (Vol. 2). Washington, DC: National Academy Press.

Institute of Medicine. (1989c). *Prevention and treatment of alcohol problems: Research opportunities* (Publication IOM-89-13). Washington, DC: National Academy Press.

Institute of Medicine. (1989d). *Research on children and adolescents with mental, behavioral, and developmental disorders: Mobilizing a national initiative*. Washington, DC: National Academy Press.

Institute of Medicine. (1990). *Broadening the base of treatment for alcohol problems*. Washington, DC: National Academy Press.

Institute of Medicine. (1991a). *The AIDS research program of the National Institutes of Health*. Washington, DC: National Academy Press.

Institute of Medicine. (1991b). *Disability in America: Toward a national agenda for prevention*. Washington, DC: National Academy Press.

Institute of Medicine. (1991c). *The second fifty years: Promoting health and preventing disability*. Washington, DC: National Academy Press.

Interagency Forum on Aging-Related Statistics. (1989). *Measuring the activities of daily living among the elderly: A guide to national surveys*. Federal Forum: A Final Report. Washington, DC: Brookings Institution.

International Center for the Disabled. (1986). *The ICD survey of disabled Americans: Bringing disabled Americans into the mainstream*. New York: Louis Harris and Associates.

Inter-University Consortium for Political and Social Research. (1981). *National crime surveys: National sample, 1973–1979*. Ann Arbor, MI: Author.

Ireys, H. T., Hauck, R. P., & Perrin, J. M. (1985). Variability among State Crippled Children's Service programs: Pluralism thrives. *American Journal of Public Health, 75*, 375–381.

Jacobs, P., & McDermott, S. (1989). Family caregiver costs of chronically ill and handicapped children: Method and literature review. *Public Health Reports, 104*, 158–163.

Jarvik, M. E. (1990). The drug dilemma: Manipulating the demand. *Science, 250*, 387–392.

Jaskulski, T., & Robinson, G. K. (1990). *The community support program: A review of a federal-state partnership*. Washington, DC: Mental Health Policy Resource Center.

Jazwiecki, T. (1986). Financing options for long-term care services. *Business and Health, 3*(5), 18–24.

Jellinek, M. S., Murphy, J. M., Bishop, S., Poitrast, F., & Quinn, S. D. (1990). Protecting severely abused and neglected children: An unkept promise. *New England Journal of Medicine, 323,* 1628–1630.

Jencks, C., & Peterson, P. E. (Eds.). (1991). *The urban underclass.* Washington, DC: Brookings Institution.

Jencks, S. F., Horgan, C., Goldman, H. H., & Taube, C. A. (1987). Bringing excluded psychiatric facilities under the Medicare prospective payment system: A review of research evidence and policy options. *Medical Care, 25*(Suppl.), S1–S51.

Jenkins, C.N.H., McPhee, S. J., Bird, J. A., & Bonilla, N. H. (1990). Cancer risks and prevention practices among Vietnamese refugees. *Western Journal of Medicine, 153,* 34–39.

Jerrell, J. M., & Hu, T. (1989). Cost-effectiveness of intensive clinical and case management compared with an existing system of care. *Inquiry, 26,* 224–234.

Jobes, D. A., Berman, A. L., & Josselson, A. R. (1987). Improving the validity and reliability of medical-legal certifications of suicide. *Suicide and Life-Threatening Behavior, 17,* 310–325.

Johnson, T. F., O'Brien, J. G., & Hudson, M. F. (Compilers). (1985). *Elder neglect and abuse: An annotated bibliography.* Bibliographies and Indexes in Gerontology, No. 1. Westport, CN: Greenwood Press.

Jones, C. L., & Battjes, R. J. (1990a). The context and caveats of prevention research on drug abuse. In C. L. Jones & R. J. Battjes (Eds.), *Etiology of drug abuse: Implications for prevention* (DHHS Publication No. ADM 90-1335, pp. 1–12). National Institute on Drug Abuse, Research Monograph Series, No. 56. Washington, DC: U.S. Government Printing Office.

Jones, C. L., & Battjes, R. J. (Eds.). (1990b). *Etiology of drug abuse: Implications for prevention* (DHHS Publication No. ADM 90-1335). National Institute on Drug Abuse, Research Monograph Series, No. 56. Washington, DC: U.S. Government Printing Office.

Jones, E. W., Densen, P. M., & Brown, S. D. (1989). Posthospital needs of elderly people at home: Findings from an eight-month follow-up study. *Health Services Research, 24,* 643–664.

Jones, K., & Vischi, T. (1979). Impact of alcohol, drug abuse, and mental health care utilization. *Medical Care, 17*(Suppl.), 1–82.

Joyce, T. (1987). The demand for health inputs and their impact on the black neonatal mortality rates in the U.S. *Social Science and Medicine, 24,* 911–918.

Joyce, T., Corman, H., & Grossman, M. (1988). A cost-effectiveness analysis of strategies to reduce infant mortality. *Medical Care, 26,* 348–360.

Justice, A. C., Feinstein, A. R., & Wells, C. K. (1989). A new prognostic staging system for the acquired immunodeficiency syndrome. *New England Journal of Medicine, 320,* 1388–1393.

Justice, B., & Justice, R. (1990). *The abusing family* (rev. ed.). New York: Plenum.

Kane, R. A., & Kane, R. L. (1988). Long-term care: Variations on a quality assurance theme. *Inquiry, 25,* 132–146.

Kane, R. L. (1990). Promoting the art of the possible in long-term care. *American Journal of Public Health, 80,* 15–16.

Kane, R. L., Kane, R. A., & Arnold, S. B. (1985). Prevention and the elderly: Risk factors. *Health Services Research, 19,* 945–1006.

Kanouse, D. E., Mathews, W. C., & Bennett, C. L. (1989). Quality-of-care issues for HIV illness: Clinical and health services research. In W. N. LeVee (Ed.), *Conference proceedings: New Perspectives on HIV-related Illnesses: Progress in Health Services Research* (DHHS Publication No. PHS 89-3449, pp. 159–169). Washington, DC: U.S. Government Printing Office.

Kaplan, H. B. (1989). Health, disease, and the social structure. In H. E. Freeman, & S. Levine (Eds.), *Handbook of medical sociology* (4th ed., pp. 46–68). Englewood Cliffs, NJ: Prentice-Hall.

Kaplan, J. (1986). Legal deterrents. *Bulletin of the New York Academy of Medicine, 62,* 601–607.

Kappel, S., Vogt, R. L., Brozicevic, M., & Kutzko, D. (1989). AIDS knowledge and attitudes among adults in Vermont. *Public Health Reports, 104,* 388–391.

Karno, M., Golding, J. M., Burnam, M. A., Hough, R. L., Escobar, J. I., Wells, K. M., & Boyer, R. (1989). Anxiety disorders among Mexican Americans and non-Hispanic whites in Los Angeles. *Journal of Nervous and Mental Disease, 177,* 202–209.

Karno, M., Hough, R. L., Burnam, M. A., Escobar, J. I., Timbers, D. M., Santana, F., & Boyd, J. H. (1987). Lifetime prevalence of specific psychiatric disorders among Mexican Americans and non-Hispanic whites in Los Angeles. *Archives of General Psychiatry, 44,* 695–701.

Katz, M. B. (1989). *The undeserving poor.* New York: Pantheon Books.

Keller, R. A., Cicchinelli, L. F., & Gardner, D. M. (1989). Characteristics of child sexual abuse treatment programs. *Child Abuse and Neglect, 13,* 361–368.

Kemper, P., Applebaum, R., & Harrigan, M. (1987). Community care demonstrations: What have we learned? *Health Care Financing Review, 8*(4), 87–100.

Kemper, P., & Murtaugh, C. M. (1991). Lifetime use of nursing homes. *New England Journal of Medicine, 324,* 595–600.

Kennedy, R. D., & Deapen, R. E. (1991). Differences between Oklahoma Indian infant mortality and other races. *Public Health Reports, 106,* 97–99.

Kessel, S. S., Kleinman, J. C., Koontz, A. M., Hogue, C.J.R., & Berendes, H. W. (1988). Racial differences in pregnancy outcomes. *Clinics in Perinatology, 15,* 745–754.

Kessler, R. C., & McRae, J. A., Jr. (1984). A note on the relationships of sex and marital status to psychological distress. *Research in Community and Mental Health, 4,* 109–130.

Khabbaz, R. F., Hartley, T. M., Lairmore, M. D., & Kaplan, J. E. (1990).

Epidemiologic assessment of screening tests for antibody to human T lymphotropic virus Type 1 (HTLV-1). *American Journal of Public Health, 80,* 190–192.

Kirp, D. L., Epstein, S., Franks, M. S., Simon, J., Conaway, D., & Lewis, J. (1989). *Learning by heart: AIDS and schoolchildren in America's communities.* New Brunswick, NJ: Rutgers University Press.

Kleinman, J. C., Fingerhut, L. A., & Prager, K. (1990). Differences in infant mortality by race, nativity status, and other maternal characteristics. *American Journal of Diseases of Children, 145,* 194–199.

Kleinman, J. C., & Kessel, S. S. (1987). Racial differences in low birth weight: Trends and risk factors. *New England Journal of Medicine, 317,* 749–753.

Kleinman, P. K., Blackbourne, B. D., Marks, S. C., Karellas, A., & Belanger, P. L. (1989). Radiologic contributions to the investigation and prosecution of cases of fatal infant abuse. *New England Journal of Medicine, 320,* 507–511.

Klerman, G. L. (1989). Psychiatric diagnostic categories: Issues of validity and measurement: An invited comment on Mirowsky and Ross. *Journal of Health and Social Behavior, 30,* 26–32.

Klerman, G. L. (1990). Paradigm shifts in the U.S.A. psychiatric epidemiology since World War II. *Social Psychiatry and Psychiatric Epidemiology, 25,* 27–32.

Knickman, J. R., Benjamin, A. E., & Duhman, N. C. (1988). *Comparing the cost effectiveness of alternative models for organizing services for persons with AIDS.* National Center for Health Services Research and Health Care Technology Assessment. Washington, DC: U.S. Government Printing Office.

Knight, B., & Walker, D. L. (1985). Toward a definition of alternatives to institutionalization for the frail elderly. *Gerontologist, 25,* 358–363.

Knitzer, J., & Olson, L. (1982). *Unclaimed children: The failure of public responsibility to children and adolescents in need of mental health services.* Washington, DC: Children's Defense Fund.

Knowles, J. (1977). Doing better and feeling worse: Health in the United States. *Daedalus, 106,* 1–278.

Knox, D. H. (1985). Spirituality: A tool in the assessment and treatment of black alcoholics and their families. In F. L. Brisbane & M. Womble (Eds.), *Treatment of black alcoholics* (pp. 31–44). New York: Haworth Press.

Knudsen, D. D. (1988). *Child protective services: Discretion, decisions, dilemmas.* Springfield, IL: Thomas.

Knudsen, D. D. (1989). Duplicate reports of child maltreatment: A research note. *Child Abuse and Neglect, 13,* 41–43.

Koff, T. H. (1988). *New approaches to health care for an aging population: Developing a continuum of chronic care services.* San Francisco: Jossey-Bass.

Koop, C. E. (1988). *The Surgeon General's letter on child sexual abuse* (HRS-MCH-88-13). Rockville, MD: Bureau of Maternal and Child Health and Resources Development.

Kosberg, J. I., Cairl, R. E., & Keller, D. M. (1990). Components of burden: Interventive implications. *Gerontologist, 30,* 236–242.

Kovar, M. G. (1986). Expenditures for the medical care of elderly people living in the community in 1980. *Milbank Quarterly, 64,* 100–132.

Kovess, V., & Fournier, L. (1990). The DISSA: An abridged self-administered version of the DIS: Approach by episode. *Social Psychiatry and Psychiatric Epidemiology, 25,* 179–186.

Kramer, A. M., Shaughnessy, P. W., Bauman, M. K., & Crisler, K. S. (1990). Assessing and assuring the quality of home health care: A conceptual framework. *Milbank Quarterly, 68,* 413–443.

Kraus, J. F., Sorenson, S. B., & Juarez, P. D. (Eds.). (1988). *Research Conference on Violence and Homicide in Hispanic Communities, September 14 and 15, 1987: Proceedings.* Office of Minority Affairs, U.S. Department of Health and Human Services. Los Angeles: UCLA Publication Services.

Krause, N. (1987). Satisfaction with social support and self-rated health in older adults. *Gerontologist, 3,* 301–308.

Kreitman, N. (1988). The two traditions in suicide research: Dublin Lecture. *Suicide and Life-Threatening Behavior, 18,* 66–72.

Kress, Y. (1989). Special issues of adult children of alcoholics. In G. W. Lawson & A. W. Lawson (Eds.), *Alcoholism and substance abuse in special populations* (pp. 139–164). Rockville, MD: Aspen.

Krout, J. A. (1983a). Correlates of service utilization among the rural elderly. *Gerontologist, 23,* 500–504.

Krout, J. A. (1983b). Knowledge and use of services by the elderly: A critical review of the literature. *International Journal of Aging and Human Development, 17,* 153–167.

Krug, S. E. (1989). Cocaine abuse: Historical, epidemiologic, and clinical perspectives for pediatricians. *Advances in Pediatrics, 36,* 369–406.

Krugman, R. D. (1989). The more we learn, the less we know "with reasonable medical certainty"? *Child Abuse and Neglect, 13,* 165–166.

Kulig, J. C. (1990). A review of the health status of Southeast Asian refugee women. *Health Care for Women International, 11,* 49–63.

Lammer, E. J., Brown, L. E., Anderka, M. T., & Guyer, B. (1989). Classification and analysis of fetal deaths in Massachusetts. *Journal of the American Medical Association, 261,* 1757–1762.

Lamphear, V. S. (1986). The psychosocial adjustment of maltreated children: Methodological limitations and guidelines for future research. *Child Abuse and Neglect, 10,* 63–69.

Langan, P. A. (1991). *Race of prisoners admitted to state and federal institutions, 1926–1986* (NCJ-125618). Washington, DC: U.S. Department of Justice, Office of Justice Programs, Bureau of Justice Statistics.

Langan, P. A., & Innes, C. A. (1986). *Preventing domestic violence against women.* Washington, DC: U.S. Department of Justice, Office of Justice Programs, Bureau of Justice Statistics.

Last, J. M. (Ed.). (1983). *A dictionary of epidemiology.* New York: Oxford University Press.

Laudicina, S. S., & Burwell, B. (1988). A profile of Medicaid home and community-based care waivers, 1985: Findings of a national survey. *Journal of Health Politics, Policy, and Law, 13,* 525–546.

Laumann, E. O., Gagnon, J. H., Michaels, S., Michael, R. T., & Coleman, J. S. (1989). Monitoring the AIDS epidemic in the United States: A network approach. *Science, 244,* 1186–1189.

Lave, J. R., & Goldman, H. H. (1990). Medicare financing for mental health care. *Health Affairs, 9*(1), 19–30.

Lawson, A. W. (1989). Substance abuse problems of the elderly: Considerations for treatment and prevention. In G. W. Lawson & A. W. Lawson (Eds.), *Alcoholism and substance abuse in special populations* (pp. 95–113). Rockville, MD: Aspen.

Lawson, G. W., & Lawson, A. W. (Eds.). (1989). *Alcoholism and substance abuse in special populations.* Rockville, MD: Aspen.

Layson, S. K. (1986). United States time-series homicide regressions with adaptive expectations. *Bulletin of the New York Academy of Medicine, 62,* 589–600.

Lazenby, H. C., & Letsch, S. W. (1990). National health expenditures, 1989. *Health Care Financing Review, 12*(2), 1–13.

Lee, E. (1988). Cultural factors in working with Southeast Asian refugee adolescents. *Journal of Adolescence, 11,* 167–179.

Leenaars, A. A. (1989). Are young adults' suicides psychologically different from those of other adults? Shneidman lecture. *Suicide and Life-Threatening Behavior, 19,* 249–263.

Lemp, G. F., Payne, S. F., Neal, D., Temelso, T., & Rutherford, G. W. (1990). Survival trends for patients with AIDS. *Journal of the American Medical Association, 263,* 402–406.

Leon, J., & Lair, T. (1990). *Functional status of the noninstitutionalized elderly: Estimates of ADL and IADL difficulties* (DHHS Publication No. PHS 90-3462). National Medical Expenditure Survey Research Findings 4, Agency for Health Care Policy and Research. Washington, DC: U.S. Government Printing Office.

Lester, D. (1988). Gun control, gun ownership, and suicide prevention. *Suicide and Life-Threatening Behavior, 18,* 176–180.

Lettieri, D. J., & Ludford, J. P. (Eds.). (1981). *Drug abuse and the American adolescent* (DHHS Publication No. ADM 81-1166). National Institute on Drug Abuse, Research Monograph Series, No. 38. Washington, DC: U.S. Government Printing Office.

Leventhal, J. M. (1987). Programs to prevent sexual abuse: What outcomes should be measured? *Child Abuse and Neglect, 11,* 169–172.

Levin, B. L., Glasser, J. H., & Jaffee, C. L., Jr. (1988). National trends in coverage and utilization of mental health, alcohol, and substance abuse services within managed health care systems. *American Journal of Public Health, 78,* 1222–1223.

Levine, C. (1990). AIDS and changing concepts of family. *Milbank Quarterly, 68*(Suppl. 1), 33–57.

Levine, D. S., & Levine, D. R. (1975). *The cost of mental illness, 1971* (DHEW Publication No. ADM 76-265). National Institute of Mental Health. Washington, DC: U.S. Government Printing Office.

Levine, D. S., & Willner, S. G. (1976). *The cost of mental illness, 1974.* National Institute of Mental Health, Statistical Note No. 125. Washington, DC: U.S. Government Printing Office.

Levine, I. S., & Haggard, L. K. (1989). Homelessness as a public health problem. In D. A. Rochefort (Ed.), *Handbook on mental health policy in the United States* (pp. 293–310). Westport, CT: Greenwood Press.

Levitan, S. A. (1990). *Programs in aid of the poor* (6th ed.). Baltimore, MD: Johns Hopkins University Press.

Lia-Hoagberg, B., Rode, P., Skovholt, C. J., Oberg, C. N., Berg, C., Mullet, S., & Choi, T. (1990). Barriers and motivators to prenatal care among low-income women. *Social Science and Medicine, 30,* 487–495.

Libow, L. S., & Starer, P. (1989). Care of the nursing home patient. *New England Journal of Medicine, 321,* 93–95.

Lieberman, E. J. (Ed.). (1975). *Mental health: The public health challenge.* Washington, DC: American Public Health Association.

Lieberman, L. R., & Orlandi, M. A. (1987). Alcohol advertising and adolescent drinking. *Alcohol Health and Research World, 12*(1), 30–33, 43.

Lindan, C. P., Hearst, N., Singleton, J. A., Trachtenberg, A. I., Riordan, N. M., Tokagawa, D. A., & Chu, G. S. (1990). Underreporting of minority AIDS deaths in San Francisco Bay area, 1985–86. *Public Health Reports, 105,* 400–405.

Lindblom, C. E. (1990). *Inquiry and change: The troubled attempt to understand and shape society.* New Haven, CT: Yale University Press.

Lindblom, C. E., & Cohen, D. K. (1979). *Usable knowledge: Social science and social problem solving.* New Haven, CT: Yale University Press.

Lindenthal, J. J., & Miller, S. I. (1989). Alcohol and drugs: A proposal to study sociocultural influences leading to alcoholism. *Medicine and Law, 8,* 37–44.

Lindsey, P. A., Jacobson, P. D., & Pascal, A. H. (1990). Medicaid home and community-based waivers for acquired immunodeficiency syndrome patients. *Health Care Financing Review, Annual Supplement,* 109–118.

Lin-Fu, J. S. (1988). Population characteristics and health care needs of Asian Pacific Americans. *Public Health Reports, 103,* 18–27.

Link, R. N., Feingold, A. R., Charap, M. H., Freeman, K., & Shelov, S. P. (1988). Concerns of medical and pediatric house officers about acquiring AIDS from their patients. *American Journal of Public Health, 78,* 455–459.

Linn, M. W., & Stein, S. (1989). Nursing homes as community mental health facilities. In D. A. Rochefort (Ed.), *Handbook on mental health policy in the United States* (pp. 267–292). Westport, CT: Greenwood Press.

Lipson, L., & Laudicina, S. S. (1991). *State home and community-based services for the aged under Medicaid: Waiver programs, optional services under the Medicaid state plan, and OBRA 1990 provisions for a new optional benefit.* Washington, DC: American Association of Retired Persons, Public Policy Institute.

Liu, K., Manton, K. G., & Liu, B. M. (1985). Home care expenses for the disabled elderly. *Health Care Financing Review, 7*(2), 51–58.

Liu, K., Manton, K. G., & Liu, B. M. (1990). Morbidity, disability, and long-term care of the elderly: Implications for insurance financing. *Milbank Quarterly, 68,* 445–450.

Lizotte, A. J. (1986). The costs of using gun control to reduce homicide. *Bulletin of the New York Academy of Medicine, 62,* 539–549.

Lorion, R. P., & Allen, L. (1989). Preventive services in mental health. In D. A. Rochefort (Ed.), *Handbook on mental health policy in the United States* (pp. 403–432). Westport, CT: Greenwood Press.

Lowe, B. F. (1988). Future directions for community-based long-term care research. *Milbank Quarterly, 66,* 552–571.

Lubitz, J., & Pine, P. (1986). Health care use by Medicare's disabled enrollees. *Health Care Financing Review, 7*(4), 19–31.

Luckey, J. W. (1987). Justifying alcohol treatment on the basis of cost savings: The "Offset" literature. *Alcohol Health and Research World, 12*(1), 8–15.

Lundgren, R. I., & Lang, R. (1989). "There is no sea, only fish": Effects of United States policy on the health of the displaced in El Salvador. *Social Science and Medicine, 28,* 697–706.

Lutterman, T. C., Mazade, N. C., Wurster, C. R., & Glover, R. W. (1988). Expenditures and revenues of state mental health agencies, 1981–1985. *Hospital and Community Psychiatry, 39,* 758–762.

Lynn, L. E., Jr., & McGeary, M.G.H. (Eds.). (1990). *Inner-city poverty in the United States.* Washington, DC: National Academy Press.

MacAdam, M., Capitman, J., Yee, D., Prottas, J., Leutz, W., & Westwater, D. (1989). Case management for frail elders: The Robert Wood Johnson Foundation's program for hospital initiatives in long-term care. *Gerontologist, 29,* 737–744.

McCall, N., Knickman, J., & Bauer, E. J. (1991). GrantWatch: Public/private partnerships: A new approach to long-term care. *Health Affairs, 10*(1), 164–176.

McCann, J. J. (1988). Long term home care for the elderly: Perceptions of nurses, physicians, and primary caregivers. *Quality Review Bulletin, 14,* 66–74.

McCaslin, R. (1988). Reframing research on service use among the elderly: An analysis of recent findings. *Gerontologist, 28,* 592–599.

McCormick, M. C. (1985). The contribution of low birth weight to infant mortality and childhood morbidity. *New England Journal of Medicine, 312,* 82–90.

Macdonald, D. I. (1987). Patterns of alcohol and drug use among adolescents. *Pediatric Clinics of North America, 34,* 275–288.

McDowall, D. (1986). Poverty and homicide in Detroit, 1926–1978. *Victims and Violence, 1,* 23–34.

McDowell, I., & Newell, C. (1987). *Measuring health: A guide to rating scales and questionnaires.* New York: Oxford University Press.

Macklin, E. D. (Ed.). (1989). *AIDS and families: Report of the AIDS Task Force: Groves Conference on Marriage and the Family.* New York: Haworth Press.

McLeer, S. V., & Anwar, R. (1989). A study of battered women presenting in an emergency department. *American Journal of Public Health, 79,* 65–66.

McLeod, J. D., & Kessler, R. C. (1990). Socioeconomic status differences in vulnerability to undesirable life events. *Journal of Health and Social Behavior, 31,* 162–172.

McMillan, A., & Gornick, M. (1984). The dually entitled elderly Medicare and Medicaid population living in the community. *Health Care Financing Review, 6*(2), 73–85.

McNellis, D. (1988). Specific federal programs for improving reproductive health care: What have we learned? In H. M. Wallace, G. Ryan, Jr., & A. C. Oglesby (Eds.), *Maternal and Child Health Practices* (3rd ed., pp. 401–407). Oakland, CA: Third Party.

McShane, D. (1988). An analysis of mental health research with American Indian youth. *Journal of Adolescence, 11,* 87–116.

Maddahian, E., Newcomb, M. D., & Bentler, P. M. (1986). Adolescents' substance use: Impact of ethnicity, income, and availability. *Advances in Alcohol and Substance Abuse, 5*(3), 63–78.

Magar, V. (1990). Health care needs of Central American refugees. *Nursing Outlook, 38,* 239–242.

Magaziner, J., & Cadigan, D. A. (1988). Community care of older women living alone. *Women and Health, 14,* 121–138.

Maiuro, R. D., & Eberle, J. E. (1989). New developments in research on aggression: An international report. *Violence and Victims, 4,* 3–15.

Maltsberger, J. T. (1986). *Suicide risk: The formulation of clinical judgment.* New York: New York University Press.

Maltsberger, J. T. (1988). Suicide danger: Clinical estimation and decision. *Suicide and Life-Threatening Behavior, 18,* 47–54.

Manton, K. G. (1989). Epidemiological, demographic, and social correlates of disability among the elderly. *Milbank Quarterly, 67*(Suppl. 2), 13–58.

Maris, R. (1986). Preface: Volume 16. *Suicide and Life-Threatening Behavior, 16.*

Markush, R. E., & Bartolucci, A. A. (1984). Firearms and suicide in the United States. *American Journal of Public Health, 74,* 123–127.

Marmor, T. R., & Gill, K. C. (1989). The political and economic context of mental health care in the United States. *Journal of Health Politics, Policy and Law, 14,* 459–475.

Marsella, A. J. (1978). Thoughts on cross-cultural studies on the epidemiology of depression. *Culture/Medicine and Psychiatry, 2,* 343–357.

Mason, J. O. (1991). Reducing infant mortality in the United States through "Healthy Start." *Public Health Reports, 106,* 479–483.

Mattson, M. R. (1984). Quality assurance: A literature review of a changing field. *Hospital and Community Psychiatry, 35,* 605–616.

Mayberry, R. M., & Lewis, R. F. (1990). Ten-year changes in birthweight distributions of black and white infants, South Carolina. *American Journal of Public Health, 80,* 724–726.

Mayfield, J. A., Rosenblatt, R. A., Baldwin, L.-M., Chu, J., & Logerfo, J. P. (1990). The relation of obstetrical volume and nursery level to perinatal mortality. *American Journal of Public Health, 80,* 819–823.

Mechanic, D. (1990). Treating mental illness: Generalist versus specialist. *Health Affairs, 9*(4), 61–75.

Mechanic, D., & Aiken, L. H. (1989a). Lessons from the past: Responding to the AIDS crisis. *Health Affairs, 9*(3), 16–32.

Mechanic, D., & Aiken, L. H. (Eds.). (1989b). *Paying for services: Promises and pitfalls of capitation.* New Directions for Mental Health Services, No. 43. San Francisco: Jossey-Bass.

Mechanic, D., Angel, R., & Davies, L. (1991). Risk and selection processes between the general and the specialty mental health sectors. *Journal of Health and Social Behavior, 32,* 49–64.

MEDSTAT. (1991, Summer). *MEDSTAT research notes.* Ann Arbor, MI: MEDSTAT Systems, Inc.

Meiners, M. R. (1984). *The state of the art in long-term care insurance* (NCHSR 84-67). Rockville, MD: National Center for Health Services Research and Health Care Technology Assessment.

Mercer, S. O. (1989). *Elder suicide: A national survey of prevention and intervention programs* (No. 8904). Washington, DC: American Association of Retired Persons, Public Policy Institute.

Mercy, J. A., & Houk, V. N. (1988). Firearm injuries: A call for science. *New England Journal of Medicine, 319,* 1283–1285.

Meyer, K. B., & Pauker, S. G. (1987). Screening for HIV: Can we afford the false positive rate? *New England Journal of Medicine, 317,* 238–241.

Miller, C. A., Fine, A., & Adams-Taylor, S. (1989). *Monitoring children's health* (2nd ed.). Washington, DC: American Public Health Association.

Miller, D. S., & Lin, E.H.B. (1988). Children in sheltered homeless families: Reported health status and use of health services. *Pediatrics, 81,* 668–673.

Miller, H. G., Turner, C. F., & Moses, L. E. (Eds.). (1990). *AIDS: The second decade.* Washington, DC: National Academy Press.

Mirowsky, J., & Ross, C. E. (1989a). Psychiatric diagnosis as reified measurement. *Journal of Health and Social Behavior, 30,* 11–25.

Mirowsky, J., & Ross, C. E. (1989b). Rejoinder—Assessing the type and severity of psychological problems: An alternative to diagnosis. *Journal of Health and Social Behavior, 30,* 38–40.

Mitchell, J. B. (1991). Physician participation in Medicaid revisited. *Medical Care, 29,* 645–653.

Momeni, J. A. (Ed.). (1989). *Homelessness in the United States: Vol. 1: State surveys.* Contributions in Sociology, No. 73. Westport, CT: Greenwood Press.

Momeni, J. A. (Ed.). (1990). *Homelessness in the United States: Vol. 2: Data and issues.* Contributions in Sociology, No. 87. Westport, CT: Greenwood Press.

Moncher, M. S., Holden, G. W., & Trimble, J. E. (1990). Substance abuse among Native-American youth. *Journal of Consulting and Clinical Psychology, 58,* 408–415.

Montgomery, K., Freeman, H. E., & Lewis, C. E. (1989). Coverage and readership of the U.S. Surgeon General's AIDS pamphlet in Los Angeles. *Medical Care, 27,* 758–761.

Montgomery, R.J.V. (1988). Respite care: Lessons from a controlled design study. *Health Care Financing Review, Annual Supplement,* 133–138.

Moon, M., Gaberlavage, G., & Newman, S. J. (Eds.). (1989). *Preserving independence, supporting needs: The role of board and care homes.* Washington, DC: American Association of Retired Persons, Public Policy Institute.

Moore, D. T. (1986). Issues and implications in genetics research. *Alcohol Health and Research World, 10*(4), 54–71.

Mor, V., Fleishman, J. A., Dresser, M., & Piette, J. (1992). Variation in health service use among HIV-infected patients. *Medical Care, 30,* 17–29.

Mor, V., Piette, J., & Fleishman, J. (1989). Community-based case management for persons with AIDS. *Health Affairs, 8*(4), 139–153.

Mor, V., Sherwood, S., & Gutkin, C. (1986). A national study of residential care for the aged. *Gerontologist, 26,* 405–417.

Moran, J. S., Janes, H. R., Peterman, T. A., & Stone, K. M. (1990). Increase in condom sales following AIDS education and publicity, United States. *American Journal of Public Health, 80,* 607–608.

Morrissey, J. P. (1989). The changing role of the public health hospital. In D. A. Rochefort (Ed.), *Handbook on mental health policy in the United States* (pp. 311–338). Westport, CT: Greenwood Press.

Morrissey, J. P., & Levine, I. S. (1987). Researchers discuss latest findings, examine needs of homeless mentally ill persons. *Hospital and Community Psychiatry, 38,* 811–812.

Moscicki, E. K. (1989). Epidemiologic surveys as tools for studying suicidal behavior: A review. *Suicide and Life-Threatening Behavior, 19,* 131–146.

Moscicki, E. K., O'Carroll, P., Rae, D. S., Locke, B. Z., Roy, A., & Regier, D. A. (1988). Suicide attempts in the epidemiologic catchment area study. *Yale Journal of Biology and Medicine, 61,* 259–268.

Mosher, J. F., & Colman, V. J. (1986). Prevention research: The model dram shop act of 1985. *Alcohol Health and Research World, 10*(4), 4–11, 35.

Mullahy, J., & Sindelar, J. (1989). Life-cycle effects of alcoholism on education, earnings, and occupation. *Inquiry, 26,* 272–282.

Munger, R. G. (1987). Sudden death in sleep of Laotian-Hmong refugees in Thailand: A case-control study. *American Journal of Public Health, 77,* 1187–1190.

Murphy, T. F. (1991). No time for an AIDS backlash. *Hastings Center Report, 21*(2), 7–11.

Murtaugh, C. M., Kemper, P., & Spillman, B. C. (1990). The risk of nursing home use in later life. *Medical Care, 28,* 952–962.

National Alliance to End Homelessness. (1988). *Housing and homelessness.* Washington, DC: Author.

National Alliance to End Homelessness. (1990). *Checklist for success: Programs to help the hungry and homeless.* Washington, DC: Author.

National Center for Education in Maternal and Child Health. (1988). *Starting early: A guide to federal resources in maternal and child health.* Washington, DC: Author.

National Center for Health Statistics [NCHS]. (1979, July). *Long-term health care: Minimum data set.* Final Report of the Technical Consultant Panel on the Long-term Health Care Data Set as Submitted to the National Committee on Vital and Health Statistics. Washington, DC: U.S. Government Printing Office.

National Center for Health Statistics. (1982). *Health, United States, 1982* (DHHS Publication No. PHS 83-1232). Washington, DC: U.S. Government Printing Office.

National Center for Health Statistics. (1983). *Health, United States, 1983* (DHHS Publication No. PHS 84-1232). Washington, DC: U.S. Government Printing Office.

National Center for Health Statistics. (1984a). *Health indicators for Hispanic, black, and white Americans* (DHHS Publication No. PHS 84-1576). Vital and Health Statistics Series 10, No. 148. Washington, DC: U.S. Government Printing Office.

National Center for Health Statistics (1984b). *Vital statistics of the United States, 1980: Vol. 1. Natality* (DHHS Publication No. PHS 85-1100). Washington, DC: U.S. Government Printing Office.

National Center for Health Statistics. (1985a). *Current estimates from the national health interview survey: United States, 1982* (DHHS Publication No. PHS 85-1578). Vital and Health Statistics Series 10, No. 150. Washington, DC: U.S. Government Printing Office.

National Center for Health Statistics. (1985b). *An inventory of alcohol, drug, and mental health data available from the National Center for Health Statistics* (DHHS Publication No. PHS 85-1319). Vital and Health Statistics Series 1, No. 17. Washington, DC: U.S. Government Printing Office.

National Center for Health Statistics. (1985c). *Vital statistics of the United States, 1980: Vol. 2. Mortality, Part A* (DHHS Publication No. PHS 85-1101). Washington, DC: U.S. Government Printing Office.

National Center for Health Statistics. (1986a). *Current estimates from the national health interview survey: United States, 1983* (DHHS Publication No. PHS 86-1582). Vital and Health Statistics Series 10, No. 154. Washington, DC: U.S. Government Printing Office.

National Center for Health Statistics. (1986b). *Current estimates from the na-*

tional health interview survey: United States, 1984 (DHHS Publication No. PHS 86-1584). Vital and Health Statistics Series 10, No. 156. Washington, DC: U.S. Government Printing Office.

National Center for Health Statistics. (1986c). *Current estimates from the national health interview survey: United States, 1985* (DHHS Publication No. PHS 86-1588). Vital and Health Statistics Series 10, No. 160. Washington, DC: U.S. Government Printing Office.

National Center for Health Statistics. (1986d). *Health, United States, 1986* (DHHS Publication No. PHS 87-1232). Washington, DC: U.S. Government Printing Office.

National Center for Health Statistics. (1986e). *Prevalence of selected chronic conditions: United States, 1979–81* (DHHS Publication No. PHS 86-1583). Vital and Health Statistics Series 10, No. 155. Washington, DC: U.S. Government Printing Office.

National Center for Health Statistics. (1986f). *Vital statistics of the United States, 1982: Vol. 2. Mortality, Part A* (DHHS Publication No. PHS 86-1122). Washington, DC: U.S. Government Printing Office.

National Center for Health Statistics. (1987). *Current estimates from the national health interview survey: United States, 1986* (DHHS Publication No. PHS 87-1592). Vital and Health Statistics Series 10, No. 164. Washington, DC: U.S. Government Printing Office.

National Center for Health Statistics. (1988a). *Current estimates from the national health interview survey: United States, 1987* (DHHS Publication No. PHS 88-1594). Vital and Health Statistics Series 10, No. 166. Washington, DC: U.S. Government Printing Office.

National Center for Health Statistics. (1988b). *Health of an aging America: Issues on data for policy analysis* (DHHS Publication No. PHS 89-1488). Vital and Health Statistics Series 4, No. 25. Washington, DC: U.S. Government Printing Office.

National Center for Health Statistics. (1988c). *Health, United States, 1987* (DHHS Publication No. PHS 88-1232). Washington, DC: U.S. Government Printing Office.

National Center for Health Statistics. (1988d). *Vital Statistics of the United States, 1985: Vol. 1. Natality* (DHHS Publication No. PHS 88-1113). Washington, DC: U.S. Government Printing Office.

National Center for Health Statistics. (1989a). *Current estimates from the national health interview survey, 1988* (DHHS Publication No. PHS 89-1501). Vital and Health Statistics Series 10, No. 173. Washington, DC: U.S. Government Printing Office.

National Center for Health Statistics. (1989b). *Health characteristics by occupation and industry of longest employment* (DHHS Publication No. PHS 89-1596). Vital and Health Statistics Series 10, No. 168. Washington, DC: U.S. Government Printing Office.

National Center for Health Statistics. (1989c). *Health, United States, 1988* (DHHS Publication No. PHS 89-1232). Washington, DC: U.S. Government Printing Office.

limiting chronic conditions among children. *American Journal of Public Health,* *76,* 178–184.

Newacheck, P. W., Budetti, P. P., & McManus, P. (1984). Trends in childhood disability. *American Journal of Public Health, 74,* 232–236.

Newacheck, P. W., & McManus, M. (1988). Financing health care for disabled children. *Pediatrics, 81,* 385–394.

Newcomer, R., Harrington, C., & Friedlob, A. (1990). Social health maintenance organizations: Assessing their initial experience. *Health Services Research, 25,* 425–454.

Nicaragua Health Study Collaborative at Harvard, CIES, and UNAN. (1989). Health effects of the war in two rural communities in Nicaragua. *American Journal of Public Health, 79,* 424–429.

Nickel, J. W. (1986, December). Should undocumented aliens be entitled to health care? *Hastings Center Report,* 19–23.

Nordlicht, S. (1986). Medical deterrents. *Bulletin of the New York Academy of Medicine, 62,* 582–588.

Norquist, G. S., Hough, R. L., Golding, J. M., & Escobar, J. I. (1990). Psychiatric disorder in male veterans and nonveterans. *Journal of Nervous and Mental Disease, 178,* 328–335.

Nyman, J. A., Cyphert, S. T., Russell, D. W., & Wallace, R. B. (1989). The ratio of impaired elderly in the community to those in nursing homes in two rural Iowa counties. *Medical Care, 27,* 920–927.

Oberg, C. N., Lia-Hoagberg, B., Hodkinson, E., Skovholt, C. J., & Vanman, R. (1990). Prenatal care comparisons among privately insured, uninsured, and Medicaid-enrolled women. *Public Health Reports, 105,* 533–535.

O'Carroll, P. W. (1989). A consideration of the validity and reliability of suicide mortality data. *Suicide and Life-Threatening Behavior, 19,* 1–16.

O'Carroll, P. W., Loftin, C., Waller, J. B., Jr., McDowall, D., Bukoff, A., Scott, R. O., Mercy, J. A., & Wiersema, B. (1991). Preventing homicide: An evaluation of the efficacy of a Detroit gun ordinance. *American Journal of Public Health, 81,* 576–581.

Office of Assistant Secretary for Planning and Evaluation. (1989). *Task I: Population profile of disability.* Washington, DC: U.S. Department of Health and Human Services, Office of Assistant Secretary for Planning and Evaluation.

Office of Assistant Secretary for Planning and Evaluation. (1990). *Task II: Federal programs for persons with disabilities.* Washington, DC: U.S. Department of Health and Human Services, Office of Assistant Secretary for Planning and Evaluation.

Office of the Attorney General. (1989). *Drug trafficking: A report to the President of the United States.* Washington, DC: U.S. Government Printing Office.

Office of Minority Health [OMH]. (1990). *Closing the gap: AIDS/HIV infection and minorities* (1990 0-860-815). Washington, DC: U.S. Government Printing Office.

Office of National Drug Control Policy. (1989). *National drug control strategy.* Washington, DC: U.S. Government Printing Office.

National Center for Health Statistics. (1989d). *The national nursing home survey: 1985 summary for the United States* (DHHS Publication No. PHS 89-1758). Vital and Health Statistics Series 13, No. 97. Washington, DC: U.S. Government Printing Office.

National Center for Health Statistics. (1989e). *Trends in low birth weight: United States, 1975–85* (DHHS Publication No. PHS 89-1926). Vital and Health Statistics Series 21, No. 48. Washington, DC: U.S. Government Printing Office.

National Center for Health Statistics. (1990a). *Advance report of final mortality statistics, 1988.* Monthly Vital Statistics Report Vol. 39, No. 7. Washington, DC: U.S. Government Printing Office.

National Center for Health Statistics. (1990b). *Advance report of final natality statistics, 1988.* Monthly Vital Statistics Report Vol. 39, No. 4. Washington, DC: U.S. Government Printing Office.

National Center for Health Statistics. (1990c). *AIDS knowledge and attitudes for April-June 1990: Provisional data from the National Health Interview Survey* (DHHS Publication No. PHS 91-1250). Advance Data No. 195. Washington, DC: U.S. Government Printing Office.

National Center for Health Statistics. (1990d). *Birth and fertility rates by education: 1980 and 1985* (DHHS Publication No. PHS 91-1927). Vital and Health Statistics Series 21, No. 49. Washington, DC: U.S. Government Printing Office.

National Center for Health Statistics. (1990e). *Current estimates from the national health interview survey, 1989* (DHHS Publication No. PHS 90-1504). Vital and Health Statistics Series 10, No. 176. Washington, DC: U.S. Government Printing Office.

National Center for Health Statistics. (1990f). *Health, United States, 1989* (DHHS Publication No. PHS 90-1232). Washington, DC: U.S. Government Printing Office.

National Center for Health Statistics. (1990g). *Vital statistics of the United States, 1987: Vol. 2. Mortality, Part A* (DHHS Publication No. PHS 90-1101). Washington, DC: U.S. Government Printing Office.

National Center for Health Statistics. (1990h). *Vital statistics of the United States, 1988: Vol. 1. Natality* (DHHS Publication No. PHS 90-1100). Washington, DC: U.S. Government Printing Office.

National Center for Health Statistics. (1991a). *Advance report of final natality statistics, 1989.* Monthly Vital Statistics Report Vol. 40, No. 8, Suppl. Washington, DC: U.S. Government Printing Office.

National Center for Health Statistics. (1991b). *Births, marriages, divorces, and deaths for 1990.* Monthly Vital Statistics Report Vol. 39, No. 12. Washington, DC: U.S. Government Printing Office.

National Center for Health Statistics. (1991c). *Health, United States, 1990* (DHHS Publication No. PHS 91-1232). Washington, DC: U.S. Government Printing Office.

National Center for Health Statistics. (1992a). *Advance report of final mortality statistics, 1989.* Monthly Vital Statistics Report, Vol. 40, No. 8, Suppl. 2. Washington, DC: U.S. Government Printing Office.

National Center for Health Statistics. (1992b). *Health, United States, 1991* (DHHS Publication No. PHS 92-1232). Washington, DC: U.S. Government Printing Office.

National Center on Child Abuse and Neglect. (1988). *Study findings: Study of national incidence and prevalence of child abuse and neglect: 1988.* Washington, DC: U.S. Government Printing Office.

National Commission on Children. (1991). *Beyond rhetoric: A new American agenda for children and families.* Washington, DC: Author.

National Commission to Prevent Infant Mortality. (1988a). *Death before life: The tragedy of infant mortality.* Washington, DC: Author.

National Commission to Prevent Infant Mortality. (1988b). *Malpractice and liability: An obstetrical crisis.* Washington, DC: Author.

National Commission to Prevent Infant Mortality. (1988c). *Prevent infant mortality: A resource directory.* Washington, DC: Author.

National Commission to Prevent Infant Mortality. (1989). *Home visiting: Opening doors for America's pregnant women and children.* Washington, DC: Author.

National Committee for Injury Prevention and Control. (1989). *Injury prevention: Meeting the challenge: A summary.* Newton, MA: Education Development Center.

National Institute on Aging [NIA]. (1989). *Dimensions of long-term care research at the National Institute on Aging: A report to the National Advisory Council on Aging.* Washington, DC: U.S. Government Printing Office.

National Institute on Drug Abuse [NIDA]. (1987). *Drug abuse and drug abuse research: Second triennial report to Congress from the Secretary, Department of Health and Human Services* (DHHS Publication No. ADM 87-1486). Washington, DC: U.S. Government Printing Office.

National Institute on Drug Abuse. (1988). *National household survey on drug abuse: Main findings 1985* (DHHS Publication No. ADM 88-1586). Washington, DC: U.S. Government Printing Office.

National Institute on Drug Abuse. (1990a). *Annual data, 1989: Data from the Drug Abuse Warning Network (DAWN)* (DHHS Publication No. ADM 90-1717). Statistical Series, Series I, No. 9. Washington, DC: U.S. Government Printing Office.

National Institute on Drug Abuse. (1990b). *National drug and alcoholism treatment unit survey (NDATUS): 1989 main findings report* (DHHS Publication No. ADM 91-1729). Washington, DC: U.S. Government Printing Office.

National Institute on Drug Abuse. (1990c). *Semiannual report: Data from the Drug Abuse Warning Network (DAWN)* (DHHS Publication No. ADM 90-1664). Statistical Series, Series G, No. 24. Washington, DC: U.S. Government Printing Office.

National Institute on Drug Abuse. (1991a). *Annual emergency room data, 1990: Data from the Drug Abuse Warning Network (DAWN)* (DHHS Publication No. ADM 90-1839). Statistical Series, Series I, No. 10-A. Washington, DC: U.S. Government Printing Office.

National Institute on Drug Abuse. (1991b). *Drug abuse and drug abuse research: Third triennial report to Congress from the Secretary, Department of Health and Human Services* (DHHS Publication No. ADM 91-1704). Washington, DC: U.S. Government Printing Office.

National Institute on Drug Abuse. (1991c). *National household survey on drug abuse: Highlights 1990* (DHHS Publication No. ADM 91-1789). Washington, DC: U.S. Government Printing Office.

National Institute on Drug Abuse. (1991d). *National household survey on drug abuse: Main findings 1990* (DHHS Publication No. ADM 91-1788). Washington, DC: U.S. Government Printing Office.

National Institute on Drug Abuse. (1991e). *National household survey on drug abuse: Population estimates 1990* (DHHS Publication No. ADM 91-1732). Washington, DC: U.S. Government Printing Office.

National Institute on Drug Abuse. (1991f). *Overview of the 1991 national household survey on drug abuse* (C-83-1-a). NIDA Capsules. Washington, DC: U.S. Government Printing Office.

National Institute on Drug Abuse. (1991g). *Summary of findings from the 1991 national household survey on drug abuse* (C-86-13). NIDA Capsules. Washington, DC: U.S. Government Printing Office.

National Institute on Drug Abuse. (1992). *Drug-related emergency room episodes: Drug abuse warning network (DAWN).* HHS News Release (May 12, 1992). Washington, DC: U.S. Government Printing Office.

National Institute of Mental Health [NIMH]. (1991). *Caring for people with severe mental disorders: A national plan of research to improve services* (DHHS Publication No. ADM 91-1762). Washington, DC: U.S. Government Printing Office.

National Maternal and Child Health Clearinghouse [NMCHC]. (1990). *Enhancing quality: Standards and indicators of quality of care for children with special health care needs.* Washington, DC: Author.

National Research Council [NRC]. (1985). *Injury in America: A continuing public health problem.* Washington, DC: National Academy Press.

National Research Council. (1988). *The aging population in the twenty-first century: Statistics for health policy.* Washington, DC: National Academy Press.

National Resource Center on Homelessness and Mental Illness. (1990). *Working with homeless children at risk for severe emotional disturbance.* Delmar, NY: Policy Research Associates.

Needleman, H. L. (1991). Childhood lead poisoning: A disease for the history texts. *American Journal of Public Health, 81,* 685–687.

Neergaard, J. A. (1990). A proposal for a foster grandmother intervention program to prevent child abuse. *Public Health Reports, 105,* 89–93.

Neighbors, H. W., Jackson, J. S., Campbell, L., & Williams, D. (1989). The influence of racial factors on psychiatric diagnosis: A review and suggestions for research. *Community Mental Health Journal, 25,* 301–311.

Newacheck, P. W., Budetti, P. P., & Halfon, N. (1986). Trends in activity-

Office for Substance Abuse Prevention [OSAP]. (1990a). *Citizen's alcohol and other drug prevention directory: Resources for getting involved* (DHHS Publication No. ADM 90-1657). Washington, DC: U.S. Government Printing Office.

Office for Substance Abuse Prevention. (1990b). *Proceedings of a National Conference on Preventing Alcohol and Drug Abuse in Black Communities, May 22–24, 1987* (DHHS Publication No. ADM 89-1648). Washington, DC: U.S. Government Printing Office.

Office of the Surgeon General. (1989). *Proceedings of the Surgeon General's Workshop on Drunk Driving.* Rockville, MD: U.S. Department of Health and Human Services, Public Health Service.

Office of Technology Assessment [OTA]. (1985). *Review of the public health service's response to AIDS: A technical memorandum* (OTA-TM-H-24). Washington, DC: U.S. Government Printing Office.

Office of Technology Assessment. (1986). *Children's mental health: Problems and services — A background paper* (OTA-BP-H-33). Washington, DC: U.S. Government Printing Office.

Office of Technology Assessment. (1987a). *The border war on drugs* (OTA-O-336). Washington, DC: U.S. Government Printing Office.

Office of Technology Assessment. (1987b). *Neonatal intensive care for low birthweight infants: Costs and effectiveness* (OTA-HCS-38). Washington, DC: U.S. Government Printing Office.

Office of Technology Assessment. (1987c). *Technology-dependent children: Hospital v. home care — A technical memorandum* (OTA-TM-H-38). Washington, DC: U.S. Government Printing Office.

Office of Technology Assessment. (1988a). *AIDS-related issues: AIDS and health insurance: An OTA survey.* Washington, DC: U.S. Government Printing Office.

Office of Technology Assessment. (1988b). *Healthy children: Investing in the future* (OTA-H-345). Washington, DC: U.S. Government Printing Office.

Office of Technology Assessment. (1989). *The use of preventive services by the elderly.* Washington, DC: U.S. Government Printing Office.

Office of Technology Assessment. (1990a). *AIDS-related issues: How has federal research on AIDS/HIV disease contributed to other fields?* Series on AIDS-Related Issues, Staff Paper No. 5. Washington, DC: U.S. Government Printing Office.

Office of Technology Assessment. (1990b). *Indian adolescent mental health* (OTA-H-446). Washington, DC: U.S. Government Printing Office.

Oktay, J. S., & Volland, P. J. (1990). Post-hospital support program for the frail elderly and their caregivers: A quasi-experimental evaluation. *American Journal of Public Health, 80,* 39–46.

Olds, D. L., Henderson, C. R., Jr., Chamberlin, R., & Tatelbaum, R. (1986). Preventing child abuse and neglect: A randomized trial of nurse home visitation. *Pediatrics, 78,* 65–78.

Olshansky, S. J., & Ault, A. B. (1986). The fourth stage of the epidemiologic transition: The age of delayed degenerative diseases. *Milbank Quarterly, 64,* 355–391.

Oppenheimer, G. M., & Padgug, R. A. (1986). AIDS: The risks to insurers, the threat to equity. *Hastings Center Report, 16*(5), 18–22.

Orbach, I. (1988). *Children who don't want to live: Understanding and treating the suicidal child.* San Francisco: Jossey-Bass.

Osgood, N. J., & McIntosh, J. L. (Eds.). (1986). *Suicide and the elderly: An annotated bibliography and review.* Westport, CT: Greenwood Press.

Padgett, D., Struening, E. L., & Andrews, H. (1990). Factors affecting the use of medical, mental health, alcohol, and drug treatment services by homeless adults. *Medical Care, 28,* 805–821.

Pagelow, M. D. (1984). *Family violence.* New York: Praeger.

Palfrey, J. S., Singer, J. D., Walker, D. K., & Butler, J. A. (1987). Early identification of children's special needs: A study in five metropolitan communities. *Journal of Pediatrics, 111,* 651–659.

Palmer, J. L., Smeeding, T., & Torrey, B. B. (Eds.). (1988). *The vulnerable.* Washington, DC: Urban Institute Press.

Panem, S. (1988). *The AIDS bureaucracy.* Cambridge, MA: Harvard University Press.

Paneth, N. (1990). Technology at birth. *American Journal of Public Health, 80,* 791–792.

Paneth, N., Kiely, J. L., Wallenstein, S., Marcus, M., Pakter, J., & Susser, M. (1982). Newborn intensive care and neonatal mortality in low-birth-weight infants: A population study. *New England Journal of Medicine, 307,* 149–155.

Partnership for the Homeless. (1987). *National growth in homelessness: Winter 1987: "Broken promises — broken lives."* New York: Author.

Partnership for the Homeless. (1989). *Moving forward: A national agenda to address homelessness in 1990 and beyond and a status report on homelessness in America.* New York: Author.

Pascal, A., Cvitanic, M., Bennett, C., Gorman, M., & Serrato, C. A. (1989). State policies and the financing of acquired immunodeficiency syndrome care. *Health Care Financing Review, 11,* 91–104.

Patrick, D. L., & Bergner, M. (1990). Measurement of health status in the 1990s. *Annual Review of Public Health, 11,* 165–183.

Patrick, D. L., & Peach, H. (Eds.). (1989). *Disablement in the community.* New York: Oxford University Press.

Payne, S. F., Rutherford, G. W., Lemp, G. F., & Clevenger, A. C. (1990). Effect of the revised AIDS case definition on AIDS reporting in San Francisco: Evidence of increased reporting in intravenous drug users. *AIDS, 4,* 335–339.

Pennbridge, J. N., Yates, G. L., David, T. G., & Mackenzie, R. G. (1990). Runaway and homeless youth in Los Angeles County, California. *Journal of Adolescent Health Care, 11,* 159–165.

Pepper Commission: U.S. Bipartisan Commission on Comprehensive Health

Care. (1990). *A call for action: Final report* (S. Prt. 101–114). Washington, DC: U.S. Government Printing Office.

Perrin, J. M., & Ireys, H. T. (1984). The organization of services for chronically ill children and their families. *Pediatric Clinics of North America, 31,* 235–257.

Petersen, L. R., White, C. R., & Premarital Screening Study Group. (1990). Premarital screening for antibodies to human immunodeficiency virus Type 1 in the United States. *American Journal of Public Health, 80,* 1087–1090.

Pfeffer, C. R. (Ed.). (1989). *Suicide among youth: Perspectives on risk and prevention.* Washington, DC: American Psychiatric Press.

Phillips, K. (1990). *The politics of rich and poor: Wealth and the American electorate in the Reagan aftermath.* New York: Random House.

Pickens, R. W., & Svikis, D. S. (Eds.). (1988). *Biological vulnerability to drug abuse* (DHHS Publication No. ADM 88-1590). National Institute on Drug Abuse, Research Monograph Series, No. 89. Washington, DC: U.S. Government Printing Office.

Piette, J., Fleishman, J. A., Mor, V., & Dill, A. (1990). A comparison of hospital and community case management programs for persons with AIDS. *Medical Care, 28,* 746–755.

Piper, J. M., Ray, W. A., & Griffin, M. R. (1990). Effects of Medicaid eligibility expansion on prenatal care and pregnancy outcome in Tennessee. *Journal of the American Medical Association, 264,* 2219–2223.

Piven, F. F., & Cloward, R. A. (1971). *Regulating the poor: The functions of public welfare.* New York: Random House.

Plant, M. A., Orford, J., & Grant, M. (1989). The effects on children and adolescents of parents' excessive drinking: An international review. *Public Health Reports, 104,* 433–442.

Poland, M. L., Ager, J. W., & Olson, J. M. (1987). Barriers to receiving adequate prenatal care. *American Journal of Obstetrics and Gynecology, 157,* 297–303.

Pollick, H. F., Rice, A. J., & Echenberg, D. (1987). Dental health of recent immigrant children in the Newcomer Schools of California. *American Journal of Public Health, 77,* 731–732.

Premo, F. H., & Wiseman, L. G. (Compilers). (1981). *Community mental health centers: Perspectives of the seventies: An annotated bibliography* (DHHS Publication No. ADM 81-1074). National Institute of Mental Health. Washington, DC: U.S. Government Printing Office.

Presidential Commission on the Human Immunodeficiency Virus Epidemic. (1988). *The report on human immunodeficiency virus epidemic.* Washington, DC: U.S. Government Printing Office.

President's Commission on Mental Health. (1978a). *Vol. 1: Report to the President.* Washington, DC: U.S. Government Printing Office.

President's Commission on Mental Health. (1978b). *Vol. 2: Appendix: Task panel reports.* Washington, DC: U.S. Government Printing Office.

President's Commission on Mental Health. (1978c). *Vol. 3: Appendix: Task panel reports.* Washington, DC: U.S. Government Printing Office.

Primm, B. J. (1990). AIDS: Today's and tomorrow's crisis. *Journal of Health Care for the Poor and Underserved, 1,* 185–195.

Public Health Reports. (1990a). CDC launches new AIDS-HIV public education campaign. *Public Health Reports, 105,* 544.

Public Health Reports. (1990b). Johnson-HUD funds provided for homeless in 9 cities. *Public Health Reports, 105,* 642–643.

Public Health Reports. (1990c). The nation's health bill for smoking: $52 billion. *Public Health Reports, 105,* 324–325.

Public Health Reports. (1991). HHS announces two new homeless health programs. *Public Health Reports, 106,* 350–351.

Public Health Service [PHS]. (1989). *Caring for our future: The content of prenatal care.* Washington, DC: U.S. Government Printing Office.

Public Health Service. (1990). *Healthy people 2000: National health promotion and disease prevention objectives: Full report, with commentary* (DHHS Publication No. PHS 91-50212). Washington, DC: U.S. Government Printing Office.

Public Health Service Task Force on Drug Abuse Data. (1990). *Report of the Public Health Service Task Force on Drug Abuse Data: Improving drug abuse statistics.* Washington, DC: Office of the Assistant Secretary for Planning and Evaluation.

Quinn, M. J., & Tomita, S. K. (1986). *Elder abuse and neglect: Causes, diagnosis, and intervention strategies.* New York: Springer.

Rand, M. R. (1990). *Handgun crime victims.* Washington, DC: U.S. Department of Justice, Office of Justice Programs, Bureau of Justice Statistics, Special Report.

Randall, T. (1990). Domestic violence intervention calls for more than treating injuries. *Journal of the American Medical Association, 264,* 939–940.

Rauschenbach, B., Frongillo, E. A., Jr., Thompson, F. E., Anderson, E.J.Y., & Spicer, D. A. (1990). Dependency on soup kitchens in urban areas of New York State. *American Journal of Public Health, 80,* 57–60.

Reamer, F. G. (1989). The contemporary mental health system: Facilities, services, personnel, and finances. In D. A. Rochefort (Ed.), *Handbook on mental health policy in the United States* (pp. 21–42). Westport, CT: Greenwood Press.

Redfield, R. R., & Tramont, E. C. (1989). Toward a better classification system for HIV infection. *New England Journal of Medicine, 320,* 1414–1416.

Regier, D. A., Boyd, J. H., Burke, J. D., Jr., Rae, D. S., Myers, J. K., Kramer, M., Robins, L. N., George, L. K., Karno, M., & Locke, B. Z. (1988). One-month prevalence of mental disorders in the United States. *Archives of General Psychiatry, 45,* 977–986.

Regier, D. A., Farmer, M. E., Rae, D. S., Locke, B. Z., Keith, S. J., Judd, L. L., & Goodwin, F. K. (1990). Comorbidity of mental disorders with alcohol and other drug abuse: Results from the epidemiologic catchment area (ECA) study. *Journal of the American Medical Association, 264,* 2511–2518.

Reich, T., Cloninger, C. R., Van Eerdewegh, P., Rice, J. P., & Mullaney, J. (1988). Secular trends in the familial transmission of alcoholism. *Alcoholism: Clinical and Experimental Research, 12,* 458–464.

Reuter, P. (1991). *On the consequences of toughness* (N-3447-DPRC). Santa Monica, CA: RAND.

Reyes, L. M., & Waxman, S. D. (1989). *A status report on hunger and homelessness in America's cities: 1989.* Washington, DC: U.S. Conference of Mayors.

Rhame, F. S., & Maki, D. G. (1989). The case for wider use of testing for HIV infection. *New England Journal of Medicine, 320,* 1248–1254.

Rice, D. P., Kelman, S., Miller, L. S., & Dunmeyer, S. (1990). *The economic costs of alcohol and drug abuse and mental illness: 1985.* San Francisco: University of California, Institute for Health and Aging.

Rice, D. P., MacKenzie, E. J., & Associates. (1989). *Cost of injury in the United States: A report to Congress, 1989.* San Francisco: University of California, Institute for Health and Aging.

Rice, T. (1987). An economic assessment of health care coverage for the elderly. *Milbank Quarterly, 65,* 488–520.

Rice, T. (1989). The use, cost, and economic burden of nursing-home care in 1985. *Medical Care, 27,* 1133–1147.

Ridgely, M. S., & Goldman, H. H. (1989). Mental health insurance. In D. A. Rochefort (Ed.), *Handbook on mental health policy in the United States* (pp. 341–361). Westport, CT: Greenwood Press.

Riley, M. W., Ory, M. G., & Zablotsky, D. (Eds.). (1989). *AIDS in an aging society: What we need to know.* New York: Springer.

Rivlin, A. M., Wiener, J. M., Hanley, R., & Spence, D. (1988). *Caring for the disabled elderly: Who will pay?* Washington, DC: Brookings Institution.

Rizzo, J. A., Marder, W. D., & Willke, R. J. (1990). Physician contact with and attitudes toward HIV-seropositive patients: Results from a national survey. *Medical Care, 28,* 251–260.

Robbins, C. (1989). Sex differences in psychosocial consequences of alcohol and drug abuse. *Journal of Health and Social Behavior, 30,* 117–130.

Robert Wood Johnson Foundation [RWJF]. (1985). *The perinatal program—what has been learned.* Special Report No. 3. Princeton, NJ: Author.

Robert Wood Johnson Foundation. (1986). *The rural infant care program.* Special Report No. 2. Princeton, NJ: Author.

Robert Wood Johnson Foundation. (1989). *Interfaith volunteer caregivers.* Special Report No. 1. Princeton, NJ: Author.

Robert Wood Johnson Foundation. (1990a). Day care center closes gap in services for disabled children. *Robert Wood Johnson Foundation—Advances, 4,* 10.

Robert Wood Johnson Foundation. (1990b). *Proceedings: AIDS Prevention and Services Workshop, February 15–16, 1990.* Princeton, NJ: Author.

Roberts, R. E., & Vernon, S. W. (1984). Minority status and psychological distress reexamined: The case of Mexican Americans. *Research in Community and Mental Health, 4,* 131–164.

Robertson, M. J., & Cousineau, M. R. (1986). Health status and access to health services among urban homeless. *American Journal of Public Health, 76,* 561–563.

Robins, L. N. (1989). Cross-cultural differences in psychiatric disorder. *American Journal of Public Health, 79,* 1479–1480.

Robins, L. N. (1990). Psychiatric epidemiology — a historic review. *Social Psychiatry and Psychiatric Epidemiology, 25,* 16–26.

Robins, L. N., Helzer, J. E., Croughan, J., & Ratcliff, K. S. (1981). National Institute of Mental Health diagnostic interview schedule: Its history, characteristics, and validity. *Archives of General Psychiatry, 38,* 381–389.

Robins, L. N., Helzer, J. E., Weissman, M. M., Orvaschel, H., Gruenberg, E., Burke, J. D., Jr., & Regier, D. A. (1984). Lifetime prevalence of specific psychiatric disorders in three sites. *Archives of General Psychiatry, 41,* 949–958.

Robinson, G. K., Meisel, J., & Guthierrez, L. (1990). *Long-term care legislation and mental illness: An analysis of current proposals.* Washington, DC: Mental Health Policy Resource Center.

Robinson, G. K., & Toff-Bergman, G. (1990). *Choices in case management: Current knowledge and practice for mental health programs.* Washington, DC: Mental Health Policy Resource Center.

Robinson, T. N., Killen, J. D., Taylor, C. B., Telch, M. J., Bryson, S. W., Saylor, K. E., Maron, D. J., Maccoby, N., & Farquhar, J. W. (1987). Perspectives on adolescent substance use: A defined population study. *Journal of the American Medical Association, 258,* 2072–2076.

Rodriguez, N. P., & Urrutia-Rojas, X. (1990). *Undocumented and unaccompanied: A mental-health study of unaccompanied, immigrant children from Central America* (IHELG Monograph 90-4). Houston, TX: University of Houston Law Center.

Rogler, L. H. (1989). The meaning of culturally sensitive research in mental health. *American Journal of Psychiatry, 146,* 296–303.

Rokaw, W. M., Mercy, J. A., & Smith, J. C. (1990). Comparing death certificate data with FBI crime reporting statistics on U.S. homicides. *Public Health Reports, 105,* 447–455.

Romeis, J. C. (1989). Caregiver strain: Toward an enlarged perspective. *Journal of Aging and Health, 1,* 188–208.

Rooks, J. P., Weatherby, N. L., Ernst, E.K.M., Stapleton, S., Rosen, D., & Rosenfield, A. (1989). Outcomes of care in birth centers: The national birth center study. *New England Journal of Medicine, 321,* 1804–1825.

Roos, N. P., & Havens, B. (1991). Predictors of successful aging: A twelve-year study of Manitoba elderly. *American Journal of Public Health, 81,* 63–68.

Ropers, R. H. (1988). *The invisible homeless: A new urban ecology.* New York: Human Sciences Press.

Rosenbaum, S., Hughes, D. C., & Johnson, K. (1988). Maternal and child health services for medically indigent children and pregnant women. *Medical Care, 26,* 315–332.

Rosenberg, M. L., Gelles, R. J., Holinger, P. C., Zahn, M. A., Stark, E., Conn, J. M., Fajman, N. N., & Karlson, T. A. (1987). Violence: Homicide, assault, and suicide. In R. W. Amler & H. B. Dull (Eds.), *Closing the gap: The burden of unnecessary illness.* New York: Oxford University Press.

Rosenberg, M. L., & Mercy, J. A. (1986). Homicide: Epidemiologic analysis at the national level. *Bulletin of the New York Academy of Medicine, 62,* 376–399.

Rosenberg, M. L., Smith, J. C., Davidson, L. E., & Conn, J. M. (1987). The emergence of youth suicide: An epidemiologic analysis and public health perspective. *Annual Review of Public Health, 8,* 417–440.

Rosenblatt, R. A. (1989). The perinatal paradox: Doing more and accomplishing less. *Health Affairs, 8,* 158–204.

Rosenfield, S. (1989). Psychiatric epidemiology: An overview of methods and findings. In D. A. Rochefort (Ed.), *Handbook on mental health policy in the United States* (pp. 45–65). Westport, CT: Greenwood Press.

Rosenheck, R., Gallup, P., Leda, C., Gorchov, L., & Errera, P. (1990, May). Help for the homeless: A progress report on the HCMI veterans program. *VA Practitioner,* pp. 53–56.

Rosenstein, M. J., Milazzo-Sayre, L. J., & Manderscheid, R. W. (1990). Characteristics of persons using specialty inpatient, outpatient, and partial care programs in 1986. In R. W. Manderscheid & M. A. Sonnenschein (Eds.), *Mental health, United States, 1990* (DHHS Publication No. ADM 90-1708, pp. 139–172). National Institute of Mental Health. Washington, DC: U.S. Government Printing Office.

Rossi, P. H. (1989). *Down and out in America: The origins of homelessness.* Chicago: University of Chicago Press.

Rossi, P. H. (1990). The old homeless and the new homelessness in historical perspective. *American Psychologist, 45,* 954–959.

Rossi, P. H., & Wright, J. D. (1987). The determinants of homelessness. *Health Affairs, 6*(1), 19–32.

Rossi, P. H., Wright, J. D., Fisher, G. A., & Willis, G. (1987). The urban homeless: Estimating composition and size. *Science, 235,* 1336–1341.

Roth, D., Bean, J., Lust, N., & Saveanu, T. (1985). *Homelessness in Ohio: A study of people in need: Statewide report.* Cincinnati, OH: Ohio Department of Mental Health, Office of Program Evaluation and Research.

Roth, L., & Fox, E. R. (1990). Children of homeless families: Health status and access to health care. *Journal of Community Health, 15,* 275–284.

Rothenberg, R. B., & Koplan, J. P. (1990). Chronic disease in the 1990s. *Annual Review of Public Health, 11,* 267–296.

Rowe, M. J., & Keintz, R. (1989). National survey of state spending for AIDS. *Intergovernmental AIDS Reports, George Washington University, 2*(3), 1–12.

Rowland, D., Lyons, B., Neuman, P., Salganicoff, A., & Taghavi, L. (1988). *Defining the functionally impaired elderly population.* Washington, DC: American Association of Retired Persons, Public Policy Institute.

Roy, A. W., Ford, A. B., & Folmar, S. J. (1990). The elderly and risk factors for institutionalization: Evidence from the Cleveland General Accounting Office (GAO) study, 1975–1984. *Journal of Applied Social Sciences, 14,* 177–195.

Rudd, M. D. (1990). An integrative model of suicidal ideation. *Suicide and Life-Threatening Behavior, 20,* 16–30.

Rumbaut, R. G., Chavez, L. R., Moser, R. J., Pickwell, S. M., & Wishik, S. M. (1988). The politics of migrant health care: A comparative study of Mexican immigrants and Indochinese refugees. *Research in the Sociology of Health Care, 7,* 143–202.

Rupp, A., Taube, C. A., Bodison, D., & Barrett, S. A. (1987). Medicaid and ambulatory mental health care: Utilization and costs. In R. W. Manderscheid & S. A. Barrett (Eds.), *Mental health, United States, 1987* (DHHS Publication No. ADM 87-1518). National Institute of Mental Health. Washington, DC: U.S. Government Printing Office.

Sable, M. R., Stockbauer, J. W., Schramm, W. F., & Land, G. H. (1990). Differentiating the barriers to adequate prenatal care in Missouri, 1987–88. *Public Health Reports, 105,* 549–555.

Sadoff, R. L. (1986). Sexual violence. *Bulletin of the New York Academy of Medicine, 62,* 466–476.

St. Clair, P. A., Smeriglio, V. L., Alexander, C. S., & Celentano, D. D. (1989). Social network structure and prenatal care utilization. *Medical Care, 27,* 823–832.

St. Clair, P. A., Smeriglio, V. L., Alexander, C. S., Connell, F. A., & Niebyl, J. R. (1990). Situational and financial barriers to prenatal care in a sample of low-income, inner-city women. *Public Health Reports, 105,* 264–267.

St. Denis, G. D., & Jaros, K. J. (Eds.). (1988). *Proceedings: Family Violence: Public Health Social Work's Role in Prevention, April 24–April 27, 1988.* Washington, DC: Bureau of Maternal and Child Health.

Sampson, R. J. (1986). The contribution of homicide to the decline of American cities. *Bulletin of the New York Academy of Medicine, 62,* 562–569.

Sanborn, C. J. (1990). Gender socialization and suicide: American Association of Suicidology Presidential Address, 1989. *Suicide and Life-Threatening Behavior, 20,* 148–155.

Sandler, R. H., & Jones, T. C. (Eds.). (1987). *Medical care of refugees.* New York: Oxford University Press.

Sardell, A. (1990). Child health policy in the U.S.: The paradox of consensus. *Journal of Health Politics, Policy and Law, 15,* 271–304.

Sargent, M. (1989). Update on programs for the homeless mentally ill. *Hospital and Community Psychiatry, 40,* 1015–1016.

Saunders, E. J. (1988). A comparative study of attitudes toward child sexual abuse among social work and judicial system professionals. *Child Abuse and Neglect, 12,* 83–90.

Savage, D. G. (1990, February 27). 1 in 4 young blacks in jail or in court control, study says. *Los Angeles Times,* p. 1.

Scallet, L. J. (1990). Paying for public mental health care: Crucial questions. *Health Affairs, 9*(1), 117–124.

Scallet, L. J., Marvelle, K., & Davidson, L. (1990). *Protection and advocacy for mentally ill individuals: Legislative history & analysis of P.L. 99-319.* Washington, DC: Mental Health Policy Resource Center.

Scanlon, W. J. (1988). A perspective on long-term care for the elderly. *Health Care Financing Review, Annual Supplement,* 7–15.

Scheffler, R. M., & Miller, A. B. (1989). Demand analysis of mental health service use among ethnic subpopulations. *Inquiry, 26,* 202–215.

Schene, P., & Bond, K. (Eds.). (1989). *Research issues in risk assessment for child protection.* Denver, CO: American Association for Protecting Children.

Scheper-Hughes, N. (Ed.). (1987). *Child survival: Anthropological perspectives on the treatment and maltreatment of children.* Dordrecht, Holland: Reidel.

Schinke, S. P., Moncher, M. S., Palleja, J., Zayer, L. H., & Schilling, R. F. (1988). Hispanic youth, substance abuse and stress: Implications for prevention research. *International Journal of Addictions, 23,* 809–826.

Schlesinger, M., & Kronebusch, K. (1990). The failure of prenatal care policy for the poor. *Health Affairs, 4,* 91–111.

Schulberg, H. C., & Burns, B. J. (1988). Mental disorders in primary care: Epidemiologic, diagnostic, and treatment research directions. *General Hospital Psychiatry, 10,* 79–87.

Schurman, R. A., Kramer, P. D., & Mitchell, J. B. (1985). The hidden mental health network. *Archives of General Psychiatry, 42,* 89–94.

Scitovsky, A. A. (1988). The economic impact of AIDS in the United States. *Health Affairs, 7,* 32–45.

Scitovsky, A. A. (1989a). Past lessons and future directions: The economics of health services delivery for HIV-related illnesses. In W. N. LaVee (Ed.), *Conference Proceedings: New Perspectives on HIV-related Illness: Progress in Health Services Research* (DHHS Publication No. PHS 89-3449, pp. 21–33). Washington, DC: U.S. Government Printing Office.

Scitovsky, A. A. (1989b). Studying the cost of HIV-related illnesses: Reflections on the moving target. *Milbank Quarterly, 67,* 318–344.

Scitovsky, A. A., & Rice, D. P. (1987). Estimates of the direct and indirect costs of acquired immunodeficiency syndrome in the United States, 1985, 1986, and 1991. *Public Health Reports, 102,* 5–17.

Scribner, R., & Dwyer, J. H. (1989). Acculturation and low birthweight among Latinos in the Hispanic HANES. *American Journal of Public Health, 79,* 1263–1267.

Sechrest, L., Freeman, H., & Mulley, A. (Eds.). (1989). *Conference Proceedings: Health Services Research Methodology: A Focus on AIDS* (DHHS Publication No. PHS 89-3439). Washington, DC: U.S. Government Printing Office.

Sedlak, A. J. (1991). *National incidence and prevalence of child abuse and neglect: 1988, Revised report.* Rockville, MD: Westat.

Segal, S. P., & Kotler, P. (1989). Community residential care. In D. A. Rochefort (Ed.), *Handbook on mental health policy in the United States* (pp. 237–265). Westport, CT: Greenwood Press.

Selby, M. L., Lee, E. S., Tuttle, D. M., & Loe, H. D., Jr. (1984). Validity of the Spanish surname infant mortality rate as a health status indicator for the Mexican American population. *American Journal of Public Health, 74,* 998–1002.

Selik, R. M., Buehler, J. W., Karon, J. M., Chamberland, M. E., & Berkelman, R. L. (1990). Impact of the 1987 revision of the case definition of acquired immune deficiency syndrome in the United States. *Journal of Acquired Immune Deficiency Syndromes, 3,* 73–82.

Selnow, G. W. (1987). Parent-child relationships and single and two parent families: Implications for substance usage. *Journal of Drug Education, 17,* 315–326.

Shadish, W. R., Jr. (1989). Critical multiplism: A research strategy and its attendant tactics. In L. Sechrest, H. Freeman, & A. Mulley (Eds.), *Conference Proceedings: Health Services Research Methodology: A Focus on AIDS* (DHHS Publication No. PHS 89-3439, pp. 5–28). Washington, DC: U.S. Government Printing Office.

Shadish, W. R., Jr., & Reis, J. (1984). A review of studies of the effectiveness of programs to improve pregnancy outcome. *Evaluation Review, 8,* 747–775.

Shapiro, E., & Tate, R. (1988). Who is really at risk of institutionalization? *Gerontologist, 28,* 237–245.

Shapiro, S., Skinner, E. A., Kessler, L. G., Von Korff, M., German, P. S., Tischler, G. L., Leaf, P. J., Benhan, L., Cottler, L., & Regier, D. A. (1984). Utilization of health and mental health services: Three epidemiologic catchment area sites. *Archives of General Psychiatry, 41,* 971–978.

Shapiro, S., Skinner, E. A., Kramer, M., Steinwachs, D. M., & Regier, D. A. (1985). Measuring need for mental health services in a general population. *Medical Care, 23,* 1033–1043.

Shaughnessy, P. W. (1985). Long-term care research and public policy. *Health Services Research, 20,* 490–499.

Shaughnessy, P. W., & Kramer, A. (1990). The increased needs of patients in nursing homes and patients receiving home health care. *New England Journal of Medicine, 322,* 21–27.

Shelp, E. E., DuBose, E. R., & Sunderland, R. H. (1990). The infrastructure of religious communities: A neglected resource for care of people with AIDS. *American Journal of Public Health, 80,* 970–972.

Shelton, T. L., Jeppson, E. S., & Johnson, B. H. (1989). *Family-centered care for children with special health care needs* (2nd ed.). Washington, DC: Association for the Care of Children's Health.

Short, P. F. (1990). *Estimates of the uninsured population, calendar year 1987* (DHHS Publication No. PHS 90-3469). National Medical Expenditure Survey Data Summary 2, Agency for Health Care Policy and Research. Washington, DC: U.S. Government Printing Office.

Short, P. F., & Leon, J. (1990). *Use of home and community services by persons ages 65 and older with functional difficulties* (DHHS Publication No. PHS 90-3466). National Medical Expenditure Survey Research Findings 5, Agency for Health Care Policy and Research. Washington, DC: U.S. Government Printing Office.

Shulsinger, E. (1990). Needs of sheltered homeless children. *Journal of Pediatric Health Care, 4*(3), 136–140.

Shy, K. K., Luthy, D. A., Bennett, F. C., & Whitfield, M. (1990). Effects of electronic fetal-heart-rate monitoring, as compared with periodic auscultation, on the neurologic development of premature infants. *New England Journal of Medicine, 322,* 588–593.

Siddharthan, K. (1990). HMO enrollment by Medicare beneficiaries in heterogeneous communities. *Medical Care, 28,* 918–927.

Silverman, H. A. (1990). Health care financing note: Use of Medicare-covered home health agency services, 1988. *Health Care Financing Review, 12*(2), 113–126.

Silverman, J. (1989). The contribution of social services to preventing youth suicide. In M. L. Rosenberg & K. Baer (Eds.), *Report of the Secretary's Task Force on Youth Suicide: Vol. 4. Strategies for the prevention of youth suicide* (DHHS Publication No. ADM 89-1624, pp. 168–170). Alcohol, Drug Abuse, and Mental Health Administration. Washington, DC: U.S. Government Printing Office.

Simon, J. L. (1991). The case for greatly increased immigration. *Public Interest, 102,* 89–118.

Singer, J. D., Butler, J. A., & Palfrey, J. S. (1986). Health care access and use among handicapped students in five public school systems. *Medical Care, 24,* 1–13.

Skogan, W. G. (1990). The polls — a review: The national crime survey redesign. *Public Opinion Quarterly, 54,* 256–272.

Slap, G. B., Vorters, D. F., Chaudhuri, S., & Centor, R. M. (1989). Risk factors for attempted suicide during adolescence. *Pediatrics, 84,* 762–772.

Sloan, J. H., Kellerman, A. L., Reay, D. T., Ferris, J. A., Koepsell, T., Rivara, F. P., Rice, C., Gray, L., & LoGerfo, J. (1988). Handgun regulations, crime, assaults, and homicide: A tale of two cities. *New England Journal of Medicine, 319,* 1256–1262.

Smeeding, T. M., & Straub, L. (1987). Health care financing among the elderly: Who really pays the bills? *Journal of Health Politics, Policy and Law, 12,* 35–52.

Smith, J. C., Mercy, J. A., & Rosenberg, M. L. (1986). Suicide and homicide among Hispanics in the Southwest. *Public Health Reports, 101,* 265–270.

Smith, P. B. (1986). Sociologic aspects of adolescent fertility and childbearing among Hispanics. *Developmental and Behavioral Pediatrics, 7,* 346–349.

Smith, S. (1989). National Center for Health Statistics data line. *Public Health Reports, 104,* 307–308.

Solnit, A. J. (1987). Child placement conflicts: New approaches. *Child Abuse and Neglect, 11,* 455–460.

Solomon, M. Z., & DeJong, W. (1989). Preventing AIDS and other STDs through condom promotion: A patient education intervention. *American Journal of Public Health, 79,* 453–458.

Somers, A. R. (1987). Insurance for long-term care: Some definitions, problems, and guidelines for action. *New England Journal of Medicine, 317,* 23–29.

Somers, S. A., & Merrill, J. C. (1991). Foundation response: Supporting states' efforts to provide long-term care insurance. *Health Affairs, 10,* 177–179.

Somervell, P. D., Leaf, P. J., Weissman, M. M., Blazer, D. G., & Bruce, M. L. (1989). The prevalence of major depression in black and white adults in five United States communities. *American Journal of Epidemiology, 130,* 725–735.

Sorenson, S. B., & Golding, J. M. (1988). Prevalence of suicide attempts in a Mexican-American population: Prevention implications of immigration and cultural issues. *Suicide and Life-Threatening Behavior, 18,* 322–333.

Southern Regional Project on Infant Mortality. (1989). *A bold step: The South acts to reduce infant mortality.* Washington, DC: Author.

Spector, W. D. (1990). Functional disability scales. In B. Spilker (Ed.), *Quality of life assessment in clinical trials* (pp. 115–129). New York: Raven Press.

Spiegler, D., Tate, D., Aitken, S., & Christian, C. (Eds.). (1989). *Alcohol use among U.S. ethnic minorities: Proceedings of a Conference on the Epidemiology of Alcohol Use and Abuse Among Ethnic Minority Groups* (DHHS Publication No. ADM 89-1435). National Institute on Alcohol Abuse Administration, Research Monograph Series, No. 18. Washington, DC: U.S. Government Printing Office.

Spilker, B., Molinek, F. R., Jr., Johnston, K. A., Simpson, R. L., Jr., & Tilson, H. H. (1990). Quality of life bibliography and indexes. *Medical Care, 28*(Suppl.), DS1–DS77.

Spitzer, W. O. (1987). State of science 1986: Quality of life and functional status as target variables for research. *Journal of Chronic Diseases, 40,* 465–471.

Spohn, P. H., Bergthold, L., & Estes, C. L. (1988). From cottages to condos: The expansion of the home health care industry under Medicare. *Home Health Care Services Quarterly, 8*(4), 25–55.

Stack, S. (1987). The sociological study of suicide: Methodological issues. *Suicide and Life-Threatening Behavior, 17,* 133–150.

Stafford, M. C., & Weisheit, R. A. (1988). Changing age patterns of U.S. male and female suicide rates, 1934–1983. *Suicide and Life-Threatening Behavior, 18,* 149–163.

Starfield, B. (1989). Preventive interventions in the health and health-related sectors with potential relevance for youth suicide. In M. L. Rosenberg & K. Baer (Eds.), *Report of the Secretary's Task Force on Youth Suicide: Vol. 4. Strategies for the prevention of youth suicide* (DHHS Publication No. ADM

89-1624, pp. 145–167). Alcohol, Drug Abuse, and Mental Health Administration. Washington, DC: U.S. Government Printing Office.

Stark, E. (1990). Rethinking homicide: Violence, race, and the politics of gender. *International Journal of Health Services, 20*, 3–26.

Stehr-Green, J. K., & Schantz, P. M. (1986). Trichinosis in Southeast Asian refugees in the United States. *American Journal of Public Health, 76*, 1238–1239.

Stein, R.E.K. (Ed.). (1989). *Caring for children with chronic illness: Issues and strategies.* New York: Springer.

Stein, R.E.K., Gortmaker, S. L., Perrin, E. C., Perrin, J. M., Pless, I. B., Walker, D. K., & Weitzman, M. (1987). Severity of illness: Concepts and measurements. *Lancet, 2*, 1506–1509.

Steinmetz, S. K. (1988). *Duty bound: Elder abuse and family care.* Sage Library of Social Research, Vol. 166. Newbury Park, CA: Sage.

Stephens, B. J. (1987). Cheap thrills and humble pie: The adolescence of female suicide attempters. *Suicide and Life-Threatening Behavior, 17*, 107–118.

Stephens, D., Dennis, E., Toomer, M., & Holloway, J. (1991). The diversity of case management needs for the care of homeless persons. *Public Health Reports, 106*, 15–19.

Stephens, R. C., Feucht, T. E., & Roman, S. W. (1991). Effects of an intervention program on AIDS-related drug and needle behavior among intravenous drug users. *American Journal of Public Health, 81*, 568–571.

Sterling, T. D., & Weinkam, J. J. (1989). Comparison of smoking-related risk factors among black and white males. *American Journal of Industrial Medicine, 15*, 319–333.

Stewart, A. L., Greenfield, S., Hays, R. D., Wells, K., Rogers, W. H., Berry, S. D., McGlynn, E. A., & Ware, J. E., Jr. (1989). Functional status and well-being of patients with chronic conditions. *Journal of the American Medical Association, 262*, 907–913.

Stoller, E. P. (1984). Self-assessment of health by the elderly: The impact of informal assistance. *Journal of Health and Social Behavior, 25*, 260–270.

Stone, R. I. (1989). The feminization of poverty among the elderly. *Women's Studies Quarterly, 17*, 20–45.

Stone, R. I., Cafferata, G. L., & Sangl, J. (1987). Caregivers of the frail elderly: A national profile. *Gerontologist, 27*, 616–626.

Stone, R. I., & Kemper, P. (1989). Spouses and children of disabled elders: How large a constituency for long-term care reform? *Milbank Quarterly, 67*, 485–506.

Stone, R. I., & Murtaugh, C. M. (1990). The elderly population with chronic functional disability: Implications for home care eligibility. *Gerontologist, 30*, 491–496.

Stone, R. I., & Short, P. F. (1990). The competing demands of employment and informal caregiving to disabled elders. *Medical Care, 28*, 513–526.

Strahan, G. W. (1990). Prevalence of selected mental disorders in nursing and related care homes. In R. W. Manderscheid & M. A. Sonnenschein (Eds.), *Mental health, United States, 1990* (DHHS Publication No. ADM 90-1708, pp. 227–240). National Institute of Mental Health. Washington, DC: U.S. Government Printing Office.

Straus, M. A. (1986). Domestic violence and homicide antecedents. *Bulletin of the New York Academy of Medicine, 62,* 446–466.

Straus, M. A., Gelles, R. J., & Steinmetz, S. K. (1981). *Behind closed doors: Violence in the American family.* Newbury Park, CA: Sage.

Straus, M. B. (Ed.). (1988). *Abuse and victimization across the life span.* Baltimore, MD: Johns Hopkins University Press.

Strauss, A., & Corbin, J. M. (1988). *Shaping a new health care system: The explosion of chronic illness as a catalyst for change.* San Francisco: Jossey-Bass.

Streiner, D. L., & Adam, K. S. (1987). Evaluation of the effectiveness of suicide prevention programs: A methodological perspective. *Suicide and Life-threatening Behavior, 17,* 93–106.

Stubbs, P. E. (1988). Head start. In H. M. Wallace, G. Ryan, Jr., & A. C. Oglesby (Eds.), *Maternal and child health practices* (3rd ed., pp. 455–462). Oakland, CA: Third Party.

Survey shows HIV reporting practices in 50 states. (1989). *American Journal of Public Health, 79,* 581.

Swartz, M., Carroll, B., & Blazer, D. (1989). In response to "Psychiatric diagnosis as reified measurement": An invited comment on Mirowsky and Ross. *Journal of Health and Social Behavior, 30,* 33–34.

Taeuber, C. M., & Siegel, P. M. (1990, November). *Counting the nation's homeless population in the 1990 Census.* Paper presented at the Conference on Enumerating Homeless Persons: Methods and Data Needs, Washington, DC.

Tatara, T. (1990). *Summaries of national elder abuse data: An exploratory study of state statistics: Based on a survey of state adult protective service and aging agencies.* Washington, DC: National Aging Resource Center on Elder Abuse.

Taube, C. A. (Ed.). (1986). Mental health services use and demand: A special supplement. *Health Services Research, 21*(2, P. II), v–vii, 241–352.

Taube, C. A. (1990). Funding and expenditures for mental illness. In R. W. Manderscheid & M. A. Sonnenschein (Eds.), *Mental health, United States, 1990* (DHHS Publication No. ADM 90-1708, pp. 216–226). National Institute of Mental Health. Washington, DC: U.S. Government Printing Office.

Taube, C. A., & Burns, B. J. (1988). Mental health services system research: The National Institute of Mental Health Program. *Health Services Research, 22,* 837–855.

Taube, C. A., Goldman, H. H., & Salkever, D. (1990). Medicaid coverage for mental illness: Balancing access and costs. *Health Affairs, 9*(1), 5–18.

Taube, C. A., Mechanic, D., & Hohmann, A. A. (Eds.). (1989). *The future of mental health services research* (DHHS Publication No. ADM 89-1600). National Institute of Mental Health. Washington, DC: U.S. Government Printing Office.

Taylor, B. M. (1989). *New directions for the national crime survey.* Technical Report. Washington, DC: U.S. Department of Justice, Office of Justice Programs, Bureau of Justice Statistics.

Taylor, D. K., & Beauchamp, C. (1988). Hospital-based primary prevention strategy in child abuse: A multilevel needs addressment. *Child Abuse and Neglect, 12,* 343–354.

Tell, E. J., Wallack, S. S., & Cohen, M. A. (1987). New directions in life care: An industry in transition. *Milbank Quarterly, 65,* 551–574.

Tesh, S. N. (1988). *Hidden arguments: Political ideology and disease prevention policy.* New Brunswick, NJ: Rutgers University Press.

Thompson, J. W., Burns, B. J., Bartko, J., Boyd, J. H., Taube, C. A., & Bourdon, K. H. (1988). The use of ambulatory services by persons with and without phobia. *Medical Care, 26,* 183–198.

Thompson, M. S., & Meyer, H. J. (1989). The costs of AIDS: Alternative methodological approaches. In L. Sechrest, H. Freeman, & A. Mulley (Eds.), *Conference proceedings: Health Services Research Methodology: A Focus on AIDS* (DHHS Publication No. PHS 89-3439, pp. 95–106). Washington, DC: U.S. Government Printing Office.

Thompson-Hoffman, S., & Storck, I. F. (Eds.). (1991). *Disability in the United States: A portrait from national data.* New York: Springer.

Tims, F. M., & Leukefeld, C. G. (Eds.). (1988). *Relapse and recovery in drug abuse* (DHHS Publication No. ADM 88-1473). National Institute on Drug Abuse, Research Monograph Series, No. 72. Washington, DC: U.S. Government Printing Office.

Tobler, N. S. (1986). Meta-analysis of 143 adolescent drug prevention programs: Quantitative outcome results of program participants compared to a control or comparison group. *Journal of Drug Issues, 16,* 537–567.

Tolan, P. (1988). Socioeconomic, family, and social stress correlates of adolescent antisocial and delinquent behavior. *Journal of Abnormal Child Psychology, 16,* 317–331.

Toole, M. J., & Waldman, R. J. (1990). Prevention of excess mortality in refugee and displaced populations in developing countries. *Journal of the American Medical Association, 263,* 3296–3302.

Torrens, P. R. (Ed.). (1985). *Hospice programs and public policy.* Chicago: American Hospital Publishing Co.

Toseland, R. W., & Rossiter, C. M. (1989). Group interventions to support family caregivers: A review and analysis. *Gerontologist, 29,* 438–448.

Trautman, P. D. (1989). Specific treatment modalities for adolescent suicide attempters. In M. R. Feinleib (Ed.), *Report of the Secretary's Task Force on Youth Suicide: Vol. 3. Prevention and interventions in youth suicide* (DHHS Publication No. ADM 89-1623, pp. 253–263). Alcohol, Drug Abuse, and Mental Health Administration. Washington, DC: U.S. Government Printing Office.

Traxler, H., & Dunaye, T. (1987). Emerging patterns in transitional care. *Health Affairs, 6,* 58–68.

Trice, H. M., & Beyer, J. M. (1984). Employee assistance programs: Blending performance-oriented and humanitarian ideologies to assist emotionally disturbed employees. *Research in Community and Mental Health, 4,* 245–297.

Trimble, J. E., Padilla, A. M., & Bell, C. S. (1987). *Drug abuse among ethnic minorities* (DHHS Publication No. ADM 87-1474). National Institute on Drug Abuse, Office of Science Monograph Series. Washington, DC: U.S. Government Printing Office.

Tucker, W. (1987). Where do the homeless come from? *National Review, 39*(18), 32.

Turner, C. F., Miller, H. G., & Moses, L. E. (Eds.). (1989). *AIDS: Sexual behavior and intravenous drug use.* Washington, DC: National Academy Press.

Turner, R. J., Grindstaff, C. F., & Phillips, N. (1990). Social support and outcome in teenage pregnancy. *Journal of Health and Social Behavior, 31,* 43–57.

Twaddle, A. C., & Hessler, R. M. (1977). *A sociology of health.* St. Louis: Mosby.

Tweed, D. L., & George, L. K. (1989). A more balanced perspective on "Psychiatric diagnosis as reified measurement": An invited comment on Mirowsky and Ross. *Journal of Health and Social Behavior, 30,* 35–37.

Tweed, J. L., Schoenbach, V. J., George, L. K., & Blazer, D. G. (1989). The effects of childhood parental death and divorce on six-month history of anxiety disorders. *British Journal of Psychiatry, 154,* 823–828.

Ulbrich, P. M., Warheit, G. J., & Zimmerman, R. S. (1989). Race, socioeconomic status, and psychological distress: An examination of differential vulnerability. *Journal of Health and Social Behavior, 30,* 131–146.

United Hospital Fund. (1990). *Homeless people and health care: An unrelenting challenge.* Paper Series No. 14. New York: United Hospital Fund of New York.

United Hospital Fund. (1991). *The challenges of AIDS.* Shaping New York's Health Care: A Report on Grantmaking, No. 1. New York: United Hospital Fund of New York.

U.S. Bureau of the Census. (1991a, June 11). *Census Bureau completes distribution of 1990 census information from summary tape file 1A.* U.S. Department of Commerce News Release. Washington, DC: U.S. Government Printing Office.

U.S. Bureau of the Census. (1991b, March 11). *Census Bureau completes distribution of 1990 redistricting tabulations to states.* U.S. Department of Commerce News Release. Washington, DC: U.S. Government Printing Office.

U.S. Bureau of the Census. (1991c). *Statistical abstract of the United States: 1991* (111th ed.). Washington, DC: U.S. Government Printing Office.

U.S. Commission on Security and Cooperation in Europe. (1990). *Staff report on homelessness in the United States.* Washington, DC: Author.

U.S. Conference of Mayors. (1991). *A status report on hunger and homelessness in America's cities: 1991.* Washington, DC: Author.

U.S. Congress, House Committee on Government Operations. (1988). *Hear-

ing (October 13, 1988): Providing shelter for the homeless on underutilized federal properties pursuant to the McKinney Homeless Assistance Act. 100th Cong., 2nd. sess. Washington, DC: U.S. Government Printing Office.

U.S. Congress, House Government Activities and Transportation Subcommittee and the Employment and Housing Subcommittee. (1989). *Joint Hearing (March 15, 1989): Implementation of the McKinney Homeless Assistance Act by the Interagency Council on the Homeless.* 101st Cong., 1st sess. Washington, DC: U.S. Government Printing Office.

U.S. Congress, House Select Committee on Aging. (1983). *Hearings (March 16, 1983): Home health care: Progress and impediments* (Comm. Publication No. 98-386). 98th Cong., 1st sess. Washington, DC: U.S. Government Printing Office.

U.S. Congress, House Select Committee on Aging. (1985). *Hearings (July 30, 1985): Twentieth anniversary of Medicare and Medicaid: Americans still at risk* (Comm. Publication No. 99-538). 99th Cong., 1st sess. Washington, DC: U.S. Government Printing Office.

U.S. Congress, House Select Committee on Aging. (1987). *Exploding the myths: Caregiving in America* (Comm. Publication No. 99-611). 100th Cong., 1st sess. Washington, DC: U.S. Government Printing Office.

U.S. Congress, House Select Committee on Aging. (1989). *Health care costs for America's elderly, 1977–88* (Comm. Publication No. 101-712). 101st Cong., 1st sess. Washington, DC: U.S. Government Printing Office.

U.S. Congress, House Select Committee on Children, Youth, and Families. (1990). *Report: No place to call home: Discarded children in America* (Report 101-395). 101st Cong., 2nd sess. Washington, DC: U.S. Government Printing Office.

U.S. Congress, Senate Committee on Labor and Human Resources. (1990). *Hearing (September 29, 1989 and May 9, 1990): Homelessness: An American tragedy* (S. Hrg. 101-806). 101st Cong., 1st sess. Washington, DC: U.S. Government Printing Office.

U.S. Congress, Senate Special Committee on Aging. (1988). *Hearings (April 18, 1988): Adult day health care: A vital component of long-term care* (Serial No. 100-20). 100th Cong., 2nd sess. Washington, DC: U.S. Government Printing Office.

U.S. Congress, Senate Subcommittee on Children, Family, Drugs, and Alcoholism. (1990). *Hearing (February 7, 1990): Street kids: Homeless and runaway youth* (S. Hrg. 101-822). 101st Cong., 2nd. sess. Washington, DC: U.S. Government Printing Office.

U.S. Department of Education in conjunction with U.S. Department of Health and Human Services. (1987). *Report to the Congress and the White House on the nature and effectiveness of federal, state, and local drug prevention/education programs.* Washington, DC: U.S. Government Printing Office.

U.S. Department of Housing and Urban Development [USDHUD]. (1984). *A report to the Secretary on the homeless and emergency shelters.* Office of Policy Development and Research. Washington, DC: U.S. Government Printing Office.

U.S. Department of Housing and Urban Development. (1988a). *A nation concerned: The first annual report of the Interagency Council on the Homeless.* Interagency Council on the Homeless. Washington, DC: U.S. Government Printing Office.

U.S. Department of Housing and Urban Development. (1988b). *SAFAH grants: Aiding comprehensive strategies for the homeless.* Office of Policy Development and Research. Washington, DC: U.S. Government Printing Office.

U.S. Department of Housing and Urban Development. (1989a). *The 1989 annual report of the Interagency Council on the Homeless.* Interagency Council on the Homeless. Washington, DC: U.S. Government Printing Office.

U.S. Department of Housing and Urban Development. (1989b). *A report on homeless assistance policy and practice in the nation's five largest cities.* Office of Policy Development and Research. Washington, DC: U.S. Government Printing Office.

U.S. Department of Housing and Urban Development. (1989c). *A report on the 1988 national survey of shelters for the homeless.* Office of Policy Development and Research. Washington, DC: U.S. Government Printing Office.

U.S. Department of Housing and Urban Development. (1990). *Report to Congress on SROs for the homeless: Section 8 Moderate Rehabilitation Program.* Office of Policy Development and Research. Washington, DC: U.S. Government Printing Office.

U.S. Department of Housing and Urban Development. (1991). *The 1990 annual report of the Interagency Council on the Homeless.* Interagency Council on the Homeless. Washington, DC: U.S. Government Printing Office.

U.S. Department of Justice. (1984a). *Attorney General's Task Force on Family Violence: Final report.* Washington, DC: U.S. Government Printing Office.

U.S. Department of Justice. (1984b). *Tracking offenders: The child victim.* Office of Justice Programs, Bureau of Justice Statistics. Washington, DC: U.S. Government Printing Office.

U.S. Department of Justice. (1988). *Report to the nation on crime and justice* (NCJ-105506) (2nd ed.). Office of Justice Programs, Bureau of Justice Statistics. Washington, DC: U.S. Government Printing Office.

University of Michigan. (1991, January 23). *1990 national high school senior drug abuse survey: Monitoring the future survey.* News and Information Services Release. Ann Arbor: Author.

University of Michigan. (1992, January 25). *1991 national high school senior drug abuse survey: Monitoring the future survey.* News and Information Services Release. Ann Arbor: Author.

Upsal, M. S. (1990). Volunteer peer support therapy for abusive and neglectful families. *Public Health Reports, 105,* 80–84.

Urrutia-Rojas, X., & Aday, L. A. (1991). A framework for community assessment: Designing and conducting a survey in an Hispanic immigrant and refugee community. *Public Health Nursing, 8*(1), 20–26.

Valdiserri, R. O., Arena, V. C., Proctor, D., & Bonati, F. A. (1989). The relationship between women's attitudes about condoms and their use: Implications for condom promotion programs. *American Journal of Public Health, 79,* 499–501.

van Steijn, P. (Ed.). (1989). *AIDS: A combined environmental and systems approach.* Amsterdam: Swets & Zeitlinger.

Vanderwagen, C., Mason, R. D., & Owan, T. C. (Eds.). (1986). *Proceedings of the Indian Health Service Alcoholism/Substance Abuse Prevention Initiative: Background, Plenary Session, and Action Plan.* Washington, DC: Health Resources and Services Administration.

Vega, W. A., Kolody, B., Hough, R. L., & Figueroa, G. (1987). Depressive symptomatology in Northern Mexico adults. *American Journal of Public Health, 77,* 1215–1218.

Vega, W. A., Scutchfield, F. D., Karno, M., & Meinhardt, K. (1985). The mental health needs of Mexican-American agricultural workers. *American Journal of Preventive Medicine, 1*(3), 47–55.

Velentgas, P., Bynum, C., & Zierler, S. (1990). The buddy volunteer commitment in AIDS care. *American Journal of Public Health, 80,* 1378–1380.

Vertrees, J. C., Manton, K. G., & Adler, G. S. (1989). Cost effectiveness of home and community-based care. *Health Care Financing Review, 10*(4), 65–78.

Viano, D. C. (1990). A blueprint for injury control in the United States. *Public Health Reports, 105,* 329–333.

Vladeck, B. C. (1980). *Unloving care: The nursing home tragedy.* New York: Basic Books.

Wagenfeld, M. O., Lemkau, P. V., & Justice, B. (Eds.). (1982). *Public mental health: Perspectives and prospects.* Newbury Park, CA: Sage.

Waldron, I., & Lye, D. (1989). Family roles and smoking. *American Journal of Preventive Medicine, 5,* 136–141.

Walker, D. K., Palfrey, J. S., Butler, J. A., & Singer, J. (1988). Use and sources of payment for health and community services for children with impaired mobility. *Public Health Reports, 103,* 411–415.

Wallace, H. M., Ryan, G. M., Jr., & Oglesby, A. C. (Eds.). (1988). *Maternal and child health practices* (3rd ed.). Oakland, CA: Third Party.

Wallace, S. P. (1990). The no-care zone: Availability, accessibility, and acceptability in community-based long-term care. *Gerontologist, 30,* 254–261.

Wallack, S. S. (1988). Recent trends in financing long-term care. *Health Care Financing Review, Annual Supplement,* 97–102.

Ward, R. A. (1985). Informal networks and well-being in later life: A research agenda. *Gerontologist, 25,* 55–61.

Ware, J. E., Jr. (1986). The assessment of health status. In L. H. Aiken & D. Mechanic (Eds.), *Applications of social science to clinical medicine and health policy* (pp. 204–228). New Brunswick, NJ: Rutgers University Press.

Ware, J. E., Jr. (1987). Standards for validating health measures: Definition and content. *Journal of Chronic Diseases, 40,* 473–480.

Ware, J. E., Jr. (1989). Measuring health and functional status in mental health services research. In C. A. Taube, D. Mechanic, & A. A. Hohmann (Eds.), *The future of mental health services research* (DHHS Publication No. ADM 89-1600, pp. 289–301). National Institute of Mental Health. Washington, DC: U.S. Government Printing Office.

Warner, K. E., & Luce, B. R. (1982). *Cost-benefit and cost-effectiveness analysis in health care: Principles, practice, and potential.* Ann Arbor, MI: Health Administration Press.

Watters, J. K., & Biernacki, P. (1989). Targeted sampling: Options for the study of hidden populations. *Social Problems, 36,* 416–430.

Weinreb, L. F., & Bassuk, E. L. (1990). Health care of homeless families: A growing challenge for family medicine. *Journal of Family Practice, 31,* 74–80.

Weinstein, M. C., & Saturno, P. J. (1989). Economic impact of youth suicides and suicide attempts. In M. L. Rosenberg & K. Baer (Eds.), *Report of the Secretary's Task Force on Youth Suicide: Vol. 4. Strategies for the prevention of youth suicide* (DHHS Publication No. ADM 89-1624, pp. 82–93). Alcohol, Drug Abuse, and Mental Health Administration. Washington, DC: U.S. Government Printing Office.

Weiss, R., & Thier, S. O. (1988). HIV testing is the answer: What's the question? *New England Journal of Medicine, 319,* 1010–1012.

Weissert, W. G., & Cready, C. M. (1989a). A prospective budgeting model for home- and community-based long-term care. *Inquiry, 26,* 114–129.

Weissert, W. G., & Cready, C. M. (1989b). Toward a model for improved targeting of aged at risk of institutionalization. *Health Services Research, 24,* 485–510.

Weissert, W. G., Cready, C. M., & Pawelak, J. E. (1988). The past and future of home- and community-based long-term care. *Milbank Quarterly, 66,* 309–388.

Weissman, M. M., Myers, J. K., Tischler, G. L., Holzer, C. E., III, Leaf, P. J., Orvaschel, H., & Brody, J. A. (1985). Psychiatric disorders (DSM-III) and cognitive impairment among the elderly in a U.S. urban community. *Acta Psychiatry Scandanavia, 71,* 366–379.

Wells, K. B., & Brook, R. H. (1989). The quality of mental health services: Past, present, and future. In C. A. Taube, D. Mechanic, & A. A. Hohmann (Eds.), *The future of mental health services research* (DHHS Publication No. ADM 89-1600, pp. 203–224). National Institute of Mental Health. Washington, DC: U.S. Government Printing Office.

Wells, K. B., Golding, J. M., Hough, R. L., Burnam, M. A., & Karno, M. (1988). Factors affecting the probability of use of general and medical health and social/community services for Mexican Americans and non-Hispanic whites. *Medical Care, 26,* 441–452.

Wells, K. B., Hough, R. L., Golding, J. M., Burnam, M. A., & Karno, M. (1987). Which Mexican-Americans underutilize health services? *American Journal of Psychiatry, 144,* 918–922.

Wells, K. B., Keeler, E., & Manning, W. G., Jr. (1990). Patterns of outpatient mental health care over time: Some implications for estimates of demand and for benefit design. *Health Services Research, 24,* 773–789.

Wells, K. B., Manning, W. G., Jr., Duan, N., Newhouse, J. P., & Ware, J. E., Jr. (1986). Sociodemographic factors and the use of outpatient mental health services. *Medical Care, 24,* 75–85.

Wells, K. B., Manning, W. G., Jr., & Valdez, R. B. (1989). *The effects of a prepaid group practice on mental health outcomes of a general population: Results from a randomized trial* (R-3834-NIMH-HFCA). Santa Monica, CA: RAND.

West, J. (Ed.). (1991). The Americans with Disability Act: From policy to practice. *Milbank Quarterly, 69*(Suppl. 1/2) Entire issue.

Westermeyer, J. (1987). Prevention of mental disorder among Hmong refugees in the United States: Lessons from the period 1976–1986. *Social Science and Medicine, 25,* 941–947.

Westermeyer, J. (1990). Methodological issues in the epidemiological study of alcohol-drug problems: Sources of confusion and misunderstanding. *American Journal of Drug and Alcohol Abuse, 16,* 47–55.

Westermeyer, J., Callies, A., & Neider, J. (1990). Welfare status and psychosocial adjustment among 100 Hmong refugees. *Journal of Nervous and Mental Disease, 178,* 300–306.

Westermeyer, J., & Neider, J. (1986). Cultural affiliation among American Indian alcoholics: Correlations and change over a ten-year period. *Annals of the New York Academy of Sciences, 472,* 179–188.

Whitaker, C. J. (1989). *The redesigned national crime survey: Selected new data.* Special Report. Washington, DC: U.S. Department of Justice, Office of Justice Programs, Bureau of Justice Statistics.

Whitcomb, D. (1985). *Prosecution of child sexual abuse: Innovations in practice.* Washington, DC: U.S. Department of Justice, Office of Justice Programs, National Institute of Justice.

White House Conference for a Drug Free America. (1988). *Final report.* Washington, DC: U.S. Government Printing Office.

Wiener, J. M., & Hanley, R. J. (1990). The bumpy road to long-term care reform. *Caring, 9*(3), 12–16.

Wiener, J. M., & Rubin, R. M. (1989). The potential impact of private long-term care financing options on Medicaid: The next thirty years. *Journal of Health Politics, Policy and Law, 14,* 327–340.

Wilk, V. A. (1986). *The occupational health of migrant and seasonal farmworkers in the United States* (2nd ed.). Washington, DC: Farmworker Justice Fund.

Williams, B. C., Phillips, E. K., Torner, J. C., & Irvine, A. A. (1990). Predicting utilization of home health resources: Important data from routinely collected information. *Medical Care, 28,* 379–391.

Williams, D. H. (1986). The epidemiology of mental illness in Afro-Americans. *Hospital and Community Psychiatry, 37,* 42–49.

Williams, K. R. (1984). Economic sources of homicide: Reestimating the effects of poverty and inequality. *American Sociological Review, 49,* 283–289.

Williams, P., Tarnopolsky, A., & Hand, D. (1980). Case definition and case identification in psychiatric epidemiology: Review and assessment. *Psychological Medicine, 10,* 101–114.

Williamson, D. F., Serdula, M. K., Kendrick, J. S., & Binkin, N. J. (1989). Comparing the prevalence of smoking in pregnant and nonpregnant women, 1985 to 1986. *Journal of the American Medical Association, 261,* 70–74.

Wilson, C. E., & Weissert, W. G. (1989). Private long-term care insurance: After coverage restrictions is there anything left? *Inquiry, 26,* 493–507.

Wilson, W. J. (1980). *The declining significance of race: Blacks and changing American institutions* (2nd ed.). Chicago: University of Chicago Press.

Wilson, W. J. (Ed.). (1989). The ghetto underclass: Social science perspectives. *Annals of the American Academy of Political and Social Science, 501.* Entire issue.

Wilson, W. J. (1990). *The truly disadvantaged: The inner city, the underclass, and public policy.* Chicago: University of Chicago Press.

Winkenwerder, W., Kessler, A. R., & Stolec, R. M. (1989). Federal spending for illness caused by the human immunodeficiency virus. *New England Journal of Medicine, 320,* 1598–1624.

Witkin, M. J., Atay, J. E., Fell, A. S., & Manderscheid, R. W. (1990). Specialty mental health system characteristics. In R. W. Manderscheid & M. A. Sonnenschein (Eds.), *Mental health, United States, 1990* (DHHS Publication No. ADM 90-1708, pp. 1–138). National Institute of Mental Health. Washington, DC: U.S. Government Printing Office.

Wolfe, B. L., & Haveman, R. (1990). Trends in the prevalence of work disability from 1962 to 1984, and their correlates. *Milbank Quarterly, 68,* 53–80.

Wood, D. L., Valdez, R. B., Hayashi, T., & Shen, A. (1990). Health of homeless children and housed, poor children. *Pediatrics, 86,* 858–866.

Worden, J. K., Flynn, B. S., Merrill, D. G., Waller, J. A., & Haugh, L. D. (1989). Preventing alcohol-impaired driving through community self-regulation training. *American Journal of Public Health, 79,* 287–290.

World Health Organization. (1948). Constitution of the World Health Organization. In *Handbook of basic documents.* Geneva: Author.

Wright, J. D. (1988). The worthy and unworthy homeless. *Society, 25*(5), 64–69.

Wright, J. D., & Weber, E. (1987). *Homelessness and health.* Washington, DC: McGraw-Hill's Healthcare Information Center.

Wurtele, S. K. (1987). School-based sexual abuse prevention programs: A review. *Child Abuse and Neglect, 11,* 483–495.

Wyatt, G. E., & Peters, S. D. (1986a). Issues in the definition of child sexual abuse in prevalence research. *Child Abuse and Neglect, 10,* 231–240.

Wyatt, G. E., & Peters, S. D. (1986b). Methodological considerations in research on the prevalence of child sexual abuse. *Child Abuse and Neglect, 10,* 241–251.

Wyatt, R. J. (1986). Scienceless to homeless. *Science, 234,* 1309.

Yankauer, A. (1990). What infant mortality tells us. *American Journal of Public Health, 80,* 653–654.

Yelin, E. H. (1986). The myth of malingering: Why individuals withdraw from work in the presence of illness. *Milbank Quarterly, 64,* 622–649.

Yelin, E. H., Greenblatt, R. M., Hollander, H., & McMaster, J. R. (1991). The impact of HIV-related illness on employment. *American Journal of Public Health, 81,* 79–84.

Yudkowsky, B. K., & Fleming, G. V. (1990). Preventive health care for Medicaid children. *Health Care Financing Review, Annual Supplement,* 89–96.

Zill, N., & Schoenborn, C. A. (1990). *Developmental learning, and emotional problems: Health of our nation's children, United States, 1988* (DHHS Publication No. PHS 91-1250). National Center for Health Statistics, Advance Data No. 190. Washington, DC: U.S. Government Printing Office.

Zimring, F. E. (1986). Gun control. *Bulletin of the New York Academy of Medicine, 62,* 615–621.

Ziter, M.L.P. (1987). Culturally sensitive treatment of black alcoholic families. *Social Work, 32,* 130–135.

Zucker, R. A., & Gomberg, E.S.L. (1986). Etiology of alcoholism reconsidered: The case for a biopsychosocial process. *American Psychologist, 41,* 783–793.

NAME INDEX

SUBJECT INDEX

369